The Other Side of Cannabis

Impact on
Mental and Physical Health

T0289772

The Other Side of Cannabis

Impact on Mental and Physical Health

Edited by

Richard Balon, M.D.

Mary K. Morreale, M.D.

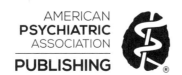

AMERICAN
PSYCHIATRIC
ASSOCIATION
PUBLISHING

If you wish to buy 50 or more copies of the same title, please go to www.appi .org/specialdiscounts for more information.

Copyright © 2025 American Psychiatric Association Publishing
ALL RIGHTS RESERVED   .

First Edition

Manufactured in the United States of America on acid-free paper

28 27 26 25 24   5 4 3 2 1
American Psychiatric Association Publishing
800 Maine Avenue SW, Suite 900
Washington, DC 20024–2812
www.appi.org

Library of Congress Cataloging-in-Publication Data
Names: Balon, Richard, author. | Morreale, Mary K, author. | American Psychiatric Association Publishing, issuing body.
Title: The other side of cannabis : impact on mental and physical health / by Richard Balon, Mary K. Morreale.
Description: First edition. | Washington, D.C. : American Psychiatric Association Publishing, [2025] | Includes bibliographical references and index.
Identifiers: LCCN 2024029196 (print) | LCCN 2024029197 (ebook) | ISBN 9781615375387 (paperback ; alk. paper) | ISBN 9781615375394 (ebook)
Subjects: MESH: Marijuana Use--adverse effects | Marijuana Use--legislation & jurisprudence | Marijuana Use--trends | Marijuana Abuse | Substance-Related Disorders | Drug and Narcotic Control | United States
Classification: LCC HV5822.M3 (print) | LCC HV5822.M3 (ebook) | NLM WM 276 | DDC 362.29/5--dc23/eng/20240724
LC record available at https://lccn.loc.gov/2024029196
LC ebook record available at https://lccn.loc.gov/2024029197

British Library Cataloguing in Publication Data

A CIP record is available from the British Library.

Contents

Contributors

Richard Balon, M.D.
Professor, Department of Psychiatry and Behavioral Neurosciences and Department of Anesthesiology, Wayne State University, Detroit, Michigan

Jasper C. Bash, M.D.
Assistant Professor, Department of Urology, Oregon Health and Science University, Portland, Oregon

Mélissa Beaudoin, M.Sc.
Department of Psychiatry and Addictology, University of Montreal, Research Center of the Institut universitaire en santé mentale de Montréal; medical student, Faculty of Medicine, McGill University, Montreal, Canada

Ashley E. Benson, M.D., M.Sc.
Assistant Professor, Division of Maternal Fetal Medicine, Department of Obstetrics and Gynecology, Oregon Health and Science University, Portland, Oregon

Benjamin J. Burwitz, Ph.D.
Associate Professor, Division of Pathobiology and Immunology, Oregon National Primate Research Center, Beaverton, Oregon

Jonathan Chevinsky, M.D.
Psychiatry Resident, Division of Addiction Psychiatry, Beth Israel Deaconess Medical Center, Boston, Massachusetts

Marco Colizzi, M.D., Ph.D.
Assistant Professor of Psychiatry, Unit of Psychiatry, Department of Medicine (DAME), University of Udine, Udine, Italy; Department of Psychosis Studies, King's College, London, United Kingdom

B. Adam Crosland, M.D., M.P.H.
Assistant Professor, Division of Maternal Fetal Medicine, Department of Obstetrics and Gynecology, Oregon Health and Science University, Portland, Oregon

Kaitlin Cuddleston, M.A.
Ferkauf Graduate School of Psychology, Yeshiva University, Bronx, New York

Joao P. De Aquino, M.D.
Assistant Professor of Psychiatry and Assistant Chief of Inpatient Psychiatry, Clinical Neuroscience Research Unit (CNRU), Yale University School of Medicine, New Haven, Connecticut; VA VISN-1 Mental Illness Research, Education, and Clinical Center (MIRECC), West Haven, Connecticut

Laura Dellazizzo, M.D., Ph.D.
Research assistant, Research Center of the Institut universitaire en santé mentale de Montréal, Montreal, Canada

Rahul J. D'Mello, M.D., Ph.D.
Assistant Professor, Division of Maternal Fetal Medicine, Department of Obstetrics and Gynecology, Oregon Health and Science University, Portland, Oregon

Alexandre Dumais, M.D., Ph.D.
Associate Clinical Professor, Department of Psychiatry and Addictology, University of Montreal, Research Center of the Institut universitaire en santé mentale de Montréal; Psychiatrist, Institut National de Psychiatrie Légale Philippe-Pinel, Montreal, Canada

Daniel Feingold, Ph.D.
Psychology Department, Achva Academic College, Achva, Israel

Sabrina Giguère, M.Sc.
Department of Psychiatry and Addictology, University of Montreal, Research Center of the Institut universitaire en santé mentale de Montréal, Montreal, Canada

David Gorelick, M.D., Ph.D.
Clinical Professor, Department of Psychiatry, University of Maryland School of Medicine, Baltimore, Maryland

Mark K. Greenwald, Ph.D.
Professor and Associate Chair for Research, Department of Psychiatry and Behavioral Neurosciences, School of Medicine, and Department of Pharmacy Practice, Eugene Applebaum College of Pharmacy and Health Sciences, Wayne State University, Detroit, Michigan

Olivia J. Hagen, B.S.
Senior Research Assistant, Division of Reproductive and Developmental Sciences, Oregon National Primate Research Center, Beaverton, Oregon

Wayne Hall, Ph.D.
Emeritus Professor, National Centre for Youth Substance Use Research, University of Queensland, Brisbane, Queensland, Australia

Sarena Hayer, M.D.
Obstetrics and Gynecology Resident, Department of Obstetrics and Gynecology, Oregon Health and Science University, Portland, Oregon

Jason C. Hedges, M.D., Ph.D.
Professor, Department of Urology, Oregon Health and Science University, Portland, Oregon

Kevin P. Hill, M.D., M.H.S.
Director of Addiction Psychiatry, Beth Israel Deaconess Medical Center; Associate Professor of Psychiatry, Harvard Medical School, Boston, Massachusetts

Onyedika J. Ilonze, M.D.
Assistant Professor, Department of Medicine, Division of Advanced Heart Failure and Transplant Cardiology, Indiana University School of Medicine, Indianapolis, Indiana

Emily H. Kim, M.A.
Ferkauf Graduate School of Psychology, Yeshiva University, Bronx, New York

David M. Ledgerwood, Ph.D.
Professor and Director, Division of Nicotine and Tobacco Research, Department of Psychiatry and Behavioral Neurosciences, Wayne State University School of Medicine, Detroit, Michigan

Janni Leung, Ph.D.
Principal Research Fellow, National Centre for Youth Substance Use Research, University of Queensland, Brisbane, Queensland, Australia

Jamie O. Lo, M.D., M.C.R.
Associate Professor, Division of Maternal Fetal Medicine, Department of Obstetrics and Gynecology, Oregon Health and Science University, Portland, Oregon

Leslie H. Lundahl, Ph.D.
Professor, Department of Psychiatry and Behavioral Neurosciences, Wayne State University School of Medicine, Detroit, Michigan

Ava D. Mandelbaum, B.S.
Department of Obstetrics and Gynecology, Oregon Health and Science University, Portland, Oregon

Jennifer A. Manuzak, Ph.D.
Assistant Professor, Division of Immunology, Tulane National Primate Research Center, Covington, Louisiana

Tanya Mehdizadeh, M.A.
Ferkauf Graduate School of Psychology, Yeshiva University, Bronx, New York

Sylvie J. Messer, Ph.D.
Clinical Psychology (Health Emphasis), Ferkauf Graduate School of Psychology, Yeshiva University, Bronx, New York

Mary K. Morreale, M.D.
Professor, Department of Psychiatry and Behavioral Neurosciences, Wayne State University School of Medicine, Detroit, Michigan

Tabitha E.H. Moses, M.S.
Department of Psychiatry and Behavioral Neurosciences, Wayne State University School of Medicine, Detroit, Michigan

Robin M. Murray, Prof., FRS
Professor, Department of Psychosis Studies, Institute of Psychiatry, Psychology and Neuroscience, King's College London, London, United Kingdom

Anahita Bassir Nia, M.D.
Assistant Professor of Psychiatry, Yale School of Medicine, New Haven; Assistant Clinical Unit Chief and Assistant Director for Training and Education, Clinical Neuroscience Research Unit (CNRU), Connecticut Mental Health Hospital, West Hartford, Connecticut

Emilie-Clare L. O'Mara, B.S.
Department of Psychiatry and Behavioral Neurosciences, Wayne State University School of Medicine, Detroit, Michigan

Robert L. Page II, Pharm.D.
Professor, Departments of Clinical Pharmacy, Physical Medicine, and Medicine, and Clinical Specialist, Division of Cardiology, Advanced Heart Failure, Schools of Pharmacy and Medicine, University of Colorado, Aurora, Colorado

Tyler Pia, Ph.D.
Clinical Psychology (Health Emphasis), Ferkauf Graduate School of Psychology, Yeshiva University, Bronx, New York

Stéphane Potvin, Ph.D.
Professor, Department of Psychiatry and Addictology, University of Montreal, Research Center of the Institut universitaire en santé mentale de Montréal, Montreal, Canada

Lucia Sideli, Ph.D.
Associate Professor of Clinical Psychiatry, Department of Human Science, LUMSA University, Rome, Italy; Department of Psychosis Studies, King's College, London, United Kingdom

Edoardo Spinazzola, Ph.D.
Research Assistant, Department of Psychosis Studies, Institute of Psychiatry, Psychology and Neuroscience, King's College London, London, United Kingdom

Daniel Stjepanović, Ph.D.
Senior Research Fellow, National Centre for Youth Substance Use Research, University of Queensland, Brisbane, Queensland, Australia

Andrea H. Weinberger, Ph.D.
Associate Professor, Ferkauf Graduate School of Psychology, Yeshiva University, Bronx, New York

Aviv Weinstein, Ph.D.
Professor, Department of Psychology and The Isadore and Ruth Kastin Chair for Brain Research, Ariel University, Science Park, Ariel, Israel

Jeremy Weleff, D.O.
Assistant Professor Adjunct in Psychiatry, Yale School of Medicine, New Haven, Connecticut

Disclosures

Marco Colizzi, M.D., Ph.D. *Consultant:* GW Pharma Ltd., GW Pharma Italy SR, F. Hoffmann-La Roche Ltd.

Joao P. De Aquino, M.D. *Consultant:* Boehringer Ingelheim; Grant/ Research Support: Jazz Pharmaceuticals.

Kevin P. Hill, M.D., M.H.S. *Author:* Hazelden, Wolters-Kluwer.

Tabitha E.H. Moses, M.S. *Grant/Research Support:* National Institutes of Health/National Institute on Drug Abuse training grant F30DA052118; *Consultant:* Wayne State University Center for Behavioral Health and Justice.

Anahita Bassir Nia, M.D. *Advisory Board:* Synendos Therapeutics.

None of remaining authors have competing interests to disclose.

1

Introduction

The Other Side of Cannabis

Richard Balon, M.D.
Mary K. Morreale, M.D.

We are both clinically oriented psychiatrists who, although not actively treating patients with substance use disorders, are very much concerned about the growing presence and tolerance of substances of abuse among our patients and in our society. We are especially concerned about substances that are promoted for their unproven health benefits and are legalized. Two substances, alcohol and tobacco, have been legalized and abused for centuries. Both had been touted as having health benefits that were later disproved. Across many societies, the battle against alcohol use disorders has had minimal to modest success. We have done a bit better with tobacco over the past several decades, seeing a significant decrease in the prevalence of tobacco smoking (U.S. Department of Health and Human Services 2014). Fortunately, society has gradually accepted that smoking tobacco is hazardous to our health. Yet we have seen an increase in vaping, especially among youth. Both battles against alcohol and tobacco abuse have been complicated by legalization, heavy promotion via advertisement, a cavalier societal attitude, legislatures who see alcohol and

1

tobacco sales as a great source of tax revenue, and lobbying by those who profit from their sales.

Unfortunately, a third substance of abuse is following a similar path of acceptance based on mostly unproven benefits, minimization of deleterious effects, and heavy promotion by those who benefit from its sales—cannabis. Cannabis has gradually risen from the low-potency counterculture joints to a legalized, much more potent substance grown and sold throughout the United States. Despite a federal law prohibiting the use, sale, and possession of cannabis containing more than 0.3% of tetrahydrocannabinol (THC), as of February 2024, the recreational use of cannabis has been legalized in 24 U.S. states, as well as in Washington, D.C., and 3 U.S. territories. Many other U.S. states allow the medical use of cannabis, and only a few states do not allow any use and sale of this substance, with some states decriminalizing possession of a small amount. Interestingly, the federal status of cannabis may also be gradually changing. A new bill introduced to the U.S. Congress in January 2023 "moves marijuana to a lower schedule of the Controlled Substances Act. Specifically, it directs the Drug Enforcement Administration to transfer marijuana from schedule I to schedule III" (H.R. 610 2023). This change in labeling implies that cannabis has less potential for abuse and dependence and is appropriate for medical use, which will likely have far-reaching consequences for health care and all of society. Nevertheless, this bill illustrates the direction our country is taking regarding cannabis. It is important to note that the United States is not alone in this trend. Many countries allow medical use of cannabis, and some countries, such as Canada, South Africa, and Uruguay, have also legalized recreational cannabis.

Cannabis is not only legalized in many states but is also heavily advertised and promoted. Examples include billboards along highways offering home delivery of cannabis, newspaper articles providing "an essential guide to buying marijuana" in a particular area, and some cannabis stores or dispensaries being built to offer a "welcoming atmosphere" similar to that of high-end, modern stores (Roberts 2023 p. 1B). The world is slowly marching toward acceptance of cannabis or, as one cannabis company executive stated, toward "fully embracing cannabis culture and communicating acceptance and inclusion" (Roberts 2023, p. 1B). In all fairness, not every community in states where cannabis is legalized allows its sale; many have opted out. Nevertheless, the direction toward acceptance is happening. We do not think that any other substance with a questionable legal status (federal vs. legal laws), deleterious effects, and abuse potential has ever been so heavily and widely promoted.

The acceptance and promotion of cannabis are occurring despite warnings in the scientific literature, namely, about the increased incidence of cannabis use and the impact of cannabis on mental and physical illness. For instance, a recent U.S. Veterans Health Administration study covering the period of 2005–2019 found that the enactment of medical cannabis laws and recreational cannabis laws played a significant role in the overall increases in cannabis use disorder (CaUD), particularly in older patients (Hasin et al. 2023). This study had some limitations, but its results suggest that the legalization of cannabis may increase the prevalence of CaUD. It is important to note in this context that the prevalence of CaUD among people who use cannabis is fairly high. According to the systematic review by Leung et al. (2020), 22% (18%–26%) of cannabis users have CaUD, 13% (8%–18%) have cannabis addiction, and 13% (10%–15%) have cannabis dependence. People who use cannabis have a one in five risk of developing a CaUD, and the risk of developing cannabis dependence increases to 33% among young people who engage in regular (weekly or daily) use of cannabis (Leung et al. 2020). Thus, it is plausible to say that the prevalence of cannabis use and CaUD will continue to rise.

In an excellent summary on cannabis and psychosis, D'Souza (2023) commented on the finding that exposure to cannabis may contribute to the risk of psychosis and schizophrenia, probably by disrupting the neurodevelopmental processes in adolescents who use cannabis. D'Souza also noted that cannabis has a negative impact on the course of schizophrenia. According to Di Forti et al. (2019), "assuming causality, if high-potency cannabis were no longer available, then 12% of first-episode psychosis could be prevented across Europe, rising to 30% in London and 50% in Amsterdam" (p. 428).

Both D'Souza (2023) and Hasin et al. (2023) warned about the opposing interests of the public health and cannabis industries and brought forward the involvement of the tobacco industry. In his poignant warning, D'Souza (2023) wrote, "In what may be an ominous development, as cigarette sales decline worldwide, the tobacco industry, with its vast experience in mass production, advertising, marketing, lobbying, and legal defense, is investing in the cannabis industry" (p. 232). Hasin et al. (2023) noted that alcohol, tobacco, and prescription opioids have undergone major shifts in public acceptance or rejection across decades and generations. Public health efforts regarding these substances have long competed with commercial interests. With cannabis increasingly legalized, similar competing public health and commercial interests are now emerging. (p. 386)

It is also important to note that the legalization of cannabis and regulation of its sales have not stopped the illicit production of this drug. In a *Wall Street Journal* article, Elinson and Vielkind (2023) wrote that legal cannabis cannot compete with the illegal market in the United States. For example, they reported that in 2022 in California, 7 years after cannabis was legalized in the state, the unlicensed sales of cannabis totaled $8.1 billion, dwarfing legal sales of $5.4 billion. In addition, the California marijuana eradication program seized more than 1.1 million plants in its first decade of operation from 1983 through 1992, whereas it seized nearly 2.2 million plants between 2021 and 2023. The state of New York seems to be heading in a similar direction. Major contributing factors to these trends include that police give little priority to fighting illegal cannabis production because more serious crimes take precedence and that the taxes on legal sales of cannabis are high. Elinson and Vielkind (2023) quoted a CEO of one cannabis company as saying, "Our No. 1 competitor is the illicit market." Thus, it is not clear whether the legalization of cannabis is going to help with controlling or decreasing the illegal production of cannabis in the United States.

The examples of widespread cannabis use—at least partially because of its legalization, the rise of illegal production despite legalization, and more evidence of the impact of cannabis on mental health—should raise more concerns among mental health professionals, legislators, and the public. We are facing a serious and growing problem that requires efforts like those developed during the antitobacco campaign. As Hasin et al. (2023) wrote,

> To inform future health and policy efforts, researchers must monitor harms related to increasing CaUD, identify whether subgroups show particular risk due to changing cannabis laws, and ensure that this knowledge is clearly communicated to policymakers, clinicians, and the public. (p. 386)

As both legalization of cannabis and the rise of illegal cannabis production continue, physicians need to be aware of the potential harms of cannabis on both physical and mental health. Without a true and comprehensive understanding of the deleterious impact of cannabis use, we will not be able to effectively educate our patients, the public, and policymakers to mitigate the risks associated with use. Thus, we put together this volume with the intention of collecting information related to the risk of cannabis use on the human body. We gathered authors from different corners of the world who share this goal. We hope that after reading this volume, readers will see that there is a side of cannabis use that is not advertised or promoted, a physically and psychiatrically detrimental side that might be darker than most of us realize.

References

Di Forti M, Quattrone D, Freeman TP, et al: The contribution of cannabis use to variation in the incidence of psychotic disorder across Europe (EU-GEI): a multicentre case-control study. Lancet Psychiatry 6(5):427–436, 2019 30902669

D'Souza DC: Cannabis, cannabinoids and psychosis: a balanced view. World Psychiatry 22(2):231–232, 2023 37159370

Elinson Z, Vielkind J: Legal cannabis can't compete. The Wall Street Journal, April 29–30, 2023, pp A1, A10

Hasin DS, Wall MM, Choi CJ, et al: State cannabis legalization and cannabis use disorder in the US Veterans Health Administration, 2005 to 2019. JAMA Psychiatry 80(4):380–388, 2023 36857036

H.R. 610, Marijuana 1-to-3 Act of 2023. 118th Congress (2023–2024). Available at: https://www.congress.gov/bill/118th-congress/house-bill/610. Accessed July 12, 2024.

Roberts A: An essential guide to buying marijuana in Metro Detroit. Detroit Free Press, July 23, 2023, pp 1B, 6B

U.S. Department of Health and Human Services: The Health Consequences of Smoking—50 Years of Progress: A Report of the Surgeon General. Atlanta, GA, U.S. Department of Health and Human Services, 2014

2

Cannabis (Marijuana)

Is It a Gateway Drug?

Wayne Hall, Ph.D.

Daniel Stjepanović, Ph.D.

Janni Leung, Ph.D.

For several decades, there has been a debate about whether cannabis use is a gateway to the use of more harmful illicit drugs (Anthony 2012). That is, does the decision by young people to use cannabis substantially increase their likelihood of using drugs such as cocaine, heroin, and methamphetamine? The gateway hypothesis received strong support from epidemiological research by Kandel (2002) and others in the 1970s, which found that cannabis use consistently preceded the use of cocaine and heroin. The hypothesis is invoked by those who oppose cannabis legalization (DuPont 2016; DuPont et al. 2018) and emphatically rejected by those who support it (Kleinig 2015; Szalavitz 2015).

In this chapter, we describe the gateway pattern of drug use and outline the major explanations offered for it. We then evaluate these explanations, considering evidence from longitudinal epidemiological studies, simulation studies, discordant twin studies, genetic

Acknowledgment: We would like to thank Tesfa Mekonen Yimer for his assistance in formatting the references and preparing the chapter for submission epidemiological studies, animal studies, and evaluations of the effects of cannabis policies on relationships between cannabis and other illicit drug use. We use a triangulation approach (Shahab et al. 2022) to assess the extent to which different types of evidence from different study designs, which are subject to independent forms of methodological imperfection, support each of the major explanations of the gateway pattern. Finally, we briefly discuss the clinical implications of the evidence and the implications for policies to reduce illicit drug use in the population.

Relationships Between Cannabis and Other Drug Use

In New York in the 1970s, Yamaguchi and Kandel (1984a, 1984b) and Kandel and Faust (1975) found a common sequence of drug use among youth in which the great majority used alcohol and tobacco before they used cannabis, and they used cannabis before using cocaine and heroin. In general, the earlier the age at which a young person first used cannabis, and the more regularly they did so during adolescence, the more likely they were to later use cocaine and heroin.

Other epidemiological studies have reported different variations in the sequence of cannabis and other substance use. Among American heroin users in the 1950s and 1960s, for example, prior involvement with cannabis was rare in those areas where cannabis was not available (Goode 1974). Among Black adolescents living in large cities, cocaine and heroin use often preceded the use of hallucinogens and "pills" (Kandel 1978). More recent studies in the United States confirmed that young people who lived in areas where cannabis was less available used other illicit drugs before using cannabis (Degenhardt et al. 2009). Among the countries that participated in the World Health Organization's World Mental Health Survey, the order in which illicit drugs were most often used varied, with national differences in their availability (Degenhardt et al. 2010). More recently, with the decline in cigarette smoking, cannabis has been reported to be a gateway to tobacco smoking (Chen et al. 2018; Reed et al. 2022).

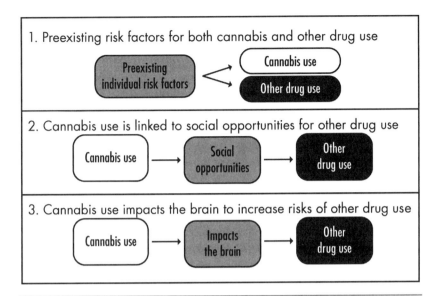

Figure 2–1. Three hypotheses on the association between cannabis and other drug use.

Explanations for the Association Between Cannabis and Other Illicit Drug Use

Hypotheses to explain patterns of cannabis use and other illicit drug use can be grouped into three broad classes, as illustrated in Figure 2–1 (Hall and Lynskey 2005; Lynskey and Agrawal 2018). The first hypothesis is that adolescents who use cannabis regularly differ from their peers who do not use cannabis in ways that make them more likely to later use other illicit drugs. These differences may include a propensity to take risks, rebelliousness, a desire to prematurely achieve adult status, and shared genetic risks of using licit and illicit drugs (Leung et al. 2020; Vanyukov et al. 2012). According to the first hypothesis, these characteristics make some young people more likely to use cannabis at an early age, to use it more often, and to later use other illicit drugs (Leung et al. 2020).

A second hypothesis is that young people who use cannabis have more social opportunities to use other illicit drugs than their peers who do not use cannabis (MacCoun and Reuter 2001; Wagner and Anthony 2002). This is because they buy cannabis from illicit markets that sell other drugs, and they affiliate with peers who use cannabis and other drugs. This hypothesis would explain why regular cannabis users are more likely than less frequent users to use other drugs—because regular users buy cannabis in larger quantities from drug dealers, often at a discounted price. Less frequent cannabis users, by contrast, typically obtain their cannabis from friends rather than directly from the illicit market.

A third hypothesis is that regular cannabis use changes brain function in ways that increase the likelihood a young person will use other illicit drugs. One variant of this hypothesis is that the pharmacological effects of regular cannabis use predispose young persons to use other drugs by sensitizing their brains to the euphoric effects (Nahas 1990; Walters 1993). A molecular variant of this hypothesis has been proposed by Kandel and Kandel (2014) to explain the association between nicotine and cocaine use.

According to the first hypothesis, the association between cannabis use and the use of other drugs is explained by common causes. The second hypothesis suggests that the illegality of cannabis use is an indirect cause that increases opportunities to use other drugs sold in the same illicit markets as cannabis, whereas the third hypothesis provides a direct causal explanation based on the pharmacological effects and brain impacts of adolescent cannabis use. Each of these hypotheses could contribute to the gateway effect, and it is possible that a combination of these factors, as well as other factors not yet identified, could play a role in explaining the relationship between the use of cannabis and the use of other illicit drugs.

Current State of Evidence on Cannabis as a Gateway Drug

Are There Shared Liabilities to Use Cannabis and Other Drugs?

A modeling study by Morral et al. (2002) is widely understood to have demonstrated that shared risk factors for drug use can potentially explain the gateway sequences of cannabis and other drug use. Their study simulated the patterns of drug use that would arise if individuals differed only in their propensity to use a variety of drugs. The authors assumed that this propensity was correlated with the opportunity to use these drugs and with the age at first use. They assumed that there was no correlation between 1) the opportunities to use or the age at first use of cannabis and 2) the opportunities to use or the age at first use of other illicit drugs. The model showed that the shared liability hypothesis predicted that cannabis use would precede the use of other drugs and that the more frequently cannabis was used, the greater the risk would be of a young person using other drugs.

The shared liability hypothesis is also empirically supported by the substantial correlations between early alcohol and illicit drug use and other nonconforming adolescent behaviors, such as dropping out of high school, early premarital sexual experience and pregnancy, and delinquency (Fergusson et al. 2015; Hall et al. 2020; Jessor and Jessor 1977; Osgood et al. 1988). These forms of behavior are, in turn, associated with rebellious attitudes and antisocial conduct in late childhood and early adolescence (Jessor and Jessor 1977; Newcomb and Bentler 1988). Regular cannabis users are more likely than peers to engage in antisocial behavior (Brook et al. 1992; McGee and Feehan 1993), be nonconformist and alienated (Brook et al. 1992; Jessor and Jessor 1978; Shedler and Block 1990), perform poorly at school (Bailey et al. 1992; Hawkins et al. 1992; Kandel and Davies 1992), and use drugs to deal with personal distress (Kaplan and Johnson 1992; Shedler and Block 1990). The more of these risk factors that adolescents have, the more likely they are to use cannabis and other drugs (Brook et al. 1992; Newcomb 1992; Scheier and Newcomb 1991).

Longitudinal studies have directly tested the hypothesis that adolescents who engage in high-risk behaviors are more likely to initiate cannabis at an early age and to use it frequently. These studies have assessed whether cannabis use predicts the use of other drugs after statistically controlling for differences in baseline risky behavior between cannabis users and nonusers (Fergusson and Horwood 2000). Early studies in the 1980s found that the relationship between cannabis use and other illicit drug use was smaller, but it persisted after controlling for preexisting adolescent behavior and attitudes, interpersonal factors, and the age at initiation into drug use (Kandel et al. 1986; O'Donnell and Clayton 1982; Robins et al. 1970; Yamaguchi and Kandel 1984b).

Fergusson and Horwood (1997, 2000) and Fergusson et al. (2002) reported a series of papers that comprehensively tested the shared liability hypothesis in a prospective study of 990 New Zealand children who were followed from birth to age 21. At each survey wave in adolescence, the researchers assessed cannabis use and a large number of potentially confounding psychosocial variables that included family background (e.g., socioeconomic status, parental relationships and substance use, childhood abuse), early adolescent characteristics and development (e.g., novelty seeking, smoking, alcohol use, conduct problems), peer substance use, and personal history of taking risks. They found a dose-response relationship between the frequency of cannabis use by age 16 and the development of a problem with cannabis, alcohol, or other substances by age 18 (Fergusson and Horwood 1997). Adolescents who initiated cannabis use at an earlier age came from lower socioeconomic status families who had a history of parental conflict and parental criminality, alcohol and drug use, and low attachment. These adolescents also had a history of conduct problems, low self-esteem, and high novelty seeking, and they affiliated with delinquent peers. Adjustments for these family and personal factors substantially reduced but did not eliminate the relationship between early cannabis use and the use of other illicit drugs.

A follow-up at age 21 found that more than a quarter of those who used cannabis also used other illicit drugs, although only 4% had used cocaine or opiates (Fergusson and Horwood 2000). The strength of these relationships was reduced after controlling for common risk factors, but a dose-response relationship was still observed: risks were 2.8 times higher (95% CI 2.4–3.1) for those who had used once or twice, and this went to up to 59.2 times higher (95% CI 36.0–97.5) for those who had used 50 times or more. This dose-response relationship was replicated using fixed effects regression to control for unobserved individual differences between early and late cannabis users in the propensity to use other drugs (Fergusson et al. 2002). They also found that the earlier cannabis was first used, the higher the risk of using other illicit drugs. A follow-up of participants at age 25 that used fixed effects regression models found that the association between the frequency of cannabis use and other drug use remained statistically significant, but its strength decreased with age (Fergusson et al. 2006).

Similar findings were observed in studies in other countries. An analysis of three waves of the U.S. National Youth Survey, a nationally representative study of 1,725 adolescents ages 11–17, found that those who used cannabis were still three to five times more likely to use other illicit drugs than those who had not, after adjusting for shared environmental triggers; personal stressors and emotions; and neighborhood, school, and family influences (Rebellon and Van Gundy 2006). Australia's Victorian Adolescent Health Cohort Study of 1,755 youth ages 15–35 found that less-than-weekly cannabis use was associated with 5.29 (95% CI 2.70–10.33) and 5.46 times (95% CI 1.62–18.42) higher odds of using amphetamines occasionally and regularly, respectively. The risks were higher if cannabis was used weekly or more often (occasional: OR 7.09, 95% CI 2.06–19.29; regular: OR 7.85, 95% CI 1.72–36.77), after adjusting for sex, psychological factors, and own and peer smoking and alcohol use (Chan et al. 2019). A follow-up study found that higher odds of other illicit drug use were found in both adolescent-onset (OR 36.8; 95% CI 17.0–80.1) and young-adult-onset (OR 20.4; 95% CI 10.7–39.1) cannabis users after adjusting for alcohol use, smoking, and psychosocial factors (Chan et al. 2021).

In a systematic review of the relationship between cannabis and subsequent opioid use, Wilson et al. (2022) summarized six epidemiological studies published between 1997 and 2020 that were conducted in the United States, Australia, and New Zealand. A meta-analysis indicated that individuals who had used cannabis had 2.76 higher odds (95% CI 2.26–3.36) of using opioids later in life. The authors highlighted that these studies were subject to serious risks of bias, which meant that there was very low certainty that cannabis use led to first-time opioid use. The authors also could not rule out the hypothesis that the association was explained by a shared propensity to use drugs because many of the studies had not comprehensively controlled for shared risk factors for cannabis and other drug use.

In summary, cohort studies suggest that a shared liability to use illicit drugs partially explains the relationship between regular cannabis use and the use of other drugs. That is, young people who regularly use cannabis differ from their peers in various ways that make them more likely to use other drugs. Controlling for these factors reduces the strength of the association but does not eliminate it, leaving open the possibility that there may be some sort of causal relationship between cannabis and other drug use. The effectiveness of controlling for indicators of the preexisting propensity to use cannabis and other drugs has been questioned by Morral et al. (2002), who argued that this approach would succeed only if the indicators were perfectly correlated with the propensity to use cannabis and other drugs. If they were not, then spurious associations could remain after controlling for the risk indicators.

Role of a Shared Genetic Vulnerability to Drug Dependence

Studies of identical (monozygotic) and nonidentical (dizygotic) twins indicate that cannabis use is influenced by environmental and genetic factors (Agrawal and Lynskey 2006; Verweij et al. 2010). There is also a genetic vulnerability to developing dependence on alcohol (Heath 1995), cannabis (Kendler and Prescott 1998), and tobacco (Han et al. 1999). A substantial part of the genetic vulnerability to all three types of drug dependence is shared, along with family and environmental risk factors (True et al. 1999). Less is known about the genetic risks of developing dependence on cocaine and heroin because the low prevalence of use of these drugs in twin studies does not allow for powerful statistical tests, but the evidence suggests that similar shared genetic factors may play a role (Kendler et al. 2003). A study of alcohol and other drug dependence in the Swedish population found that these substance use disorders shared a substantial common genetic component (Kendler et al. 2023). A review of family, adoption, and twin studies also found converging evidence for genetic influences on addiction (Agrawal and Lynskey 2008).

An Australian discordant twin study by Lynskey et al. (2003) provided a test of whether shared genetic factors explained the association between cannabis and other illicit drug use. Lynskey and colleagues examined the relationship between cannabis and other illicit drug use in 136 monozygotic and 175 dizygotic discordant twin pairs—that is, twin pairs in which one twin had and the other had not used cannabis before age 17. If the association between cannabis and other drug use was attributable to a shared environment, then discordant twins raised together should not differ in their use of other drugs. Similarly, if the association was due to shared genetic vulnerability to drug dependence, then there should be no difference in the use of other illicit drugs between monozygotic twins who did and did not use cannabis. These researchers found that the twin who had used cannabis before age 17 was more likely to have also used sedatives, hallucinogens, stimulants, and opioids than the co-twin who had not. Twins who had used cannabis were also more likely to report symptoms of abuse or dependence on cannabis and other drugs than their co-twins who did not use cannabis. These relationships persisted after controlling for other nonshared environmental factors that were associated with an increased risk of developing drug abuse or dependence. They also persisted when the analysis was confined to twin pairs in which both had used cannabis at some time in their lives.

Two later attempted replications of the Lynskey et al. (2003) study produced conflicting results. Both analyzed data from the U.S. nationally representative National Longitudinal Study of Adolescent Health (Cleveland and Wiebe 2008; Lessem et al. 2006). Lessem et al. (2006) tested three aspects of the gateway hypothesis: 1) whether there was an association between early cannabis use and later illicit drug use (N=18,286), 2) whether the association remained after adjusting for familial factors in 360 sibling pairs, and 3) whether the association remained after adjusting for genetic and environmental factors among discordant pairs. This study improved on that of Lynskey et al. (2003), which relied on retrospective self-reports of cannabis use that were susceptible to recall bias. After controlling for important confounding factors, Lessem et al. (2006) found that twins who used cannabis were still more likely to use other illicit drugs (OR 1.83; 95% CI 1.58, 2.13).

Cleveland and Wiebe (2008) tested the gateway effect theory by using three waves of longitudinal data from same-sex twin pairs. This study overcame two limitations of the Lynskey et al. (2003) study; namely, Cleveland and Wiebe (2008) did not restrict their study to discordant twin pairs, which would threaten the generalizability of the results, and did not rely on retrospective self-reports. They hypothesized that if the effect was genetic, within-pair differences in cannabis use would not predict differences in drug use between monozygotic twins, but they could explain initial and later differences in cannabis and illicit drug use between dizygotic twins. They found that earlier cannabis use predicted later illicit drug use only in dizygotic twins (B=0.22, P<0.05). There was no evidence of a gateway effect in genetically identical monozygotic twins (B=0.01, P>0.05). The authors argued that the frequency of cannabis use and later use of other illicit drugs reflect a genetically influenced behavioral trajectory rather than a gateway effect of cannabis use.

Mendelian randomization studies provide a novel genetic strategy to test whether associations are causal or not. Reed et al. (2022) used bidirectional Mendelian randomization from European ancestry genome-wide association summary data to test whether there was a causal relationship between smoking and alcohol use and cannabis, cocaine, and opioid use. Some bidirectional effects were found, such as from smoking initiation to cannabis use (OR 1.34), and vice versa (i.e., cannabis use to smoking initiation; OR 1.39). Cannabis use was not significantly associated with alcohol use in either direction. They did not test whether cannabis use was associated with cocaine and opioid use.

Overall, studies on the genetics of cannabis and other drug use and dependence indicate that shared genetic factors may partially explain the association between cannabis use and the use of other illicit drugs. An association nonetheless persists after adjustment for shared genetic factors in most of these studies, again suggesting a causal relationship between cannabis and other illicit drug use. Larger genetic studies, especially those using Mendelian randomization, are needed to better understand the role that genetic factors play in the relationship between cannabis and other illicit drug use.

Is Cannabis Use Linked to Social Opportunities for Other Drug Use?

Role of Illicit Drug Markets

According to another hypothesis, individuals who regularly use cannabis will have more opportunities to use other drugs because they purchase cannabis from the same illicit markets and affiliate with other drug users (Cohen 1972; Goode 1974). Wagner and Anthony (2002) reported on one of the very few comparisons of opportunities to use tobacco, alcohol, cannabis, and cocaine between cannabis users and nonusers among young adults ages 12–25 in the 1991–1994 U.S. National Household Surveys of Drug Abuse. They found that opportunities to use cocaine were strongly related to cannabis, alcohol, and tobacco use: only 13% of young people who had not used alcohol, tobacco, or cannabis reported an opportunity to use cocaine, compared with 26% of alcohol and tobacco users, 51% of cannabis-only users, and 75% of those who had used all three drugs. Those who had used cannabis were 15 times more likely to accept an offer to use cocaine than those who had not. These relationships did not change when young people who used cocaine within a year of their first opportunity to use were excluded from the analysis. These studies did not measure propensity to use illicit drugs, so it is difficult to exclude the possibility that personal characteristics may explain these associations.

In the Netherlands, the drug market explanation of the gateway pattern of cannabis use provided the rationale for a policy that aimed to separate the illicit markets for cannabis from those of other drugs (MacCoun and Reuter 2001). In the mid-1970s, the Dutch government chose not to enforce criminal penalties for personal possession and use of cannabis, and they later tolerated the sale of small quantities of cannabis in "coffee shops" (Korf 2019; MacCoun and Reuter 2001). The effect that this policy had provides a test of the hypothesis that the gateway pattern is explained by shared illicit markets (MacCoun and Reuter 2001). MacCoun and Reuter cited one cross-sectional survey by Cohen and Sas (1997) that assessed the strength of the association between cannabis and cocaine use among young people in the Netherlands in the 1990s. Cohen and Sas found that a smaller proportion of Dutch than American youth had used cocaine, but Dutch youth who had used cannabis were still more likely to use cocaine than were youth who had not.

No longitudinal studies have evaluated the effects of Dutch cannabis policy on the relationship between cannabis use and cocaine and heroin use. Analyses of cross-sectional studies have been reported by van Ours (2003), who analyzed patterns of cannabis and cocaine use in surveys of drug use conducted in Amsterdam between 1987 and 1997. van Ours found a typical gateway sequence that he attributed to a shared liability to use of cannabis and cocaine. MacCoun (2011) analyzed European survey data for the period 1998–2008 to assess whether Dutch youth who used cannabis were more or less likely than other European youth to have used cocaine. He found very similar rates of cocaine use among cannabis users in the Netherlands and elsewhere in Europe. A study of Dutch twins who were discordant for cannabis use also found that the twin who had used cannabis was more likely to have used other illicit drugs (Lynskey and Agrawal 2018). All of the available evidence suggests that the gateway pattern of cannabis use in the Netherlands has persisted, although perhaps attenuated, despite a policy of attempting to separate the cannabis market from other illicit drug markets.

Does Cannabis Use Cause Other Drug Use?

Cannabis use could potentially be a cause of other drug use if its regular use produces cognitive or neurobiological changes that increase the likelihood of using other drugs. A quasi-experimental co-twin design found that frequent cannabis use during adolescence was associated with poorer executive functions and general cognitive ability in early adulthood, but most of the associations between cannabis use and poorer cognitive function were weak (Ross et al. 2020). A systematic review of prospective epidemiological studies found associations between cannabis use and cognitive impairments and evidence of cognitive recovery following cessation of cannabis use (Lorenzetti et al. 2020).

Animal Studies of the Gateway Pattern of Drug Use

For ethical and practical reasons, we cannot randomly assign young people to use cannabis or not in order to assess whether the association between early and regular cannabis use and later illicit drug use is explained by personal characteristics and social contexts. We can, however, conduct experimental studies in which we randomly assign animals to receive either cannabis or a placebo and then assess whether the cannabis-exposed animals, as adults, are more likely to use cocaine and heroin than the animals exposed to the placebo.

This is a promising approach because animal studies have identified possible mechanisms by which cannabis use could increase the use of other illicit drugs. The endocannabinoid system undergoes profound changes during adolescence in humans and other animals and is thought to therefore be sensitive to the deleterious effects of cannabis and other drug use. This is reflected in the persistent alterations in behavioral measures of motivation, emotion, memory, and cognition (Kruse et al. 2019; Renard et al. 2017), and these effects are more pronounced in adolescence than after adult cannabinoid exposure (Quinn et al. 2008). Animal studies (e.g., Tanda et al. 1997) also indicate that shared neural pathways are involved in the rewarding effects of cannabis, cocaine, heroin, and nicotine (MacCoun 1998), all of which act directly or indirectly on the dopaminergic neurotransmitter systems in the reward centers in the midbrain (Gardner 1999).

Furthermore, animal studies indicate that the cannabinoid and opioid receptors have similar signal transduction systems (Cichewicz 2004; Viganò et al. 2005) and are expressed in several brain regions that have antinociceptive effects (Cichewicz 2004; Woodhams et al. 2015), and the cannabinoid 2 (CB_2) receptor has been shown to indirectly stimulate opioid receptors in afferent pathways (Ibrahim et al. 2005). Mutant mice in which the cannabinoid 1 (CB_1) receptor had been knocked out showed diminished place learning, were less likely to self-administer morphine, and showed reduced extracellular dopamine following morphine microdialysis (Befort 2015). Third, studies indicate that corticotropin-releasing factor, a key mediator of stress, is intimately involved in producing withdrawal symptoms from alcohol, opioids, cocaine, and cannabinoids (Rodríguez de Fonseca et al. 1997; Zorrilla et al. 2014).

However, the relationships between cannabinoids and opioids and their receptor systems are not clear-cut. Stopponi et al. (2014) exposed male rats to tetrahydrocannabinol (THC) during adolescence and found increased stress reinstatement of heroin seeking in adulthood. Importantly, however, they did not find any differences in the acquisition or maintenance of heroin self-administration. This finding may be a result of the relatively high dose of THC that was used (2.5 mg/kg). Indeed, studies that examined lower doses found increased heroin administration and behavioral responses to cocaine (Ellgren et al. 2007; Friedman et al. 2019). These discordant findings highlight the potential importance of cannabinoid dose as a mediating factor in susceptibility to other drug use.

Additional examples of the difficulty in drawing clear, translatable conclusions from animal studies include the works of Cadoni et al. (2001) and Lamarque et al. (2001). These studies found cross-sensitivity between cannabinoids and opioids and stimulant drugs in rats, providing some evidence that would suggest a direct path between cannabinoids and other drugs. However, in Lamarque et al.'s (2001) study, this was observed only in a strain of rats that were highly responsive to drug effects, indicating the mediating role of vulnerability. More studies of this type would be useful.

These inconsistencies highlight the difficulty in assessing the usefulness of animal models to understand human drug use. Some of the inconsistencies in preclinical studies are likely due to the variation in the cannabinoids employed, their dosage, dosing schedule, and washout period and the sex and developmental stage of the animals. Additionally, some of the common methodological practices in animal studies do not resemble how humans use cannabis. Synthetic cannabinoids are used in animal studies instead of the phytocannabinoids THC and cannabidiol (CBD) that are used predominantly by humans, hampering translation. Animal studies predominantly use systemic injections of pure THC, which has a different pharmacokinetic profile from the oral or inhalation routes typically used by humans. The dose of cannabinoids used also varied significantly across studies, ranging from 0.3 mg/kg up to 10 mg/kg THC (Poulia et al. 2020; Rubino et al. 2008). The duration of washout periods is critical to allow withdrawal syndromes to subside so that any effects of adolescent drug exposure can be isolated. Most studies have used only male animals, but when sex is examined directly, there are marked differences between male and female rats in their metabolism of THC, and interactions between sex and dose differ in the effects of THC on behavior, neural activity, and functional connectivity (see Ruiz et al. 2021 for one example).

Last, cross-sensitization between cannabinoids and opioids is typically investigated in only one direction, whereas the effect appears to be symmetrical. That is, animals that were administered opioids were cross-sensitive to cannabinoids and vice versa (Cadoni et al. 2001, 2008), suggesting that if opioids were more readily available than cannabis, they could be a gateway to cannabis use.

Effect of Delaying Cannabis Use on Other Illicit Drug Use

If cannabis use is a cause of the use of other illicit drugs, then preventing or delaying the former among adolescents should reduce the latter (Botvin and Griffin 2016; Pentz and Li 2002; Polich et al. 1984). Implementation of programs designed to prevent adolescent tobacco use and delay alcohol use resulted in reduced tobacco use, heavy alcohol use, and cannabis use (Botvin et al. 2002). For several reasons, however, these studies have not been able to provide compelling evidence that delaying cannabis use reduces the use of heroin and cocaine.

First, it has been difficult to demonstrate any effects of these programs on the use of cocaine and heroin because such use is rare in representative samples of adolescents (Gerstein and Green 1993; Manski et al. 2001). Second, even if the gateway hypothesis were correct, the most effective drug prevention programs have only modest effects on cannabis use and so would produce smaller reductions in the use of other illicit drugs (Caulkins et al. 1999). These features mean that very large sample sizes are needed to provide adequate statistical power to detect any effect that delaying cannabis use may have on the use of other drugs.

Deleterious Effects

If cannabis is a gateway to the use of other illicit drugs, its major deleterious effect would be to increase the use of cocaine, opioids, and methamphetamines, as well as the serious adverse effects that regular use of these drugs can produce (Darke et al. 2019). In 2022, there were more than 100,000 overdose deaths involving opioids and other illicit drugs in the United States (Centers for Disease Control and Prevention 2023). In addition, polydrug addiction is associated with greater risks of adverse psychiatric and physical health problems than cannabis use alone (Connor et al. 2014). These negative consequences include mental disorders, blood-borne viruses and infections, cancers, and other medical complications; deficits in cognitive functioning; and addiction treatment complications (Connor et al. 2014, 2021; Robertson 2022).

Studies of the effects of cannabis legalization in the United States have generally found that the frequency of cannabis use has increased among adult users, along with a minor increase in the number of adult cannabis users (Anderson and Rees 2023; Chiu et al. 2021; French et al. 2022; Hollingsworth et al. 2022). Adolescent cannabis use has not consistently increased after legalization (Anderson and Rees 2023; Chiu et al. 2021; French et al. 2022; Hollingsworth et al. 2022). Survey data have been inconclusive on the impacts of cannabis legalization on the prevalence of use of cocaine and heroin and other opioids among adults (Anderson and Rees 2023). Cannabis legalization has occurred during a period in which there have been steep increases in opioid overdose deaths in the United States. This was fueled by the liberalization of opioid prescribing in the 1990s, followed by increased trafficking of heroin and fentanyl into the United States from Mexico during the 2000s and 2010s (Stein et al. 2023). One study compared arrests for cocaine and opioid possession offenses in Washington State, where cannabis was legalized, with those in a synthetic cohort of the remaining states and found a reduction in these other drug arrests in Washington State (Wu and Cullenbine 2024). The authors interpreted this study as suggestive evidence of a reduction in the use of these drugs after cannabis legalization. It is open to a different interpretation: namely, that the police have reduced their attention to all drug possession offenses in Washington State since adult cannabis was legalized.

Beneficial Effects

Cannabis use would be beneficial if it reduced rather than increased the use of illicit drugs that are more harmful. A Canadian cohort study of street-involved youth ages 14–26 conducted between 2005 and 2015 challenged the hypothesis that cannabis is a gateway drug because it revealed that those who used cannabis daily had a lower, rather than higher, risk of initiating injecting drug use (adjusted hazard ratio 0.66; 95% CI 0.45–0.98) (Reddon et al. 2018).

On a population level, opioids are currently causing the largest number of illnesses and deaths after tobacco and alcohol. There could be potential health benefits if individuals who use these drugs were to use only cannabis. In the United States, during an epidemic of opioid overdose deaths, research has focused on a possible reverse gateway effect in which the use of cannabis replaces opioids for pain management or opioid dependence (Wadsworth et al. 2022). Interest in the hypothesis was initially sparked by reports of decreased opioid use among patients with chronic pain who used cannabis (Boehnke et al. 2016) and by a study reporting that U.S. states with medical cannabis programs had lower opioid overdose mortality rates than states that did not (Bachhuber et al. 2014). However, a later extension of the same time series data found that the association disappeared when a longer time series was analyzed (Shover et al. 2019), and a review of epidemiological studies did not find strong support for the hypothesis (Campbell et al. 2018). A recent analysis of household survey data found that those who used opioids did so *more often* on days when they used cannabis, both in individuals who did and did not have pain, suggesting that cannabis was *not* used as a substitute for opioids (Gorfinkel et al. 2021). Additionally, a more recent analysis of U.S. opioid mortality rate data indicated that the increase in the opioid mortality rate was higher in jurisdictions where cannabis was legalized than in those that had not legalized cannabis between 2010 and 2020 (Bleyer et al. 2022). Overall, the evidence does not strongly support the hypothesis that increased access to cannabis after adult legalization reduced opioid-related harms in the U.S. population.

If the gateway pattern arises from shared illicit markets for cannabis and other drugs, then the legalization of adult cannabis use could reduce access to and use of these other drugs. To date, analyses of survey data on the prevalence of drug use have consistently found an increase in the frequency of use among adult cannabis users but inconclusive results on trends in the prevalence of cocaine and heroin use (Chiu et al. 2021; Hollingsworth et al. 2022). It remains to be seen if the situation changes as adult cannabis legalization under full commercialization is implemented in many Canadian provinces and in more U.S. states.

Clinical Significance and Recommendations

The clinical significance of the gateway hypothesis depends on its underlying explanation. If cannabis use and the use of other illicit drugs reflect a shared liability to use drugs, then cannabis use initiated in adolescence will still predict young persons who are at increased risk of using other drugs. These young people would be a high priority for monitoring drug use and for using educational and clinical interventions to prevent them from becoming regular users of cannabis and harder drugs such as cocaine and opioids. However, a systematic review of universal school-based programs for preventing drug use did not find consistent effectiveness in reducing cannabis or other drug use (Faggiano et al. 2014). Some studies have found that broad programs of social competence and social influence interventions resulted in lower drug use, whereas others have reported no differences compared with usual curricula or no intervention.

If the association between cannabis and other drug use arises from shared social opportunities and increased involvement in illicit markets, then policies that separate the cannabis market from these illicit drug markets could reduce the use of other drugs. As indicated previously, this was the rationale for the de facto legalization of cannabis use and small-scale sales in the Netherlands, but evaluations of Dutch cannabis policy have not provided convincing evidence that this goal has been achieved. A similar claim about the benefits of adult cannabis legalization remains to be evaluated in Canada and many U.S. states. As discussed, studies to date do not suggest that increased adult access to cannabis has so far reduced opioid-related harms in the population (Shover et al. 2019).

Finally, if the relationship between cannabis and other illicit drug use is at least in part causal, then interventions that reduce cannabis use should reduce the use of other drugs, and public health and school-based interventions would be recommended. On the basis of this hypothesis, a policy that may increase the prevalence of cannabis use, such as the legalization of cannabis for recreational use (Zellers et al. 2023), would also increase the prevalence of cocaine, opioid, and methamphetamine use. If this were the case, then countries that decide to legalize adult cannabis use would need to implement strategies to minimize cannabis use among youth (Fischer et al. 2020).

Conclusion

Although the gateway effect of cannabis use is widely accepted, we cannot simply say that cannabis use causes individuals to use other illicit drugs. The mechanisms behind this association probably reflect the contributions of shared liabilities, social environment, and pharmacological effects in ways that remain to be elucidated.

Key Points

- A common sequence of drug use in the United States in the 1970s was one in which the use of cannabis followed that of alcohol and tobacco and preceded the use of cocaine and opioids. The earlier cannabis use was initiated and the more frequently it was used, the more likely a young person was to use other illicit drugs. The sequence largely reflected the availability of different illicit drugs in the community.
- There is a consistent, strong association between regular, especially daily, cannabis use and the use of other drugs that needs to be explained. A shared liability to use various illicit drugs partially explains the association.
- Regular cannabis users have more opportunities to use cocaine at an earlier age and are more likely to take these opportunities than are peers who have not used cannabis.
- Animal studies provide suggestive evidence that regular cannabis use in adolescent animals can increase the chances of adult animals using other illicit drugs.
- The relative contributions of shared liabilities, social environment, and the pharmacological effects of cannabis to the increased risk of using other drugs among regular cannabis users remain to be elucidated.

References

Agrawal A, Lynskey MT: The genetic epidemiology of cannabis use, abuse and dependence. Addiction 101(6):801–812, 2006 16696624

Agrawal A, Lynskey MT: Are there genetic influences on addiction: evidence from family, adoption and twin studies. Addiction 103(7):1069–1081, 2008 18494843

Anderson DM, Rees DI: The public health effects of legalizing marijuana. J Econ Lit 61(1):86–143, 2023

Anthony JC: Steppingstone and gateway ideas: a discussion of origins, research challenges, and promising lines of research for the future. Drug Alcohol Depend 123(Suppl 1):S99–S104, 2012 22572210

Bachhuber MA, Saloner B, Cunningham CO, et al: Medical cannabis laws and opioid analgesic overdose mortality in the United States, 1999–2010. JAMA Intern Med 174(10):1668–1673, 2014 25154332

Bailey SL, Flewelling RL, Rachal JV: Predicting continued use of marijuana among adolescents: the relative influence of drug-specific and social context factors. J Health Soc Behav 33(1):51–65, 1992 1619258

Befort K: Interactions of the opioid and cannabinoid systems in reward: insights from knockout studies. Front Pharmacol 6:6, 2015 25698968

Bleyer A, Barnes B, Finn K: United States marijuana legalization and opioid mortality epidemic during 2010–2020 and pandemic implications. J Natl Med Assoc 114(4):412–425, 2022 35469600

Boehnke KF, Litinas E, Clauw DJ: Medical cannabis use is associated with decreased opiate medication use in a retrospective cross-sectional survey of patients with chronic pain. J Pain 17(6):739–744, 2016 27001005

Botvin GJ, Griffin KW: Prevention of substance abuse, in APA Handbook of Clinical Psychology, Vol 3: Applications and Methods. Edited by Norcross JC, VandenBos GR, Freedheim DK. Washington, DC, American Psychological Association, 2016, pp 485–509

Botvin GJ, Scheier LM, Griffin KW: Preventing the onset and developmental progression of adolescent drug use: implications for the gateway hypothesis, in Stages and Pathways of Drug Involvement: Examining the Gateway Hypothesis. Edited by Kandel DB. New York, Cambridge University Press, 2002, pp 115–138

Brook JS, Cohen P, Whiteman M, et al: Psychosocial risk factors in the transition from moderate to heavy use or abuse of drugs, in Vulnerability to Drug Abuse. Edited by Glantz MD, Pickens RW. Washington, DC, American Psychological Association, 1992, pp 359–388

Cadoni C, Pisanu A, Solinas M, et al: Behavioural sensitization after repeated exposure to delta 9-tetrahydrocannabinol and cross-sensitization with morphine. Psychopharmacology (Berl) 158(3):259–266, 2001 11713615

Cadoni C, Valentini V, Di Chiara G: Behavioral sensitization to delta 9-tetrahydrocannabinol and cross-sensitization with morphine: differential changes in accumbal shell and core dopamine transmission. J Neurochem 106(4):1586–1593, 2008 18513369

Campbell G, Hall W, Nielsen S: What does the ecological and epidemiological evidence indicate about the potential for cannabinoids to reduce opioid use and harms? A comprehensive review. Int Rev Psychiatry 30(5):91–106, 2018 30522342

Caulkins JP, Rydell CP, Everingham SMS, et al: An Ounce of Prevention, a Pound of Uncertainty: The Cost-Effectiveness of School-Based Drug Prevention Programs. Santa Monica, CA, RAND, 1999

Centers for Disease Control and Prevention: Provisional data shows U.S. drug overdose deaths top 100,000 in 2022. Washington, DC, Centers for Disease Control and Prevention, 2023. Available at: https://blogs.cdc.gov /nchs/2023/05/18/7365. Accessed May 23, 2023.

Chan GCK, Butterworth P, Becker D, et al: Longitudinal patterns of amphetamine use from adolescence to adulthood: a latent class analysis of a 20-year prospective study of Australians. Drug Alcohol Depend 194:121–127, 2019 30419406

Chan GCK, Becker D, Butterworth P, et al: Young-adult compared to adolescent onset of regular cannabis use: a 20-year prospective cohort study of later consequences. Drug Alcohol Rev 40(4):627–636, 2021 33497516

Chen JC, Green KM, Arria AM, et al: Prospective predictors of flavored e-cigarette use: a one-year longitudinal study of young adults in the U.S. Drug Alcohol Depend 191:279–285, 2018 30165328

Chiu V, Leung J, Hall W, et al: Public health impacts to date of the legalisation of medical and recreational cannabis use in the USA. Neuropharmacology 193:108610, 2021 34010617

Cichewicz DL: Synergistic interactions between cannabinoid and opioid analgesics. Life Sci 74(11):1317–1324, 2004 14706563

Cleveland HH, Wiebe RP: Understanding the association between adolescent marijuana use and later serious drug use: gateway effect or developmental trajectory? Dev Psychopathol 20(2):615–632, 2008 18423097

Cohen P, Sas A: Cannabis Use, A Stepping Stone to Other Drugs? The Case of Amsterdam. Amsterdam, Centre for Drug Research (CEDRO), University of Amsterdam, 1997. Available at: http://www.cedro-uva.org/lib/cohen .cannabis.html. Accessed July 18, 2024.

Cohen S: Drug use: religion and secularization. Am J Psychiatry 129(1):97, 1972 5034192

Connor JP, Gullo MJ, White A, et al: Polysubstance use: diagnostic challenges, patterns of use and health. Curr Opin Psychiatry 27(4):269–275, 2014 24852056

Connor JP, Stjepanović D, Le Foll B, et al: Cannabis use and cannabis use disorder. Nat Rev Dis Primers 7(1):16, 2021 33627670

Darke S, Lappin J, Farrell MP: The Clinician's Guide to Illicit Drugs and Health. London, Silverback, 2019

Degenhardt L, Chiu WT, Conway K, et al: Does the "gateway" matter? Associations between the order of drug use initiation and the development of drug dependence in the National Comorbidity Study Replication. Psychol Med 39(1):157–167, 2009 18466664

Degenhardt L, Dierker L, Chiu WT, et al: Evaluating the drug use "gateway" theory using cross-national data: consistency and associations of the order of initiation of drug use among participants in the WHO World Mental Health Surveys. Drug Alcohol Depend 108(1–2):84–97, 2010 20060657

DuPont RL: Marijuana has proven to be a gateway drug. The New York Times, April 26, 2016. Available at: https://www.nytimes.com/roomfordebate/2016/04/26/is-marijuana-a-gateway-drug/marijuana-has -proven-to-be-a-gateway-drug. Accessed July 18, 2024.

DuPont RL, Han B, Shea CL, et al: Drug use among youth: national survey data support a common liability of all drug use. Prev Med 113:68–73, 2018 29758306

Ellgren M, Spano SM, Hurd YL: Adolescent cannabis exposure alters opiate intake and opioid limbic neuronal populations in adult rats. Neuropsychopharmacology 32(3):607–615, 2007 16823391

Faggiano F, Minozzi S, Versino E, et al: Universal school-based prevention for illicit drug use. Cochrane Database Syst Rev 2014(12):CD003020, 2014 25435250

Fergusson DM, Horwood LJ: Early onset cannabis use and psychosocial adjustment in young adults. Addiction 92(3):279–296, 1997 9219390

Fergusson DM, Horwood LJ: Does cannabis use encourage other forms of illicit drug use? Addiction 95(4):505–520, 2000 10829327

Fergusson DM, Horwood LJ, Swain-Campbell N: Cannabis use and psychosocial adjustment in adolescence and young adulthood. Addiction 97(9):1123–1135, 2002 12199828

Fergusson DM, Boden JM, Horwood LJ: Cannabis use and other illicit drug use: testing the cannabis gateway hypothesis. Addiction 101(4):556–569, 2006 16548935

Fergusson DM, Boden JM, Horwood LJ: Psychosocial sequelae of cannabis use and implications for policy: findings from the Christchurch Health and Development Study. Soc Psychiatry Psychiatr Epidemiol 50(9):1317–1326, 2015 26006253

Fischer B, Russell C, Boyd N: A century of cannabis control in Canada: a brief overview of history, context and policy frameworks from prohibition to legalization, in Legalizing Cannabis: Experiences, Lessons and Scenarios. Edited by Decorte T, Lenton S, Wilkins C. London, Routledge, 2020, pp 89–115

French MT, Zukerberg J, Lewandowski TE, et al: Societal costs and outcomes of medical and recreational marijuana policies in the United States: a systematic review. Med Care Res Rev 79(6):743–771, 2022 35068253

Friedman AL, Meurice C, Jutkiewicz EM: Effects of adolescent Δ9-tetrahydrocannabinol exposure on the behavioral effects of cocaine in adult Sprague-Dawley rats. Exp Clin Psychopharmacol 27(4):326–337, 2019 30932503

Gardner EL: Cannabinoid interaction with brain reward systems, in Marihuana and Medicine. Edited by Nahas GG, Sutin KM, Harvey DJ, et al. Totowa, NJ, Humana Press, 1999, pp 187–205

Gerstein DR, Green LW (eds): Preventing Drug Abuse: What Do We Know? Washington, DC, National Academy Press, 1993

Goode E: Marijuana use and the progression to dangerous drugs, in Marijuana: Effects on Human Behavior. Edited by Miller LL. New York, Academic Press, 1974, pp 303–338

Gorfinkel LR, Stohl M, Greenstein E, et al: Is cannabis being used as a substitute for non-medical opioids by adults with problem substance use in the United States? A within-person analysis. Addiction 116(5):1113–1121, 2021 33029914

Hall W, Leung J, Lynskey M: The effects of cannabis use on the development of adolescents and young adults. Annu Rev Dev Psychol 2:461–483, 2020

Hall WD, Lynskey M: Is cannabis a gateway drug? Testing hypotheses about the relationship between cannabis use and the use of other illicit drugs. Drug Alcohol Rev 24(1):39–48, 2005 16191720

Han C, McGue MK, Iacono WG: Lifetime tobacco, alcohol and other substance use in adolescent Minnesota twins: univariate and multivariate behavioral genetic analyses. Addiction 94(7):981–993, 1999 10707437

Hawkins JD, Catalano RF, Miller JY: Risk and protective factors for alcohol and other drug problems in adolescence and early adulthood: implications for substance abuse prevention. Psychol Bull 112(1):64–105, 1992 1529040

Heath AC: Genetic influences on alcoholism risk: a review of adoption and twin studies. Alcohol Health Res World 19(3):166–171, 1995 31798109

Hollingsworth A, Wing C, Bradford AC: Comparative effects of recreational and medical marijuana laws on drug use among adults and adolescents. J Law Econ 65(3):515–554, 2022

Ibrahim MM, Porreca F, Lai J, et al: CB2 cannabinoid receptor activation produces antinociception by stimulating peripheral release of endogenous opioids. Proc Natl Acad Sci USA 102(8):3093–3098, 2005 15705714

Jessor R, Jessor SL: Problem Behavior and Psychosocial Development: A Longitudinal Study of Youth. New York, Academic Press, 1977

Jessor R, Jessor SL: Theory testing in longitudinal research on marijuana use, in Longitudinal Research on Drug Use: Empirical Findings and Methodological Issues. Edited by Kandel DB. New York, John Wiley, 1978, pp 41–72

Kandel DB: Convergences in prospective longitudinal surveys of drug use in normal populations, in Longitudinal Research on Drug Use: Empirical Findings and Methodological Issues. Edited by Kandel DB. New York, John Wiley, 1978, pp 3–39

Kandel DB (ed): Stages and Pathways of Drug Involvement: Examining the Gateway Hypothesis. New York, Cambridge University Press, 2002

Kandel DB, Davies M: Progression to regular marijuana involvement: phenomenology and risk factors for near-daily use, in Vulnerability to Drug Abuse. Edited by Glantz MD, Pickens RW. Washington, DC, American Psychological Association, 1992, pp 211–253

Kandel D, Faust R: Sequence and stages in patterns of adolescent drug use. Arch Gen Psychiatry 32(7):923–932, 1975 1156108

Kandel DB, Davies M, Karus D, et al: The consequences in young adulthood of adolescent drug involvement: an overview. Arch Gen Psychiatry 43(8):746–754, 1986 3729669

Kandel ER, Kandel DB: Shattuck lecture: a molecular basis for nicotine as a gateway drug. N Engl J Med 371(10):932–943, 2014, 25184865

Kaplan HB, Johnson RJ: Relationships between circumstances surrounding initial illicit drug use and escalation of drug use: moderating effects of gender and early adolescent experiences, in Vulnerability to Drug Abuse. Edited by Glantz MD, Pickens RW. Washington, DC, American Psychological Association, 1992 pp 299–358

Kendler KS, Prescott CA: Cannabis use, abuse, and dependence in a population-based sample of female twins. Am J Psychiatry 155(8):1016–1022, 1998 9699687

Kendler KS, Jacobson KC, Prescott CA, et al: Specificity of genetic and environmental risk factors for use and abuse/dependence of cannabis, cocaine, hallucinogens, sedatives, stimulants, and opiates in male twins. Am J Psychiatry 160(4):687–695, 2003 12668357

Kendler KS, Ohlsson H, Sundquist J, et al: The interrelationship of the genetic risks for different forms of substance use disorder in a Swedish national sample: a top-down genetic analysis. J Stud Alcohol Drugs 84(3):361–367, 2023 36971740

Kleinig J: Ready for retirement: the gateway drug hypothesis. Subst Use Misuse 50(8–9):971–975, 2015 25774577

Korf DJ: Cannabis Regulation in Europe: Country Report Netherlands. Amsterdam,Transnational Institute, 2019

Kruse LC, Cao JK, Viray K, et al: Voluntary oral consumption of Δ9-tetrahydrocannabinol by adolescent rats impairs reward-predictive cue behaviors in adulthood. Neuropsychopharmacology 44(8):1406–1414, 2019 30965351

Lamarque S, Taghzouti K, Simon H: Chronic treatment with delta(9)-tetrahydrocannabinol enhances the locomotor response to amphetamine and heroin: implications for vulnerability to drug addiction. Neuropharmacology 41(1):118–129, 2001 11445192

Lessem JM, Hopfer CJ, Haberstick BC, et al: Relationship between adolescent marijuana use and young adult illicit drug use. Behav Genet 36(4):498–506, 2006 16565887

Leung J, Hall W, Degenhardt L: Adolescent cannabis use disorders, in Adolescent Addiction: Epidemiology, Assessment, and Treatment, 2nd Edition. Edited by Essau CA, Delfabbro PH. San Diego, CA, Academic Press, 2020, pp 111–135

Lorenzetti V, Hoch E, Hall W: Adolescent cannabis use, cognition, brain health and educational outcomes: a review of the evidence. Eur Neuropsychopharmacol 36:169–180, 2020 32268974

Lynskey MT, Agrawal A: Denise Kandel's classic work on the gateway sequence of drug acquisition. Addiction 113(10):1927–1932, 2018 29575218

Lynskey MT, Heath AC, Bucholz KK, et al: Escalation of drug use in early-onset cannabis users vs co-twin controls. JAMA 289(4):427–433, 2003 12533121

MacCoun R: In What Sense (If Any) Is Marijuana a Gateway Drug? FAS Drug Policy Anal Bull 4. Washington, DC, Federation of American Scientists, 1998

MacCoun RJ: What can we learn from the Dutch cannabis coffeeshop system? Addiction 106(11):1899–1910, 2011 21906196

MacCoun RJ, Reuter P: Drug War Heresies: Learning from Other Vices, Times, and Places. Cambridge, UK, Cambridge University Press, 2001

Manski CF, Pepper JV, Petrie CV (eds): Informing America's Policy on Illegal Drugs: What We Don't Know Keeps Hurting Us. Washington, DC, National Academy Press, 2001

McGee R, Feehan M: Cannabis use among New Zealand adolescents. NZ Med J 106(961):345, 1993 8341482

Morral AR, McCaffrey DF, Paddock SM: Reassessing the marijuana gateway effect. Addiction 97(12):1493–1504, 2002 12472629

Nahas GG: Keep Off the Grass. Middlebury, VT, Paul Eriksson, 1990

Newcomb MD: Understanding the multidimensional nature of drug use and abuse: the role of consumption, risk factors, and protective factors, in Vulnerability to Drug Abuse. Edited by Glantz MD, Pickens RW. Washington, DC, American Psychological Association, 1992, pp 255–297

Newcomb MD, Bentler PM: Consequences of Adolescent Drug Use: Impact on the Lives of Young Adults. Thousand Oaks, CA, Sage, 1988

O'Donnell JA, Clayton RR: The stepping-stone hypothesis: marijuana, heroin, and causality. Chem Depend 4(3):229–241, 1982 6985447

Osgood DW, Johnston LD, O'Malley PM, et al: The generality of deviance in late adolescence and early adulthood. Am Sociol Rev 53(1):81–93, 1988

Pentz MA, Li C: The gateway theory applied to prevention, in Stages and Pathways of Drug Involvement: Examining the Gateway Hypothesis. Edited by Kandel DB. New York, Cambridge University Press, 2002, pp 139–157

Polich JM, Ellickson PL, Reuter P, et al: Strategies for Controlling Adolescent Drug Use. Santa Monica, CA, RAND, 1984

Poulia N, Delis F, Brakatselos C, et al: Escalating low-dose Δ9 -tetrahydrocannabinol exposure during adolescence induces differential behavioral and neurochemical effects in male and female adult rats. Eur J Neurosci 52(1):2681–2693, 2020 31626712

Quinn HR, Matsumoto I, Callaghan PD, et al: Adolescent rats find repeated Δ(9)-THC less aversive than adult rats but display greater residual cognitive deficits and changes in hippocampal protein expression following exposure. Neuropsychopharmacology 33(5):1113–1126, 2008 17581536

Rebellon CJ, Van Gundy K: Can social psychological delinquency theory explain the link between marijuana and other illicit drug use? A longitudinal analysis of the gateway hypothesis. J Drug Issues 36(3):515–539, 2006

Reddon H, DeBeck K, Socias ME, et al: Cannabis use is associated with lower rates of initiation of injection drug use among street-involved youth: a longitudinal analysis. Drug Alcohol Rev 37(3):421–428, 2018 29430806

Reed ZE, Wootton RE, Munafò MR: Using Mendelian randomization to explore the gateway hypothesis: possible causal effects of smoking initiation and alcohol consumption on substance use outcomes. Addiction 117(3):741–750, 2022 34590374

Renard J, Szkudlarek HJ, Kramar CP, et al: Adolescent THC exposure causes enduring prefrontal cortical disruption of GABAergic inhibition and dysregulation of sub-cortical dopamine function. Sci Rep 7(1):11420, 2017 28900286

Robertson R: Book review: The Pocket Guide to Drugs and Health. By Shane Darke, Julia Lappin, and Michael Farrell, United Kingdom: Silverback Publishing, 2021, ISBN: 9781912141180. Addiction 117(7):2124–2125, 2022

Robins L, Darvish HS, Murphy GE: The long-term outcome for adolescent drug users: a follow-up study of 76 users and 146 nonusers, in The Psychopathology of Adolescence. Edited by Zubin J, Freedman AM. New York, Grune and Stratton, 1970

Rodríguez de Fonseca F, Carrera MR, Navarro M, et al: Activation of corticotropin-releasing factor in the limbic system during cannabinoid withdrawal. Science 276(5321):2050–2054, 1997 9197270

Ross JM, Ellingson JM, Rhee SH, et al: Investigating the causal effect of cannabis use on cognitive function with a quasi-experimental co-twin design. Drug Alcohol Depend 206:107712, 2020 31753729

Rubino T, Vigano D, Realini N, et al: Chronic delta 9-tetrahydrocannabinol during adolescence provokes sex-dependent changes in the emotional profile in adult rats: behavioral and biochemical correlates. Neuropsychopharmacology 33(11):2760–2771, 2008 18172430

Ruiz CM, Torrens A, Castillo E, et al: Pharmacokinetic, behavioral, and brain activity effects of Δ9-tetrahydrocannabinol in adolescent male and female rats. Neuropsychopharmacology 46(5):959–969, 2021 32927465

Scheier LM, Newcomb MD: Psychosocial predictors of drug use initiation
    and escalation: an expansion of the multiple risk factors hypothesis using
    longitudinal data. Contemp Drug Probl 18:31–73, 1991
Shahab L, Brown J, Boelen L, et al: Unpacking the gateway hypothesis of
    e-cigarette use: the need for triangulation of individual- and population-
    level data. Nicotine Tob Res 24(8):1315–1318, 2022 35137222
Shedler J, Block J: Adolescent drug use and psychological health: a
    longitudinal inquiry. Am Psychol 45(5):612–630, 1990 2350080
Shover CL, Davis CS, Gordon SC, et al: Association between medical
    cannabis laws and opioid overdose mortality has reversed over time.
    Proc Natl Acad Sci U S A 116(26):12624–12626, 2019 31182592
Stein BD, Kilmer B, Taylor J, et al (eds): America's Opioid Ecosystem: How
    Leveraging System Interactions Can Help Curb Addiction, Overdose,
    and Other Harms. Santa Monica, CA, RAND, 2023
Stopponi S, Soverchia L, Ubaldi M, et al: Chronic THC during adolescence
    increases the vulnerability to stress-induced relapse to heroin seeking in
    adult rats. Eur Neuropsychopharmacol 24(7):1037–1045, 2014 24412506
Szalavitz M: Once and for all, marijuana is not a gateway drug. VICE,
    October 13, 2015. Available at: https://www.vice.com/en/article/9bgn7a/
    why-marijuana-is-not-a-gateway-drug-1013. Accessed July 18, 2024.
Tanda G, Pontieri FE, Di Chiara G: Cannabinoid and heroin activation of
    mesolimbic dopamine transmission by a common mu1 opioid receptor
    mechanism. Science 276(5321):2048–2050, 1997 9197269
True WR, Heath AC, Scherrer JF, et al: Interrelationship of genetic and
    environmental influences on conduct disorder and alcohol and
    marijuana dependence symptoms. Am J Med Genet 88(4):391–397, 1999
    10402507
van Ours JC: Is cannabis a stepping-stone for cocaine? J Health Econ
    22(4):539–554, 2003 12842314
Vanyukov MM, Tarter RE, Kirillova GP, et al: Common liability to addiction
    and "gateway hypothesis": theoretical, empirical and evolutionary
    perspective. Drug Alcohol Depend 123(Suppl 1):S3–S17, 2012 22261179
Verweij KJH, Zietsch BP, Lynskey MT, et al: Genetic and environmental
    influences on cannabis use initiation and problematic use: a meta-
    analysis of twin studies. Addiction 105(3):417–430, 2010 20402985
Viganò D, Rubino T, Parolaro D: Molecular and cellular basis of cannabinoid
    and opioid interactions. Pharmacol Biochem Behav 81(2):360–368, 2005
    15927245
Wadsworth E, Hines LA, Hammond D: Legal status of recreational cannabis
    and self-reported substitution of cannabis for opioids or prescription
    pain medication in Canada and the United States. Subst Abus 43(1):943–
    948, 2022 35420977

Wagner FA, Anthony JC: Into the world of illegal drug use: exposure opportunity and other mechanisms linking the use of alcohol, tobacco, marijuana, and cocaine. Am J Epidemiol 155(10):918–925, 2002 11994231

Walters E: Marijuana: An Australian Crisis. Malvern, VIC, Australia, E. Walters, 1993

Wilson J, Mills K, Freeman TP, et al: Weeding out the truth: a systematic review and meta-analysis on the transition from cannabis use to opioid use and opioid use disorders, abuse or dependence. Addiction 117(2):284–298, 2022 34264545

Woodhams SG, Sagar DR, Burston JJ, et al: The role of the endocannabinoid system in pain, in Pain Control. Edited by Schaible H-G. Berlin, Springer Berlin Heidelberg, 2015, pp 119–143

Wu G, Cullenbine RR: Recreational marijuana legalization and drug-related offenses in Washington State: an interrupted time series analysis with a combination of synthetic controls. J Exp Criminol 20:395–420, 2024

Yamaguchi K, Kandel DB: Patterns of drug use from adolescence to young adulthood II: sequences of progression. Am J Public Health 74(7):668–672, 1984a 6742252

Yamaguchi K, Kandel DB: Patterns of drug use from adolescence to young adulthood: III. Predictors of progression. Am J Public Health 74(7):673–681, 1984b 6742253

Zellers SM, Ross JM, Saunders GRB, et al: Impacts of recreational cannabis legalization on cannabis use: a longitudinal discordant twin study. Addiction 118(1):110–118, 2023 36002928

Zorrilla EP, Logrip ML, Koob GF: Corticotropin releasing factor: a key role in the neurobiology of addiction. Front Neuroendocrinol 35(2):234–244, 2014 24456850

3

Cannabis Perspective Across the Lifespan

Childhood and Adolescence, Adult Age, and Older Adult Age

Sylvie J. Messer, Ph.D.

Tyler Pia, Ph.D.

Tanya Mehdizadeh, M.A.

Kaitlin Cuddleston, M.A.

Emily H. Kim, M.A.

Andrea H. Weinberger, Ph.D.

Cannabis is a mind-altering substance derived from the plant *Cannabis sativa*, which includes the psychoactive constituent Δ^9-tetrahydrocannabinol (Δ^9-THC) (Drug Enforcement Administration 2017; Hall and Solowij 1998). Cannabis acts on receptors in the brain that influence feelings of pleasure, memory, thought, concentration, perception, and coordinated movement (Drug Enforcement Administration

2017). Research on the long-term effects of cannabis use, both beneficial and deleterious, has been generating interest in recent years because of the availability of emerging longitudinal data and a shift in attitudes toward cannabis use. Cannabis use has been increasing as a result of changes in legalization and reduction of stigma; according to the U.S. 2020 National Survey on Drug Use and Health (NSDUH), 17.9% of people age 12 or older used cannabis in the past year, and the highest percentage of use was among young adults ages 18–25 (Substance Abuse and Mental Health Services Administration 2021). There is also evidence that the potency of cannabis has been increasing over time, which has corresponded to an increase in cannabis-related emergency department visits, particularly among adolescents (ElSohly et al. 2016). Although cannabis use is most common in young adults, individuals across the lifespan use cannabis, and there are substantial differences in the effects of cannabis use in adolescents, adults, and older adults. In this chapter, we review the current state of the evidence surrounding cannabis use across the lifespan (childhood and adolescence, adult age, and older adult age) and findings regarding the beneficial and deleterious effects of cannabis use related to each of these lifespan groups.

Current State of Evidence

Childhood and Adolescence

Cannabis is the most common illicit substance that is used or misused among adolescents (Simpson and Magid 2016). According to epidemiological data from the Substance Abuse and Mental Health Services Administration (SAMHSA) in 2014, about 1.2 million individuals ages 12–17 used cannabis for the first time within the prior year. Cannabis use was estimated to be 6.5% for individuals ages 12–17 (McClure et al. 2020), and 5.8% of individuals in this age range reported daily cannabis use (Simpson and Magid 2016). More specifically, 35.1% of twelfth graders in the United States reported having used cannabis within the past year, and one in eight adolescents had been approached by someone selling cannabis (Simpson and Magid 2016). According to epidemiological data from 2020, 2.7% of adolescents between ages 12 and 17 met diagnostic criteria for cannabis use disorder (CaUD) within 1 year (Center for Behavioral Health Statistics and Quality 2015). Regarding trends over time, there was a modest increase in past-month and past-year cannabis use from 2017 to 2019 and a significant increase in daily use among high school students during this period (Hammond et al. 2021). It is worth noting that cannabis use may be affected by changes in legalization status. There is a dearth of studies examining legalization and cannabis use among adolescents. In Colorado, cannabis use was approved for recreational purposes in 2012, and since then, it has accounted for 76% of adolescent substance treatment referrals (LeNoue et al. 2017). However, Hammond et al. (2021) found that legalization did not affect cannabis use trends among youth in the United States.

Several treatment options to address cannabis use are available for adolescents, and these are critical because 35%–75% of adolescents report experiencing withdrawal symptoms during attempts to reduce or abstain from cannabis use (Simpson and Magid 2016). Simpson and Magid (2016) reported that motivational enhancement with cognitive-behavioral therapy and the Adolescent Community Reinforcement Approach are the most effective treatments for CaUD because these treatments help to provide adolescents with insight into the consequences and benefits of discontinuing use. Prevention messages in school were also found to significantly decrease the likelihood of adolescents engaging in substance use. Pharmacological interventions such as *N*-acetylcysteine that target the brain region (e.g., ventral tegmental area) responsible for drug-seeking behavior also aided in cannabis use reduction. Interestingly, male adolescents tended to have more positive treatment outcomes than did female adolescents (McClure et al. 2020), including in states where cannabis was legalized (LeNoue et al. 2017).

Adult Age

Cannabis use in adults has increased in recent years. The United Nations estimated that 3.9% of the global adult population used cannabis in 2018 (Connor et al. 2021). The prevalence of past-year cannabis use varied significantly by country and region, with estimates as high as 12.4% in North America, West Africa, and Central Africa and as low as 1.8% across Asia (Connor et al. 2021; Steigerwald et al. 2020). According to NSDUH data from 2002 to 2017, the prevalence of adult cannabis use increased from 10.4% to 15.3% (~33% increase), and the prevalence of daily or near-daily use increased from 1.9% to 4.2% (~200% increase; Compton et al. 2019).

Studies suggest that the legalization of medicinal or recreational cannabis use in the United States has led to both an increase in cannabis use among adults and a shift in attitudes about cannabis use (Carliner et al. 2017; Chiu et al. 2021; Hall and Lynskey 2020). Namely, harm and risk perceptions of cannabis use seem to be decreasing nationwide despite increases in cannabis-related adverse health consequences, including CaUDs, fatal crashes, and emergency department visits (Carliner et al. 2017; Hasin 2018; Steigerwald et al. 2020). In addition to a decrease in the perceived harm of cannabis use, the price of cannabis has reduced significantly, which may have also contributed to increased use by giving individuals easier access to cannabis (Chiu et al. 2021).

Few changes in the characteristics of adults who use cannabis have been reported in recent years. In a study that examined the relationship between changes in cannabis use and changes in legal status, Cerdá et al. (2020) found that the increases in cannabis use and past-year CaUD occurred primarily among individuals 26 years or older, whereas cannabis use and CaUD prevalence among young adults ages 18–25 remained stable. Over a 12-year period (2002–2014), past-year cannabis use in the United States increased regardless of sex, age, race/ethnicity, income, education, marital status, or geographical region (Chiu et al. 2021). Although the legalization of cannabis use was partially motivated by racial disparities in the legal consequences of possession and use of cannabis, evidence suggests that individuals who engage in daily use continue to be disproportionately Black or Native American and of lower socioeconomic status (Jeffers et al. 2021). Frequent and daily use were also more common among young adults compared with middle-aged adults and among males compared with females (Jeffers et al. 2021).

Research has been done to compare the characteristics of individuals who use cannabis recreationally and individuals who use cannabis medicinally. For example, Turna et al. (2020) found a 60:40 split between individuals who used cannabis recreationally versus those who used it medicinally. In addition, more than 80% of individuals who used cannabis medicinally also used it recreationally. Compared with individuals who used cannabis only recreationally, individuals who used it for medicinal purposes were older, reported lower income, and endorsed greater use of other substances.

Although evidence indicates that the prevalence of cannabis use has increased over time in the United States, the evidence of changes in the prevalence of CaUD is inconsistent (e.g., Compton et al. 2019; Hasin et al. 2019). According to NSDUH data, the prevalence of CaUD from 2002 to 2017 did not increase overall; however, according to data from the National Epidemiologic Survey on Alcohol and Related Conditions, the prevalence of CaUD did increase overall from 2001–2002 to

2012–2013, with significant increases in states with medical cannabis laws (0.7% greater than in states that did not pass medical cannabis laws) (Compton et al. 2019; Leung et al. 2018). According to NSDUH data, significantly greater increases in the prevalence of CaUD were found for men compared with women, adults ages 18–29 compared with adults ages 35 and older, Black individuals compared with White individuals, and individuals at lower income levels compared with individuals at higher income levels (Hasin et al. 2019).

Older Adults

Cannabis use in older adults, generally defined as people ages 50–65 and older (Han and Palamar 2020; Hasin et al. 2019; Javanbakht et al. 2022), is increasing across the United States. In a study that included adults age 50 and older, 7.6% reported recent cannabis use (Javanbakht et al. 2022). Another national U.S. study indicated that approximately 9.0% of adults ages 50–64 and 2.9% of adults age 65 and older reported past-year cannabis use (Han and Palamar 2018). Nationally representative surveys showed a trend toward an increase in cannabis use, with one study showing a 75% relative increase from 2015 to 2018 (Han and Palamar 2020). This study found that the prevalence of adults age 65 and older who reported past-year cannabis use increased significantly from 2.4% to 4.2% ($P=0.001$) (Han and Palamar 2020). Likewise, from 2006 to 2015, cannabis use among older adults increased significantly from 0.56% to 2.44%, a relative increase of 336% (Le and Palamar 2019). Although the prevalence of cannabis use is increasing among older adults, the rate of change in use is significantly lower in adults age 65 and older than among younger populations (Hasin et al. 2019).

Various characteristics appear to be associated with the prevalence of and trends in cannabis use in older adults. Regarding prevalence, many studies have shown that cannabis use is more prevalent in older adults who are male, college-educated, unmarried, and of lower socioeconomic status (Hudson and Hudson 2021). In one sample, the prevalence of cannabis use (7.6%) was significantly higher than that of tobacco use (4.0%) and was greater among those taking psychotropic medications compared with those not taking psychotropic medications ($P<0.01$; Javanbakht et al. 2022). Other evidence indicates that older adults using cannabis are more likely to have an alcohol use disorder (AUD), be nicotine dependent, use cocaine, and misuse opioids compared with older adults not using cannabis (Han and Palamar 2018). Individuals with medical conditions such as respiratory and neurological conditions also had increased odds of cannabis use (Javanbakht et al. 2022).

Regarding trends in cannabis use, older adults receiving mental health treatment and those reporting past-year alcohol use showed significant increases in cannabis use from 2015 to 2018 (Han and Palamar 2020). Although studies found that cannabis use was more prevalent in males, another study showed a significant trend of greater increases in older adult females using cannabis (93.3% relative increase; $P<0.01$) compared with older adult males (58.3% relative increase; $P<0.05$) (Han and Palamar 2020).

Similar to the trends in cannabis use, CaUD in older adults also appears to be increasing (Hasin et al. 2019). The prevalence of past-year CaUD in adults older than 65 was 0.0% in 2001–2002 compared with 0.3% in 2012–2013 (Hasin et al. 2015). Among older adults ages 50–69 who were admitted to an inpatient unit, approximately 14.2% had symptoms that met criteria for a CaUD, and among adults age 70 and older, 0.4% had symptoms that met criteria for a CaUD (Charilaou et al. 2017). Although the prevalence of CaUD is increasing in older adults, they still have the lowest risk of developing CaUD compared with other age groups, with one study showing the risk being 4.5% for older adults compared with 41.1% for young adults (Leung et al. 2020).

Deleterious Effects

Childhood and Adolescence

Cannabis is the most commonly used drug in adolescence, with more than 20% of adolescents in the United States reporting monthly cannabis use (Choo et al. 2014); use in this population continues to increase over time, with significant increases specifically seen during the coronavirus disease 2019 (COVID-19) pandemic (Hammond et al. 2021). Adolescence is a critical period of development, and during this time, the brain and body are particularly vulnerable to the negative effects of cannabis, resulting in adverse impacts on cerebral development, physical health, and mental health (Lubman et al. 2015; Rubino and Parolaro 2008; Tuvel et al. 2023).

Cannabis use in adolescence has been linked with several deleterious effects on cognitive functioning and brain structure (Jacobus and Tapert 2014). Deficits in cognitive domains related to attention, learning, memory, and executive functioning have been found in adolescents who use cannabis (Fontes et al. 2011; Jacobus and Tapert 2014; Medina et al. 2007; Tapert et al. 2002; for reviews, see National Academies of Sciences, Engineering, and Medicine 2017 and Volkow et al. 2016). Such neurocognitive deficits are linked with structural changes in gray matter tissue, alterations of white matter structures, and abnormalities in neural function (Ashtari et al. 2009; Jacobus and Tapert 2014; Scott et al. 2019). Cognitive deficits in adolescents who use cannabis persist beyond abstinence and may persist into adulthood with heavy usage (Medina et al. 2007; Pope et al. 2003). Both an earlier age at initiation of cannabis use (before age 15) and heavy cannabis use are associated with greater cognitive deficits (Jacobus and Tapert 2014).

Cannabis use in adolescents is also linked with a number of physical health consequences, including increased risk of respiratory problems, cardiovascular issues, and sleep disturbances (Tuvel et al. 2023). Smoking cannabis is associated with coughing, wheezing, and shortness of breath (Taylor et al. 2000). In severe cases, smoking cannabis can lead to chronic bronchitis and other respiratory infections (Taylor et al. 2000; Tuvel et al. 2023). The use of cannabis can also affect the cardiovascular system, causing increases in heart rate and, in rare cases, acute cardiovascular events such as myocardial infarction, atrial fibrillation, and stroke (Rezkalla and Kloner 2019; Tuvel et al. 2023). Sleep disturbances, including insomnia, shorter total time spent sleeping, and later bedtimes are also noted in adolescents who use cannabis (Roane and Taylor 2008; Troxel et al. 2015).

The use of cannabis during adolescence is associated with adverse effects on mental health, including an increased risk of developing mental disorders and a decreased average age at onset of mental disorders (Di Forti et al. 2014; Meier et al. 2012; Silins et al. 2014; for a review, see National Academies of Sciences, Engineering, and Medicine 2017). It is correlated with an increased risk of developing depressive symptoms and mood disorders (Brook et al. 2011), and earlier onset of cannabis use is associated with a significantly higher risk of suicidal behaviors (Gobbi et al. 2019). Cannabis use in adolescence affects mental health well into adulthood and is linked with an increased risk of developing depression and suicidal behavior later in life, even in adults with no prior mental health history (Gobbi et al. 2019). Additionally, robust evidence suggests associations between psychotic disorders and the use of cannabis in adolescence. Cannabis use in adolescence is correlated with a significantly increased risk of developing schizophrenia and other psychotic disorders, regardless of frequency of use (Godin and Shehata 2022), as well as the early onset of psychotic disorders, particularly in individuals who have a predisposition for psychosis and those who use cannabis heavily (Bagot et al. 2015). Last, evidence indicates that cannabis use in adolescence is associated with the use of cigarettes, use of other drugs, and substance use disorders (SUDs). For example, youth who initiated cannabis use before age 14 were more likely to use other drugs such as tobacco and cocaine at an earlier age (Hawke et al. 2020), and youth who used cannabis were more likely to initiate both cigarette and electronic cigarette use over a 1-year period (Weinberger et al. 2021).

Adult Age

Despite the ubiquity of cannabis use in adulthood, its use in this age group is associated with many negative mental and medical consequences (National Academies of Sciences, Engineering, and Medicine 2017; Volkow et al. 2014, 2016). Long-term cannabis use in adults is correlated with respiratory disorders, vascular conditions, reproductive health issues, and an increased risk of motor vehicle collisions (Volkow et al. 2014). The most common way of ingesting cannabis among adults is smoking, which is associated with numerous respiratory issues, including inflammation of airways and chronic symptoms of bronchitis such as coughing and wheezing. Cannabis use is also linked with an increased risk of vascular conditions such as myocardial infarction and stroke during intoxication. Strong evidence suggests that cannabis use has a negative impact on reproductive health in people of both sexes and is associated with changes in reproductive hormones, disruptions in the menstrual cycle, and abnormal spermatogenesis (Lo et al. 2022). Additionally, cannabis use is correlated with substantial impairment in driving ability, which increases the risk of involvement in a motor vehicle accident twofold and may lead to physical injury or death (Hartman and Huestis 2013; Ramaekers et al. 2004).

Evidence suggests that cannabis use in adulthood is linked with an increased risk of serious psychological distress and various mental health disorders, including psychosis, depression, bipolar disorder, anxiety, and externalizing disorders (Hasin and Walsh 2020; Lowe et al. 2019; van der Pol et al. 2013; Weinberger et al. 2019), as well as cigarette use, other drug use, and SUDs (Hasin and Walsh 2020; Weinberger et al. 2016, 2020). Compared with lower-frequency use of cannabis, higher-frequency use is associated with worse mood and anxiety disorders symptomatology (Lowe et al. 2019). Individuals diagnosed with CaUD report a higher prevalence of any mental health disorder, and internalizing disorders such as mood and anxiety disorders are also more prevalent (van der Pol et al. 2013).

Older Adult Age

Cannabis remains the most commonly used illicit substance among older adults, and specific negative consequences appear to be related to cannabis use in this population. Aging may increase susceptibility to adverse events associated with any drug, including cannabis, because of differences in pharmacokinetics that may lead to an increase in drug serum levels; therefore, drug interactions with cannabis may exacerbate various negative effects on older adults' physical and mental health functioning (Lloyd and Striley 2018). For example, adverse events (e.g., sedation) in older adults were more common among individuals who used cannabis compared with individuals not using cannabis (Ameri 1999; van den Elsen et al. 2014).

Cannabis use in older adults has also been shown to be associated with several consequences across a broad range of medical areas, including oral disease (Le and Palamar 2019), injury, cardiovascular disease, respiratory problems, metabolic syndrome, and cancer (Lloyd and Striley 2018). Cannabis use is a potential risk factor for several different oral diseases, such as periodontal diseases; moreover, older adults who use both cannabis and tobacco have a significantly greater incidence of adverse effects in the oral cavity compared with those only using tobacco (Le and Palamar 2019). Physical injury is also a concern for older adults who use cannabis. Car accidents and slips and falls are prevalent in this population because of a decline in cognitive processing speed and visual skills, which are known to decrease as one ages (Lloyd and Striley 2018).

Individuals who report current and lifetime use of cannabis are more likely to be diagnosed with both SUDs and AUD (Lloyd and Striley 2018). Additionally, various other mental health diagnoses are strongly correlated with cannabis use (versus no use) in older adults. Some of the primary disorders that are particularly prevalent in older adults who use cannabis include major depressive disorder, anxiety disorders, PTSD, and schizophrenia (Lloyd and Striley 2018). More frequent and chronic use of cannabis is linked with an increased risk of developing both affective and psychotic symptoms (Hudson and Hudson 2021). Furthermore, evidence suggests that it may negatively affect recovery among older adults who are seeking treatment for mental health and substance use problems (Lloyd and Striley 2018).

Beneficial Effects
Childhood and Adolescence

Compared with studies on the deleterious effects of cannabis use, substantially less literature has examined its beneficial effects. Nonetheless, several beneficial effects have been identified. Previous research investigating the medicinal use of cannabis among youth and adolescents has revealed positive findings. Typically, cannabidiol (CBD), which is the nonpsychoactive component of the cannabis plant, is used for the medical treatment of children and adolescents.

Among a sample of 74 Israeli children and adolescents with intractable epilepsy who were treated with CBD-enriched medical cannabis oil for an average of 6 months, the CBD treatment showed a significant effect on seizure load (Tzadok et al. 2016). Most patients (89%) reported a reduction in seizure frequency. Fifty-nine percent of patients reported additional positive effects of the treatment, including improvements in communication, behavior, motor skills, and sleep. CBD-enriched medical cannabis was also found to be effective for refractory epilepsy among children and adolescents, with most patients (56%) reporting a reduction in seizure frequency following CBD treatment (Hausman-Kedem et al. 2018). The findings of these studies align with an earlier study on pediatric treatment-resistant epilepsy, which found that 84% of parents reported a reduction in their child's seizure frequency while the child took CBD-enriched cannabis, in addition to observed improvements in mood (79%), alertness (74%), and sleep (68%) and decreased self-stimulation (32%) (Porter and Jacobson 2013).

A pilot study conducted by Libzon et al. (2018) on the use of medical cannabis for children with complex motor disorder found that a CBD-enriched 5% oil formulation of cannabis was associated with significant improvement in dystonia and spasticity, sleep quality, pain severity, and quality of life after 5 months of treatment administration. Likewise, a retrospective study conducted in Germany found that children with dystonia and spasticity responded positively to synthetic THC and demonstrated either improved symptom management or reduced use of other medications causing negative side effects (Kuhlen et al. 2016). A case study of a 12-year-old boy with Tourette's disorder who was treated with a combination of cannabis-based medicines also found that the treatment resulted in an immediate marked reduction in motor tics and premonitory urges as well as a significant improvement in overall impairment based on self-ratings and parent and clinician reports (Szejko et al. 2019).

A scoping review on the use of medicinal cannabis for the management of behaviors related to autism spectrum disorder in children and adolescents revealed substantial behavioral and symptom improvements associated with its use, with 61%–93% of participants across all eight studies showing improvement (Fletcher et al. 2022). Specifically, reported improvements were related to self-injurious behaviors, repetitive behaviors, sleep, hyperactivity, cognition, communication, mood, and anxiety.

Several studies also explored the use of medicinal cannabis for chemotherapy-induced nausea and vomiting (CINV) in children. Results from three randomized controlled trials (RCTs) revealed that THC was more effective at reducing CINV than were other pharmaceutical medications such as domperidone, prochlorperazine, and metoclopramide (Chan et al. 1987; Dalzell et al. 1986; Ekert et al. 1979). Accordingly, medicinal cannabis was found to be associated with a reduction in nausea and vomiting and an increase in appetite among children with a neurological diagnosis and children with a cancer diagnosis (Doherty et al. 2020). However, research on the medical use of cannabis among children is ongoing, and its efficacy should be carefully evaluated over the long term (Rieder 2016).

Adult Age

Approximately 81% of adults in the United States report believing that cannabis has at least some benefits (Keyhani et al. 2018). The most commonly reported benefits of cannabis use are pain management (66%), treatment of various diseases (e.g., epilepsy, multiple sclerosis; 48%), and relief from anxiety, stress, or depression (47%). Beyond these beliefs, research investigating the use of cannabis among adult populations has suggested several beneficial effects related to its use.

First, adults using medical cannabis widely use it for pain management. One study found that 65% of respondents reported taking cannabis for pain relief, and 80% of these respondents reported cannabis to be very or extremely helpful in relieving pain; most respondents taking pain medications also reported reducing or stopping the use of those medications (Bachhuber et al. 2019). Moreover, several RCTs have demonstrated cannabis to be an effective treatment for pain (Hill 2015). Notably, a systematic review of the medical use of cannabinoids for the treatment of chronic pain found that among 2,454 adults with a variety of health conditions causing chronic pain (e.g., neuropathic pain, cancer pain, diabetic peripheral neuropathy, fibromyalgia, HIV-associated sensory neuropathy) across 28 RCTs, cannabinoids were associated with a greater reduction in pain than was placebo (Whiting et al. 2015). Another systematic review that investigated the medical use of cannabinoids for the treatment of nonmalignant neuropathic, chronic, and cancer pain found that across 15 RCTs, a greater number of patients taking cannabinoids reported a 30% pain reduction than did those taking placebo (Allan et al. 2018). Several clinical studies have also suggested that cannabis-based medications are effective in alleviating some of the symptoms associated with multiple sclerosis, including chronic pain (Koppel et al. 2014; Rog et al. 2005; Whiting et al. 2015). Furthermore, a cross-sectional survey of patients using medical cannabis found that most patients reported it to be more effective than opioid-based and non-opioid-based medications for pain management (Reiman et al. 2017). Among patients using opioids, 97% reported that they were able to take fewer opioids when they also used cannabis, and 81% reported that cannabis by itself was more effective than opioids. Comparably, among patients using non-opioid-based pain medications, 96% reported that they were able to take less of their non-opioid-based medications when they used cannabis, and 92% reported that cannabis was more effective than their non-opioid-based pain medications.

Studies have also examined the use of recreational and medicinal cannabis to mitigate risk factors of cardiovascular disease (Goyal et al. 2017). Specifically, epidemiological studies of U.S. adults report a lower prevalence of obesity and diabetes among people using cannabis compared with those not using cannabis (Le Strat and Le Foll 2011; Rajavashisth et al. 2012). In a U.S. study of 4,657 adults ages 20–59 who completed the U.S. National Health and Nutrition Examination Survey between 2005 and 2010, current cannabis use was associated with lower levels of fasting insulin, lower insulin resistance, and a smaller waist circumference (Penner et al. 2013). A double-blind, controlled study in the United Kingdom examined the use of CBD for the treatment of nicotine dependence and found a 40% reduction in cigarette smoking among the treatment group given a CBD inhaler compared with the placebo group (Morgan et al. 2013).

A literature review on the acute and long-term effects of cannabinoid use has highlighted evidence of the therapeutic effects of CBD on psychological function (Cohen et al. 2019). Specifically, a neuroimaging study performed by Crippa et al. (2009) assessed the impact of an acute CBD treatment on patients with social anxiety and found that CBD treatment decreased symptoms of subjective anxiety. Likewise, a double-blind RCT in patients with social anxiety found that patients who received CBD treatment reported lower ratings of subjective anxiety during a simulated public speaking task, as well as lower cognitive impairments and mental distress, compared with the group of patients who received a placebo and a control group without social anxiety (Bergamaschi et al. 2011). For the treatment of PTSD, CBD treatment has also been associated with a decrease in stress and anxiety symptoms (Fraser 2009; Greer et al. 2014; Roitman et al. 2014).

Regarding the treatment of psychosis, a double-blind randomized study investigating the efficacy of CBD compared with a conventional antipsychotic in attenuated psychosis found that CBD treatment led to significant clinical improvement with fewer negative side effects than did the antipsychotic treatment (Leweke et al. 2012). A study comparing patients with schizophrenia who received CBD treatment or a placebo along with their ongoing antipsychotic medications found that patients who received the CBD treatment reported fewer positive symptoms of psychosis after 6 weeks of treatment compared with the placebo group (McGuire et al. 2018). Additionally, a case report found a significant decrease in psychotic symptoms following CBD monotherapy among six patients with Parkinson's disease (Zuardi et al. 2009).

In a study of adult patients undergoing emetogenic chemotherapy, patients preferred a combination of cannabis-based medicines (THC and CBD) and reported less CINV compared with patients receiving the standard antiemetics (Grimison et al. 2020). Several studies also have found improved sleep and reduced use of sleep medication among adults using medical cannabis (Bachhuber et al. 2019; Cranford et al. 2017; Piper et al. 2017).

Hammersley and Leon (2006) administered a self-report questionnaire to 176 university students (ages 17–45) in the United Kingdom to assess the experiences of those using recreational cannabis. Notably, students using cannabis reported several positive effects, including increased feelings of relaxation, happiness, and excitement, as well as heightened creativity and imagination. Respondents also reported greater enjoyment of music, art, sex, and their surroundings. These findings map onto previous research on the psychotropic effects of cannabis consumption, which include mild euphoria, relaxation, and a general pleasant feeling (D'Souza et al. 2004).

Older Adult Age

A number of medical problems are being targeted with the use of cannabis in older adults. However, this research is greatly affected by government and policy regulations that control clinical trials of cannabinoids. Despite this barrier, older adults use cannabis for a variety of medicinal purposes, including the treatment of pain and arthritis (Ware et al. 2010), spasticity, sleep problems, depression (Beedham et al. 2020), anxiety (Bergamaschi et al. 2011), nausea (Smith et al. 2015), cancer-associated anorexia (Jatoi et al. 2002), and movement disorders (Chagas et al. 2014). Cannabinoids have been shown to be effective compared with placebo in treating symptoms associated with CINV (Smith et al. 2015). Some evidence suggests that cannabis may relieve anxiety, and anxiety disorders are common in older age populations (Wolitzky-Taylor et al. 2010); preliminary evidence has suggested that CBD but not THC may reduce symptoms associated with anxiety (Bergamaschi et al. 2011; Fusar-Poli et al. 2009).

Watson et al. (2022) investigated resting-state functional connectivity among older adults and found stronger connections among certain brain regions in older adults who used cannabis than among older adults who did not use cannabis. Specifically, the researchers found a connection between the anterior cerebellar regions and the hippocampal structures, and stronger connections in these regions may prevent typical age-related decline. These results suggest some beneficial effects of cannabis in the aging brain. However, further research is warranted to understand these effects longitudinally while considering the quantity, frequency, potency, and duration of use.

Clinical Significance and Recommendations

The increase in cannabis use prevalence and frequency over time has shed light on both the negative consequences of cannabis use and the potential benefits that cannabis use has for the treatment of certain medical and psychiatric conditions. With the recent legalization of cannabis in many U.S. states and Canada, a shift in attitudes has been leading people to increasingly view cannabis use as low risk. It is important to revisit the potential clinical implications of increasing acceptability and promotion of cannabis use.

As we have discussed, the prevalence of cannabis use has been increasing among all age groups, and evidence indicates that there are differences by age in the characteristics of individuals who use cannabis. Additionally, the limited research on cannabis use in childhood, adolescence, and older age thus far suggests that different effects of cannabis should be considered depending on the age group; in younger individuals, there are neurodevelopmental concerns to consider alongside the medical and psychological concerns shared by all age groups. As individuals grow older, they are at an increased risk of experiencing adverse interactions because the number of medications an individual is taking typically increases over time. Older individuals are also at an increased risk of physical injury due to a decline in cognitive processing speed and visual acuity, which typically occur as one ages. Cannabis use is associated with an increased risk of medical and psychological concerns across all age groups. For all age groups, it is also important to recognize the increasing prevalence of CaUD.

There is limited formal research on the clinical utility of cannabis because of its previous illicit legal status. The available research suggests that cannabis, or components of cannabis such as CBD, may have some use for the treatment of various ailments, including pain, nausea, and vomiting, as well as the alleviation of some psychiatric symptoms. Even in the absence of empirical data, prescriptions for cannabis have been available in recent years in the United States, and anecdotal evidence has suggested that individuals report benefits from cannabis beyond recreational use.

The evidence is mixed concerning the safety, efficacy, and clinical utility of cannabis use among all age groups. Although some evidence demonstrates positive effects of cannabis use for both medical and mental illnesses, a growing body of evidence appears to indicate risks of use within these domains. Additionally, future research is called for to understand how the legalization status of cannabis affects the prevalence of use across the lifespan and how it may be implicated in changes in prevalence of CaUDs and treatment options.

Conclusion

Cannabis is a psychoactive drug that is commonly used across the lifespan; however, the effects of its use differ substantially depending on the user's developmental stage. Adolescence is a critical period of development when youth are particularly vulnerable to the effects of cannabis. Despite widespread popularity, cannabis use during adolescence is associated with an increased risk of respiratory and cardiovascular issues and neurocognitive deficits, as well as an increased risk of depressive symptoms and mood disorders and a lower age at onset of psychosis and schizophrenia. Limited literature has addressed the beneficial effects of cannabis use for adolescents, although there is evidence that cannabis has positive effects on various medical and mental health conditions, including epilepsy, movement disorders, pain, and autism spectrum disorder.

Among adults, long-term cannabis use is associated with respiratory disorders (when cannabis is smoked), reproductive issues, and cardiovascular diseases. Additionally, cannabis use in adults is associated with an increased risk of developing depression, anxiety, bipolar disorders, and psychosis. However, it may be beneficial for adults in treating chronic pain, nicotine dependence, and social anxiety, as well as mitigating risk factors for cardiovascular disorders.

In older adults, cannabis use is associated with oral disease, injury, cardiovascular disease, respiratory problems, metabolic syndrome, and mental health issues such as depression, anxiety, and schizophrenia. Older adults use cannabis for medicinal purposes, including the treatment of pain, arthritis, spasticity, sleep, nausea, cancer-associated anorexia, and movement disorders.

For all developmental stages, further research is necessary to understand the effects of cannabis use across the lifespan while considering the quantity, frequency, potency, and duration of use.

Key Points

- Cannabis is the most commonly used and misused illicit substance among adolescents, and cannabis use trends among youth have not been affected by cannabis legalization in the United States.
- Cannabis use among adolescents is linked with abnormal brain development, cognitive deficits, and an increased risk of medical problems (e.g., respiratory problems) and mental health problems (e.g., mood disorders and psychotic disorders).
- Among youth, cannabidiol-enriched medical cannabis has been linked with significant symptom improvement for a number of neurological disorders, including epilepsy syndromes,

movement disorders, and autism spectrum disorder, as well as chemotherapy-induced nausea and vomiting (CINV).

- Studies suggest that cannabis legalization is associated with an increased prevalence of cannabis use and a positive shift in attitudes toward cannabis among adult populations.
- The prevalences of cannabis use and cannabis use disorder (CaUD) have increased among older adults; however, older adults have the lowest risk of developing CaUD compared with younger age groups.
- Cannabis use among older adults is associated with an increased susceptibility to adverse events (e.g., slips and falls), physical health problems, and mental health problems.
- Adult and older adult populations report several beneficial effects of cannabis use, including improvements in pain management, sleep, spasticity, mood, CINV, cardiovascular health, stress, and anxiety.

References

Allan GM, Finley CR, Ton J, et al: Systematic review of systematic reviews for medical cannabinoids: pain, nausea and vomiting, spasticity, and harms. Can Fam Physician 64(2):e78–e94, 2018 29449262

Ameri A: The effects of cannabinoids on the brain. Prog Neurobiol 58(4):315–348, 1999 10368032

Ashtari M, Cervellione K, Cottone J, et al: Diffusion abnormalities in adolescents and young adults with a history of heavy cannabis use. J Psychiatr Res 43(3):189–204, 2009 19111160

Bachhuber M, Arnsten JH, Wurm G: Use of cannabis to relieve pain and promote sleep by customers at an adult use dispensary. J Psychoactive Drugs 51(5):400–404, 2019 31264536

Bagot KS, Milin R, Kaminer Y: Adolescent initiation of cannabis use and early onset psychosis. Subst Abus 36(4):524–533, 2015 25774457

Beedham W, Sbai M, Allison I, et al: Cannabinoids in the older person: a literature review. Geriatrics (Basel) 5(1):2, 2020 31941020

Bergamaschi MM, Queiroz RHC, Chagas MHN, et al: Cannabidiol reduces the anxiety induced by simulated public speaking in treatment-naïve social phobia patients. Neuropsychopharmacology 36(6):1219–1226, 2011 21307846

Brook JS, Lee JY, Brown EN, et al: Developmental trajectories of marijuana use from adolescence to adulthood: personality and social role outcomes. Psychol Rep 108(2):339–357, 2011 21675549

Carliner H, Brown QL, Sarvet AL, et al: Cannabis use, attitudes, and legal status in the U.S.: a review. Prev Med 104:13–23, 2017 28705601

Center for Behavioral Health Statistics and Quality: 2014 National Survey on Drug Use and Health: Methodological Summary and Definitions. Rockville, MD, Substance Abuse and Mental Health Services Administration, 2015

Cerdá M, Mauro C, Hamilton A, et al: Association between recreational marijuana legalization in the United States and changes in marijuana use and cannabis use disorder from 2008 to 2016. JAMA Psychiatry 77(2):165–171, 2020 31722000

Chagas MHN, Zuardi AW, Tumas V, et al: Effects of cannabidiol in the treatment of patients with Parkinson's disease: an exploratory double-blind trial. J Psychopharmacol 28(11):1088–1098, 2014 25237116

Chan HSL, Correia JA, MacLeod SM: Nabilone versus prochlorperazine for control of cancer chemotherapy-induced emesis in children: a double-blind, crossover trial. Pediatrics 79(6):946–952, 1987 3035479

Charilaou P, Agnihotri K, Garcia P, et al: Trends of cannabis use disorder in the inpatient: 2002 to 2011. Am J Med 130(6):678–687.e7, 2017 28161344

Chiu V, Leung J, Hall W, et al: Public health impacts to date of the legalisation of medical and recreational cannabis use in the USA. Neuropharmacology 193:108610, 2021 34010617

Choo EK, Benz M, Zaller N, et al: The impact of state medical marijuana legislation on adolescent marijuana use. J Adolesc Health 55(2):160–166, 2014 24742758

Cohen K, Weizman A, Weinstein A: Positive and negative effects of cannabis and cannabinoids on health. Clin Pharmacol Ther 105(5):1139–1147, 2019 30703255

Compton WM, Han B, Jones CM, et al: Cannabis use disorders among adults in the United States during a time of increasing use of cannabis. Drug Alcohol Depend 204:107468, 2019 31586809

Connor JP, Stjepanović D, Le Foll B, et al: Cannabis use and cannabis use disorder. Nat Rev Dis Primers 7(1):16, 2021 33627670

Cranford JA, Arnedt JT, Conroy DA, et al: Prevalence and correlates of sleep-related problems in adults receiving medical cannabis for chronic pain. Drug Alcohol Depend 180:227–233, 2017 28926791

Crippa JA, Zuardi AW, Martín-Santos R, et al: Cannabis and anxiety: a critical review of the evidence. Hum Psychopharmacol 24(7):515–523, 2009 19693792

Dalzell AM, Bartlett H, Lilleyman JS: Nabilone: an alternative antiemetic for cancer chemotherapy. Arch Dis Child 61(5):502–505, 1986 3013104

Di Forti M, Sallis H, Allegri F, et al: Daily use, especially of high-potency cannabis, drives the earlier onset of psychosis in cannabis users. Schizophr Bull 40(6):1509–1517, 2014 24345517

Doherty M, Power L, Attala M, et al: Use of oral cannabis extracts in the pediatric palliative care setting: a retrospective chart review. Palliat Med 34(3):435–437, 2020 32103704

Drug Enforcement Administration: Drugs of Abuse: A DEA Resource Guide. Washington, DC, Drug Enforcement Administration, U.S. Department of Justice, 2017

D'Souza DC, Perry E, MacDougall L, et al: The psychotomimetic effects of intravenous delta-9-tetrahydrocannabinol in healthy individuals: implications for psychosis. Neuropsychopharmacology 29(8):1558–1572, 2004 15173844

Ekert H, Waters KD, Jurk IH, et al: Amelioration of cancer chemotherapy-induced nausea and vomiting by delta-9-tetrahydrocannabinol. Med J Aust 2(12):657–659, 1979 231736

ElSohly MA, Mehmedic Z, Foster S, et al: Changes in cannabis potency over the last 2 decades (1995–2014): analysis of current data in the United States. Biol Psychiatry 79(7):613–619, 2016 26903403

Fletcher S, Pawliuk C, Ip A, et al: Medicinal cannabis in children and adolescents with autism spectrum disorder: a scoping review. Child Care Health Dev 48(1):33–44, 2022 34403168

Fontes MA, Bolla KI, Cunha PJ, et al: Cannabis use before age 15 and subsequent executive functioning. Br J Psychiatry 198(6):442–447, 2011 21628706

Fraser GA: The use of a synthetic cannabinoid in the management of treatment-resistant nightmares in posttraumatic stress disorder (PTSD). CNS Neurosci Ther 15(1):84–88, 2009 19228182

Fusar-Poli P, Crippa JA, Bhattacharyya S, et al: Distinct effects of delta9-tetrahydrocannabinol and cannabidiol on neural activation during emotional processing. Arch Gen Psychiatry 66(1):95–105, 2009 19124693

Gobbi G, Atkin T, Zytynski T, et al: Association of cannabis use in adolescence and risk of depression, anxiety, and suicidality in young adulthood: a systematic review and meta-analysis. JAMA Psychiatry 76(4):426–434, 2019 30758486

Godin SL, Shehata S: Adolescent cannabis use and later development of schizophrenia: an updated systematic review of longitudinal studies. J Clin Psychol 78(7):1331–1340, 2022 35018649

Goyal H, Awad HH, Ghali JK: Role of cannabis in cardiovascular disorders. J Thorac Dis 9(7):2079–2092, 2017 28840009

Greer GR, Grob CS, Halberstadt AL: PTSD symptom reports of patients evaluated for the New Mexico Medical Cannabis Program. J Psychoactive Drugs 46(1):73–77, 2014 24830188

Grimison P, Mersiades A, Kirby A, et al: Oral THC:CBD cannabis extract for refractory chemotherapy-induced nausea and vomiting: a randomised, placebo-controlled, Phase II crossover trial. Ann Oncol 31(11):1553–1560, 2020 32801017

Hall W, Lynskey M: Assessing the public health impacts of legalizing recreational cannabis use: the US experience. World Psychiatry 19(2):179–186, 2020 32394566

Hall W, Solowij N: Adverse effects of cannabis. Lancet 352(9140):1611–1616, 1998 9843121

Hammersley R, Leon V: Patterns of cannabis use and positive and negative experiences of use amongst university students. Addict Res Theory 14(2):189–205, 2006

Hammond D, Wadsworth E, Reid JL, et al: Prevalence and modes of cannabis use among youth in Canada, England, and the US, 2017 to 2019. Drug Alcohol Depend 219:108505, 2021 33421799

Han BH, Palamar JJ: Marijuana use by middle-aged and older adults in the United States, 2015–2016. Drug Alcohol Depend 191:374–381, 2018 30197051

Han BH, Palamar JJ: Trends in cannabis use among older adults in the United States, 2015–2018. JAMA Intern Med 180(4):609–611, 2020 32091531

Hartman RL, Huestis MA: Cannabis effects on driving skills. Clin Chem 59(3):478–492, 2013 23220273

Hasin DS: US epidemiology of cannabis use and associated problems. Neuropsychopharmacology 43(1):195–212, 2018 28853439

Hasin D, Walsh C: Cannabis use, cannabis use disorder, and comorbid psychiatric illness: a narrative review. J Clin Med 10(1):15, 2020 33374666

Hasin DS, Saha TD, Kerridge BT, et al: Prevalence of marijuana use disorders in the United States between 2001–2002 and 2012–2013. JAMA Psychiatry 72(12):1235–1242, 2015 26502112

Hasin DS, Shmulewitz D, Sarvet AL: Time trends in US cannabis use and cannabis use disorders overall and by sociodemographic subgroups: a narrative review and new findings. Am J Drug Alcohol Abuse 45(6):623–643, 2019 30870044

Hausman-Kedem M, Menascu S, Kramer U: Efficacy of CBD-enriched medical cannabis for treatment of refractory epilepsy in children and adolescents—an observational, longitudinal study. Brain Dev 40(7):544–551, 2018 29674131

Hawke LD, Wilkins L, Henderson J: Early cannabis initiation: substance use and mental health profiles of service-seeking youth. J Adolesc 83:112–121, 2020 32768740

Hill KP: Medical marijuana for treatment of chronic pain and other medical and psychiatric problems: a clinical review. JAMA 313(24):2474–2483, 2015 26103031

Hudson A, Hudson P: Risk factors for cannabis-related mental health harms in older adults: a review. Clin Gerontol 44(1):3–15, 2021 32862795

Jacobus J, Tapert SF: Effects of cannabis on the adolescent brain. Curr Pharm Des 20(13):2186–2193, 2014 23829363

Jatoi A, Windschitl HE, Loprinzi CL, et al: Dronabinol versus megestrol acetate versus combination therapy for cancer-associated anorexia: a North Central Cancer Treatment Group study. J Clin Oncol 20(2):567–573, 2002 11786587

Javanbakht M, Takada S, Akabike W, et al: Cannabis use, comorbidities, and prescription medication use among older adults in a large healthcare system in Los Angeles, CA 2019–2020. J Am Geriatr Soc 70(6):1673–1684, 2022 35234291

Jeffers AM, Glantz S, Byers A, et al: Sociodemographic characteristics associated with and prevalence and frequency of cannabis use among adults in the US. JAMA Netw Open 4(11):e2136571, 2021 34846523

Keyhani S, Steigerwald S, Ishida J, et al: Risks and benefits of marijuana use: a national survey of US adults. Ann Intern Med 169(5):282–290, 2018 30039154

Koppel BS, Brust JCM, Fife T, et al: Systematic review: efficacy and safety of medical marijuana in selected neurologic disorders: report of the Guideline Development Subcommittee of the American Academy of Neurology. Neurology 82(17):1556–1563, 2014 24778283

Kuhlen M, Hoell JI, Gagnon G, et al: Effective treatment of spasticity using dronabinol in pediatric palliative care. Eur J Paediatr Neurol 20(6):898–903, 2016 27506815

Le A, Palamar JJ: Oral health implications of increased cannabis use among older adults: another public health concern? J Subst Use 24(1):61–65, 2019 30524195

LeNoue SR, Salomonsen-Sautel S, Min SJ, et al: Marijuana commercialization and adolescent substance treatment outcomes in Colorado. Am J Addict 26(8):802–806, 2017 29064160

Le Strat Y, Le Foll B: Obesity and cannabis use: results from 2 representative national surveys. Am J Epidemiol 174(8):929–933, 2011 21868374

Leung J, Chiu CYV, Stjepanović D, et al: Has the legalisation of medical and recreational cannabis use in the USA affected the prevalence of cannabis use and cannabis use disorders? Curr Addict Rep 5(4):403–417, 2018

Leung J, Chan GCK, Hides L, et al: What is the prevalence and risk of cannabis use disorders among people who use cannabis? A systematic review and meta-analysis. Addict Behav 109:106479, 2020 32485547

Leweke FM, Piomelli D, Pahlisch F, et al: Cannabidiol enhances anandamide signaling and alleviates psychotic symptoms of schizophrenia. Transl Psychiatry 2(3):e94, 2012 22832859

Libzon S, Schleider LB-L, Saban N, et al: Medical cannabis for pediatric moderate to severe complex motor disorders. J Child Neurol 33(9):565–571, 2018 29766748

Lloyd SL, Striley CW: Marijuana use among adults 50 years or older in the 21st century. Gerontol Geriatr Med 4:2333721418781668, 2018 29977980

Lo JO, Hedges JC, Girardi G: Impact of cannabinoids on pregnancy, reproductive health, and offspring outcomes. Am J Obstet Gynecol 227(4):571–581, 2022 35662548

Lowe DJE, Sasiadek JD, Coles AS, et al: Cannabis and mental illness: a review. Eur Arch Psychiatry Clin Neurosci 269(1):107–120, 2019 30564886

Lubman DI, Cheetham A, Yücel M: Cannabis and adolescent brain development. Pharmacol Ther 148:1–16, 2015 25460036

McClure EA, Baker NL, Hood CO, et al: Cannabis and alcohol co-use in a smoking cessation pharmacotherapy trial for adolescents and emerging adults. Nicotine Tob Res 22(8):1374–1382, 2020 31612956

McGuire P, Robson P, Cubala WJ, et al: Cannabidiol (CBD) as an adjunctive therapy in schizophrenia: a multicenter randomized controlled trial. Am J Psychiatry 175(3):225–231, 2018 29241357

Medina KL, Hanson KL, Schweinsburg AD, et al: Neuropsychological functioning in adolescent marijuana users: subtle deficits detectable after a month of abstinence. J Int Neuropsychol Soc 13(5):807–820, 2007 17697412

Meier MH, Caspi A, Ambler A, et al: Persistent cannabis users show neuropsychological decline from childhood to midlife. Proc Natl Acad Sci U S A 109(40), E2657–E2664, 2012 22927402

Morgan CJA, Das RK, Joye A, et al: Cannabidiol reduces cigarette consumption in tobacco smokers: preliminary findings. Addict Behav 38(9):2433–2436, 2013 23685330

National Academies of Sciences, Engineering, and Medicine: The Health Effects of Cannabis and Cannabinoids: The Current State of Evidence and Recommendations for Research. Washington, DC, National Academies Press, 2017

Penner EA, Buettner H, Mittleman MA: The impact of marijuana use on glucose, insulin, and insulin resistance among US adults. Am J Med 126(7):583–589, 2013 23684393

Piper BJ, DeKeuster RM, Beals ML, et al: Substitution of medical cannabis for pharmaceutical agents for pain, anxiety, and sleep. J Psychopharmacol 31(5):569–575, 2017 28372506

Pope HG Jr, Gruber AJ, Hudson JI, et al: Early onset cannabis use and cognitive deficits: what is the nature of the association? Drug Alcohol Depend 69(3):303–310, 2003 12633916

Porter BE, Jacobson C: Report of a parent survey of cannabidiol-enriched cannabis use in pediatric treatment-resistant epilepsy. Epilepsy Behav 29(3):574–577, 2013 24237632

Rajavashisth TB, Shaheen M, Norris KC, et al: Decreased prevalence of diabetes in marijuana users: cross-sectional data from the National Health and Nutrition Examination Survey (NHANES) III. BMJ Open 2(1):e000494, 2012 22368296

Ramaekers JG, Berghaus G, van Laar M, et al: Dose related risk of motor vehicle crashes after cannabis use. Drug Alcohol Depend 73(2):109–119, 2004 14725950

Reiman A, Welty M, Solomon P: Cannabis as a substitute for opioid-based pain medication: patient self-report. Cannabis Cannabinoid Res 2(1):160–166, 2017 28861516

Rezkalla S, Kloner RA: Cardiovascular effects of marijuana. Trends Cardiovasc Med 29(7):403–407, 2019 30447899

Rieder MJ: Is the medical use of cannabis a therapeutic option for children? Paediatr Child Health 21(1):31–34, 2016 26941559

Roane BM, Taylor DJ: Adolescent insomnia as a risk factor for early adult depression and substance abuse. Sleep 31(10):1351–1356, 2008 18853932

Rog DJ, Nurmikko TJ, Friede T, et al: Randomized, controlled trial of cannabis-based medicine in central pain in multiple sclerosis. Neurology 65(6):812–819, 2005 16186518

Roitman P, Mechoulam R, Cooper-Kazaz R, et al: Preliminary, open-label, pilot study of add-on oral Δ9-tetrahydrocannabinol in chronic post-traumatic stress disorder. Clin Drug Investig 34(8):587–591, 2014 24935052

Rubino T, Parolaro D: Long lasting consequences of cannabis exposure in adolescence. Mol Cell Endocrinol 286(1–2 Suppl 1), S108–S113, 2008 18358595

Scott JC, Rosen AFG, Moore TM, et al: Cannabis use in youth is associated with limited alterations in brain structure. Neuropsychopharmacology 44(8):1362–1369, 2019 30780151

Silins E, Horwood LJ, Patton GC, et al: Young adult sequelae of adolescent cannabis use: an integrative analysis. Lancet Psychiatry 1(4):286–293, 2014 26360862

Simpson AK, Magid V: Cannabis use disorder in adolescence. Child Adolesc Psychiatr Clin N Am 25(3):431–443, 2016 27338965

Smith LA, Azariah F, Lavender VT, et al: Cannabinoids for nausea and vomiting in adults with cancer receiving chemotherapy. Cochrane Database Syst Rev 2015(11):CD009464, 2015 26561338

Steigerwald S, Cohen BE, Vali M, et al: Differences in opinions about marijuana use and prevalence of use by state legalization status. J Addict Med 14(4):337–344, 2020 31821192

Substance Abuse and Mental Health Services Administration: Key Substance Use and Mental Health Indicators in the United States: Results From the 2020 National Survey on Drug Use and Health (HHS Publ No PEP21-07-01-003, NSDUH Series H-56). Rockville, MD, Center for Behavioral Health Statistics and Quality, Substance Abuse and Mental Health Services Administration, 2021

Szejko N, Jakubovski E, Fremer C, et al: Vaporized cannabis is effective and well-tolerated in an adolescent with Tourette syndrome. Med Cannabis Cannabinoids 2(1):60–63, 2019 34676335

Tapert SF, Granholm E, Leedy NG, et al: Substance use and withdrawal: neuropsychological functioning over 8 years in youth. J Int Neuropsychol Soc 8(7):873–883, 2002 12405538

Taylor DR, Poulton R, Moffitt TE, et al: The respiratory effects of cannabis dependence in young adults. Addiction 95(11):1669–1677, 2000 11219370

Troxel WM, Ewing B, D'Amico EJ: Examining racial/ethnic disparities in the association between adolescent sleep and alcohol or marijuana use. Sleep Health 1(2):104–108, 2015 26436131

Turna J, Balodis I, Munn C, et al: Overlapping patterns of recreational and medical cannabis use in a large community sample of cannabis users. Compr Psychiatry 102:152–188, 2020 32653594

Tuvel AL, Winiger EA, Ross JM: A review of the effects of adolescent cannabis use on physical health. Child Adolesc Psychiatr Clin N Am 32(1):85–105, 2023 36410908

Tzadok M, Uliel-Siboni S, Linder I, et al: CBD-enriched medical cannabis for intractable pediatric epilepsy: the current Israeli experience. Seizure 35:41–44, 2016 26800377

van den Elsen GA, Ahmed AI, Lammers M, et al: Efficacy and safety of medical cannabinoids in older subjects: a systematic review. Ageing Res Rev 14:56–64, 2014 24509411

van der Pol P, Liebregts N, de Graaf R, et al: Mental health differences between frequent cannabis users with and without dependence and the general population. Addiction 108(8):1459–1469, 2013 23530710

Volkow ND, Baler RD, Compton WM, et al: Adverse health effects of marijuana use. N Engl J Med 370(23):2219–2227, 2014 24897085

Volkow ND, Swanson JM, Evins AE, et al: Effects of cannabis use on human behavior, including cognition, motivation, and psychosis: a review. JAMA Psychiatry 73(3):292–297, 2016 26842658

Ware MA, Wang T, Shapiro S, et al: Smoked cannabis for chronic neuropathic pain: a randomized controlled trial. CMAJ 182(14):E694–E701, 2010 20805210

Watson KK, Bryan AD, Thayer RE, et al: Cannabis use and resting state functional connectivity in the aging brain. Front Aging Neurosci 14:804–890, 2022 35221994

Weinberger AH, Platt J, Goodwin RD: Is cannabis use associated with an increased risk of onset and persistence of alcohol use disorders? A three-year prospective study among adults in the United States. Drug Alcohol Depend 161:363–367, 2016 26875671

Weinberger AH, Pacek LR, Sheffer CE, et al: Serious psychological distress and daily cannabis use, 2008 to 2016: potential implications for mental health? Drug Alcohol Depend 197:134–140, 2019 30825793

Weinberger AH, Delnevo CD, Wyka K, et al: Cannabis use is associated with increased risk of cigarette smoking initiation, persistence, and relapse among adults in the United States. Nicotine Tob Res 22(8):1404–1408, 2020 31112595

Weinberger AH, Zhu J, Lee J, et al: Cannabis use and the onset of cigarette and e-cigarette use: a prospective, longitudinal study among youth in the United States. Nicotine Tob Res 23(3):609–613, 2021 32835370

Whiting PF, Wolff RF, Deshpande S, et al: Cannabinoids for medical use: a systematic review and meta-analysis. JAMA 313(24):2456–2473, 2015 26103030

Wolitzky-Taylor KB, Castriotta N, Lenze EJ, et al: Anxiety disorders in older adults: a comprehensive review. Depress Anxiety 27(2):190–211, 2010 20099273

Zuardi AW, Crippa JA, Hallak JE, et al: Cannabidiol for the treatment of psychosis in Parkinson's disease. J Psychopharmacol 23(8):979–983, 2009 18801821

4

Cannabis Use and Adolescent Psychosocial Function

Leslie H. Lundahl, Ph.D.

David M. Ledgerwood, Ph.D.

Emilie-Clare L. O'Mara, B.S.

Cannabis use, especially among youth and young adults, has been thought to negatively affect the transition to adulthood and the assumption of adult roles (e.g., relationships, employment, educational attainment, independence from parents). In popular literature, this phenomenon has been referred to as a "failure to launch." Whereas *emerging adulthood* describes a tendency to explore job possibilities and options (Arnett 2000; Edwards and Hertel-Fernandez 2010), often within periods of leaving and returning to parental homes (Shulman et al. 2005), *failure to launch* refers to declining independent living and economic self-sufficiency in the transition to adulthood (Bell et al. 2007; Lebowitz 2016). It is further characterized by passivity and impairments in mental health (e.g., depression, anxiety), discipline, motivation, resilience, and executive function. Adolescence and emerging adulthood represent a time of tremendous neural and behavioral change (Giedd 2015), with substantial growth in both brain function and structure that underlie cognitive development. It is also a time when the skills required to function as an adult in society undergo rapid development. As a result, exposure to cannabis and other substances during this vulnerable period can interfere with psychological, social, and academic functioning to a greater extent than it might at later developmental periods (Jacobus et al. 2015), thus delaying or even preventing the skill acquisition necessary for taking on adult roles. In this chapter, we examine whether cannabis may be directly contributing to impairments in the transition to adulthood by focusing on research that explores the potential effects of cannabis use on motivation, academic achievement, social functioning, emotional functioning, and mental health.

Deleterious Effects of Cannabis on Psychosocial Development and Function

Cannabis and Emotional Development

Clinicians, parents, policymakers, and others have often been concerned that early cannabis use may lead to various emotional problems among youth and young adults. Although there is no research on failure to launch per se as it relates to cannabis use and emotional problems, deficits in normative emotional development or the development of mental health difficulties might prevent youth from achieving independence in adulthood. In this chapter, we answer the following questions: To what extent are cannabis use and mental health problems or deficits in emotional development associated among youth? And to what extent does early cannabis use predict later mental health problems or emotional development deficits among youth? Because the correlational nature of these questions precludes determining if cannabis use causes emotional problems, it is important to consider that the interrelationship between cannabis use and emotional development may not be unidirectional but reciprocal. Nevertheless, we focus primarily on studies that explore the association between cannabis use and emotional development longitudinally, which provides the clearest picture of whether and how early cannabis use might lead to later emotional and mental health problems.

Cannabis Use and Emotional Problems Among Youth

Relatively few studies have explored the interrelationship between youth cannabis use and emotional development per se. On the other hand, several studies have explored the relationship between cannabis use and the subsequent development of mental health problems such as depression, anxiety, externalizing problems, substance use, and psychosis.

Very few studies have examined emotional self-regulation, personality, and other factors associated with early cannabis use, Brook et al. (2016) assessed cannabis use at an average age of 14 years and subsequently assessed developmental trajectories of these participants at a mean age of 43 years. They found that participants with trajectories reflecting chronic/heavy or chronic/occasional cannabis use experienced significant emotional dysregulation, and chronic/heavy use was associated with greater sensation seeking in mid-adulthood. Another study examining cannabis use and cannabis use disorder (CaUD) at age 17 found that youth with CaUD experienced significantly greater negative emotionality (as measured by the Multidimensional Personality Questionnaire) compared with cannabis nonusers but no differences when compared with those who used cannabis but did not have CaUD (Foster et al. 2018). This study also revealed that cannabis users with CaUD and those without CaUD exhibited lower behavioral constraint (reflecting cautiousness, planfulness [i.e., how carefully people think about achieving their goals], endorsement of traditional social values, and avoidance of danger) than did nonusers.

Several large-scale studies have examined the interrelationship between cannabis use and mental health problems among youth. One cross-sectional study of Canadian youth revealed that cannabis use was associated with depression and anxiety, but this relationship was no longer significant after controlling for flourishing (a general measure of overall psychological well-being) (Butler et al. 2019). A longitudinal study of 927 Australian fifth-grade students followed over six waves between ages 12 and 19 years revealed that youth who had early onset of cannabis use experienced the greatest number of adjustment problems as young adults, including antisocial behavior, violence, cannabis- and alcohol-related harms, and tobacco use, compared with youth who abstained from cannabis (Scholes-Balog et al. 2016). Youth with lateronset of cannabis use also experienced elevated harms related to cannabis and other substance use compared with youth who abstained.

Patton et al. (2002) examined cannabis use in a 6-year longitudinal study in Australia and revealed that daily cannabis use among young females was associated with a fivefold increase in depression and anxiety. Furthermore, weekly or more frequent cannabis use among teenagers predicted a twofold increased risk for later depression and anxiety. However, early depression and anxiety did not predict later cannabis use. Another longitudinal examination of alcohol and cannabis use trajectories from early adolescence to young adulthood revealed that poorer school performance and commitment, lower self-esteem, poorer family relations, poorer peer pressure resistance, greater sensation seeking, positive marijuana expectancies, and increased incidence of conduct disorder were predictive of cannabis use, with a roughly linear relationship between early-onset, later-onset, and nonuser groups (Flory et al. 2004).

Several studies have specifically revealed that early cannabis use is predictive of depression and anxiety. A large-scale meta-analysis of 11 longitudinal studies (*N*=23,317) found that adolescent cannabis use was linked with the later development of depression and suicidality but not with anxiety disorder (Gobbi et al. 2019). Another large-scale meta-analysis examining 14 longitudinal studies with 76,058 participants found that cannabis use was correlated with a modestly increased risk of developing depression and heavy cannabis use was associated with a moderately increased risk, but the authors also noted a need for further research into cumulative exposure and study-specific factors (Lev-Ran et al. 2014). Additional studies confirmed associations between cannabis use in adolescence and subsequent depression and/or anxiety (e.g., Capaldi et al. 2022; Schaefer et al. 2021).

Studies have also revealed that early cannabis use is linked with aggressive, antisocial, or oppositional behavior (Brook et al. 2011; Fergusson et al. 2002; Foster et al. 2018; Schaefer et al. 2021); attention difficulties (Capaldi et al. 2022; Foster et al. 2018); substance misuse (Fergusson et al. 2002; Foster et al. 2018; Schaefer et al. 2021); and sleep problems (Troxel et al. 2021). Younger use of cannabis is also associated with increased suicidality (Fergusson et al. 2002). Finally, there is also evidence to support that mental health difficulties related to adolescent cannabis use may continue into mid-adulthood (Brook et al. 2011, 2016; Capaldi et al. 2022). Overall, adolescence may represent a critical period during which the developing brain is particularly susceptible to the harmful effects of cannabis on mental health (Lubman et al. 2015).

Despite the relatively consistent findings, not all studies have identified clear-cut relationships between cannabis use and subsequent mental health problems. One examination of 264 men from low socioeconomic backgrounds assessed at ages 17, 20, and 22 revealed a correlation between cannabis use and depressive symptoms but only modest support that cannabis led to later depression in this population (Womack et al. 2016). Meier et al. (2015) found that among an upper-middle-class American high school sample, persistent cannabis use across 4 years of high school was associated with increased externalizing mental health symptoms (e.g., delinquency), but these associations were no longer significant after controlling for persistent alcohol and tobacco use. Cannabis use was not correlated with greater internalizing symptoms (e.g., anxiety, depression) in this sample.

Some evidence supports the interrelationship between cannabis use and depression at the level of brain function. Mechanistically, for example, there is evidence that cannabinoid receptors play a role in emotional expression. Animal studies with cannabinoid 1 (CB_1) receptor knockout mice have shown that CB_1 receptor availability may be associated with aggressive and depressive responses during stressful tasks (e.g., Martin et al. 2002). Rodent studies have also demonstrated the role of CB_1 receptor antagonists in the modulation of emotion (anxiety, depression) (e.g., Griebel et al. 2005).

Human studies demonstrate that brain function plays a role in the interrelationship between early cannabis use and subsequent psychopathology. One study of 16- to 18-year-old cannabis users found associations between cannabis use and depression symptoms, as well as an interaction between cannabis use and brain white matter volume, with greater white matter volume being associated with lower depression scores among cannabis users but not nonusers (Medina et al. 2007). Several studies also indicate that CB_1 receptors play a role in parts of the brain involved with regulating mood (e.g., Hungund et al. 2004; Vinod et al. 2005).

Heitzeg et al. (2015) examined brain functioning longitudinally during an emotionally arousing task among young adults who were initially assessed in their early teens. They found that individuals who were heavy cannabis users in adolescence (compared with minimal users) did not differ in emotional functioning in their early teen years but experienced significantly greater negative emotionality and less resiliency in early adulthood. Neuroimaging revealed that heavy cannabis users in adolescence demonstrated less activation in emotional processing regions, including the right insula, prefrontal

cortex, and occipital cortex, when presented with words with negative emotional connotations and less activation in the right inferior
parietal lobe in response to positive words. Amygdala activation was
relatively reduced in response to words with both negative and positive emotional valence. Additional brain findings were noted that supported the researchers' conclusion that cannabis use during teenage
years might negatively affect later emotional processing. Overall, findings from imaging studies align with those from longitudinal studies
that show adolescence may represent a critical period for the harmful
effects of cannabis.

A controversial issue that has received substantial study over the
past two decades concerns whether cannabis use can lead to the development of psychotic disorders, including schizophrenia. Several studies have demonstrated significant relationships between adolescent
cannabis use and later psychosis (e.g., Capaldi et al. 2022; Moore et al.
2007), but this literature is also not clear-cut in terms of whether early
cannabis use causes the later onset of schizophrenia or other psychotic
disorders. For example, Volkow et al. (2016) argued in their review that
compelling scientific evidence supports a mechanistic link between
cannabis use and schizophrenia. On the other hand, Ksir and Hart 2016
contended that the research evidence supports the assertion that cannabis use does not cause psychotic disorders but that early and heavy
cannabis use is more likely to occur in individuals who are vulnerable to developing psychosis (as well as other significant mental health
and psychosocial problems). Importantly, the research literature is consistent in finding that cannabis use predicts later persistent psychotic
disorders and is associated with earlier onset of psychotic disorders,
as well as that evidence indicates a biological link between long-term,
heavy cannabis use and the development of psychotic symptoms (for
reviews, see Hasan et al. 2020; Volkow et al. 2016). Thus, individuals
who use cannabis at an early age, particularly heavy users or those
who use high-potency products, may experience significantly worse
psychosocial outcomes than do nonusers, especially if they have an
underlying vulnerability to psychosis.

Emotional Problems and Adverse Events As a Predictor of Adolescent Cannabis Use

The self-medication hypothesis states that individuals with underlying emotional vulnerability might use substances to manage their
symptoms (Khantzian 1997). This hypothesis has been controversial

(Lembke 2012); it suggests that childhood or adolescent development of mental health symptoms might predict a greater prevalence of cannabis use in adolescence.

Studies exploring whether early emotional problems might predict subsequent cannabis use have reported mixed findings. A review by Degenhardt et al. (2003) found little evidence for early depression being a predictor of later cannabis use. Patton et al. (2002) found that among a longitudinal Australian cohort, early cannabis use was associated with the subsequent development of depression and anxiety, but early depression and anxiety did not predict subsequent cannabis use. Heitzeg et al. (2015) reported no differences between 13-year-olds who went on to become heavy cannabis users and control subjects in negative emotionality or resiliency despite finding group differences during young adulthood. Nevertheless, these findings are not universal, and a small number of studies have found that early mental health experiences predict later use. For example, experience of trauma and adverse events in childhood may be associated with greater cannabis use; Gonçalves et al. (2023) found that exposure to four or more adverse childhood experiences was related to regular cannabis use and regular co-use of alcohol and cannabis in adolescence and young adulthood.

Social Functioning and Social Roles

Social development refers to the acquisition of interpersonal skills, the formation of relationships, and the ability to navigate diverse social contexts (McNeely and Blanchard 2009). In this process, adolescents transition from limited childhood roles to the broader roles of young adulthood. During adolescence, a shift from the family to peers occurs, reflecting a move toward independence, and peer approval, rejection, and pressure become central determinants of behavior (Steinberg and Morris 2001). Teens begin to explore romantic relationships, develop a sense of identity, and take pride in their accomplishments and goals. In addition to developing cognitive skills in school, they are also learning to relate to peers, adjust their behavior in response to social feedback, and resolve conflict.

Although chronic cannabis use is thought to interfere with normative social development, few empirical studies have addressed the relationship between cannabis and social development per se. Several studies on the impact of adolescent cannabis use on social functioning and social roles have been published, but the results are inconsistent. A systematic review of 16 longitudinal studies examining the effects of cannabis use on psychosocial outcomes revealed an inconsistent link between cannabis use and social functioning as indicated by antisocial behaviors, including conduct disorder, delinquency, or involvement with police (Macleod et al. 2004).

More recently, Brook et al. (2016) followed 548 individuals longitudinally from ages 14 years to 43 years to assess the impact of various cannabis use trajectories on psychosocial outcomes over time. They found that individuals classified as chronic/heavy users (i.e., started use early, used weekly by late adolescence, and continued weekly use through their early forties), increasing users (i.e., started late, increased to weekly or daily use by late adolescence or their early thirties, and continued through early forties), and chronic/occasional users (i.e., started late, used less than monthly, and continued through early forties) were more likely than nonusers to engage in unconventional behavior, defined as rebellion, delinquency, antisocial behaviors, and tolerance of deviance. The authors posited that these findings reveal that chronic and increasing use of cannabis interferes with adolescent and adult development.

Other studies have shown a significant correlation between cannabis use and negative relationships with others. Cannabis use in adolescence appears to be associated with negative social outcomes. For example, data from twelfth graders in the Monitoring the Future study indicated that high school seniors who reported using cannabis on 40 or more occasions were more likely to report impaired relationships with parents, teachers, and job supervisors, as well as more contact with police (Palamar et al. 2014). It is noteworthy, however, that alcohol-related negative social outcomes were worse than those reported with cannabis. In a study of juvenile offenders, Chassin et al. (2010) found that adolescent cannabis use was inversely related to psychosocial maturity in young adulthood. This form of maturity is characterized by perspective-taking, responsibility, and temperance and is thought to be important for successfully navigating social relationships and making a transition into adult roles.

Higher-frequency cannabis use (i.e., >20 times) in adolescence has been associated with parenting outside of marriage (Green and Ensminger 2006) and increased difficulty with partner and peer relationships (Brook et al. 2002; Foster et al. 2018). Foster et al. (2018) found that adolescents who reported weekly cannabis use experienced more parent-child conflict and had fewer prosocial and more antisocial peers compared with nonusers. In addition to a higher risk of conflict in partner and peer relationships, cannabis use was linked with rebelliousness and lower engagement in productive activities (e.g., having gone to school, been in the military, or worked full time) in a sample of Black and Puerto Rican young adults (Brook et al. 2002).

Taken together, support for a direct link between cannabis use and impaired social functioning or decreased involvement in developmentally appropriate social roles is fairly limited. Although some studies have found an association between cannabis use and negative interpersonal relationships, the paucity of high-quality research makes it difficult to draw definitive conclusions. Some evidence indicates that more frequent and persistent cannabis use, especially during adolescence, may be linked with some negative social consequences. However, whether cannabis use directly contributes to impaired social functioning or a failure to engage in age-appropriate social roles remains unclear.

Cannabis and Academic Achievement

Cannabis can have negative effects on attention, learning, and memory that can persist after the acute effects of the drug have dissipated (Schweinsburg et al. 2008) and even up to 1 year after cessation of cannabis use (Meier et al. 2012). Because these impairments can have implications for academic and professional performance, an important question is whether cannabis use has effects on educational achievement (e.g., reaching one's potential in academics, professional life, or other life domains).

Several prospective longitudinal studies have examined the links between cannabis use and academic achievement. In such studies, multiple assessments of cannabis use and educational performance are made over time. Potential confounds (e.g., sex, age at first cannabis use, family history) are included in statistical analyses to assess whether prior cannabis use is associated with subsequent educational performance when potential covariates are considered. Many of these studies demonstrated that students who used cannabis had poorer academic outcomes compared with those who did not use cannabis. For example, in their study of nearly 1,000 youth followed from birth to age 16 years, Fergusson et al. (1996) found that using cannabis prior to age 15 was associated with a threefold greater likelihood of dropping out of school at age 15–16. Results from a follow-up with this same cohort indicated that nearly 36% of youth who had used cannabis on 10 or more occasions between ages 15 and 16 did not complete high school compared with 17% who had not used cannabis (Fergusson and Horwood 1997). Similar findings from an Australian longitudinal study showed that individuals who started cannabis use prior to age 17 were significantly less likely to graduate from high school or to complete undergraduate degrees compared with nonusers (Silins et al. 2014). They also were more likely to have CaUD, use other illicit substances, and report more suicide attempts. It is important to note that any of these other factors also could contribute to lower academic functioning. Finally, using data from the Minnesota Twin Family Study, Schaefer et al. (2021) found that greater cannabis use during adolescence was consistently associated with lower grade point average (GPA) and motivation to perform academically and with a greater likelihood of academic problem behaviors and school discipline problems. The authors concluded that adolescent cannabis use has potentially causal negative effects on academic functioning in adolescence.

Some studies have reported only indirect links between cannabis use and educational attainment. In a study using longitudinal growth curve modeling to examine cannabis use and GPA over 4 years of college, Arria et al. (2013) found an indirect path in which cannabis use led to increased absences from class, which resulted in a lower GPA. A direct path from cannabis use to lower GPA was not observed. Moreover, an inverse relationship between past-month cannabis use and the likelihood of graduating from college was not significant when analyses were adjusted for age and parental education level (Braun et al. 2000).

The age at which cannabis use is initiated may be important in determining educational outcomes. In a study involving 6,000 participants from three Australian cohort studies, Horwood et al. (2010) found that starting use prior to age 18 was associated with a lower likelihood of completing high school, attending college, and earning a college degree compared with individuals who had not used cannabis prior to that age. Moreover, pooled odds ratios indicated that the educational attainment of individuals who initiated cannabis use prior to age 15 was 1.9–2.9 times worse than that of those who had not started cannabis use prior to age 18. These findings remained significant even after controlling for confounding factors. Similarly, Green and Ensminger (2006) followed a community sample (N=530) of Black individuals from age 6 to age 32–33 and found that those who reported cannabis use on 20 or more occasions prior to age 17 were more likely to drop out of high school. Finally, analyses of data from the French Trajectoires Epidémiologiques en Population (TEMPO) cohort study comparing early cannabis use initiation (at age 16 or earlier) with late initiation (after age 16) indicated that early initiators were less likely to graduate from high school (Melchior et al. 2017). This association was stronger among young females compared with young males.

Cannabis use patterns also appear to have an effect because greater frequency and persistence of cannabis use have been linked with lower academic performance. Degenhardt et al. (2010) found that in a sample of Australian students (N=1,943), those who reported weekly or near-weekly cannabis use during adolescence had poorer post-school outcomes at age 24 compared with those who never used cannabis, although adjustment for cigarette use and other demographic variables reduced the strength of this association. Similarly, occasional cannabis use was also associated with a greater risk of dropping out of school, but this correlation was nonsignificant after controlling for tobacco use. Conversely, analysis of data from the Minnesota Twin Family Study comparing weekly cannabis users with and without a diagnosis of CaUD with nonusers revealed that weekly users, regardless of CaUD status, experienced more academic problems (e.g., lower GPA, negative attitudes about school) than did nonusers (Foster et al. 2018). Regular use, again irrespective of CaUD diagnosis, was also associated with lower educational attainment in adulthood. Finally, in their study of 662 youth from the Victoria Healthy Youth Survey, Thompson et al. (2019) reported lower educational attainment in young adults who reported early onset and persistently high or increasingly frequent cannabis use during the transition from adolescence to young adulthood.

As is the case with social and emotional functioning, the link between cannabis use and negative educational outcomes is correlational, and other factors likely play a shared role in both cannabis use and academic achievement. In addition to cannabis use patterns and age at first use as described previously, compelling evidence indicates that other substance use, especially tobacco and alcohol, is likely a confounding variable in studies of cannabis and educational outcomes. For example, Macleod et al. (2004) noted in their systematic review that the strength of the association between cannabis use and negative educational outcomes was notably reduced after controlling for alcohol and tobacco use. A more recent study by Maggs et al. (2015) indicated that individuals who used cannabis frequently at ages 19–20 years were less likely than infrequent or nonusers to earn a college degree, even after controlling for multiple confounding and risk factors. However, controlling for prior alcohol and tobacco use at age 18 reduced this finding to nonsignificance. Similar results were reported by Mokrysz et al. (2016), who analyzed data from the Avon Longitudinal Study of Parents and Children (N=2,235 adolescents) and found that heavy cannabis use at age 15 predicted lower academic performance at age 16. However, after controlling for other substance use (particularly cigarettes), academic performance was not affected by cannabis use at age 15. The authors stated the importance of considering other factors, such as concurrent tobacco and alcohol use, when interpreting the effects of cannabis on academic performance.

The mixed findings that have been presented underlie the lack of consensus on whether cannabis use limits academic achievement. Indeed, after controlling for shared familial factors of other substance use, the associations between cannabis use and academic achievement often disappear (Schaefer et al. 2021). According to Fergusson and Horwood (1997), some of the effects of cannabis use on educational performance and other social outcomes may depend more on the social context in which cannabis use occurs than on cannabis-specific neurophysiological effects. For example, teens who purchase and use cannabis may be in a peer group that does not engage in normative behavior, such as focusing on achievement, gaining employment, or placing value on interpersonal relationships. Thus, some of the apparent cannabis-related effects on academic performance may be explained by associations with delinquent or substance-using peers (Brook et al. 2016). Overall, stronger evidence is needed to address the role of cannabis in educational outcomes (Macleod et al. 2004; Volkow et al. 2014).

Cannabis and Employment

Several studies have shown that cannabis use over extended periods of time is associated with occupational difficulties. Compared with nonusers, cannabis users have been found to be less likely to be employed, or if employed, they tend to be in lower-prestige occupations (Braun et al. 2000), earn lower incomes (Ringel et al. 2007), or be less successful at work (Green and Ensminger 2006). Braun et al. (2000) interpreted these results as reflecting that cannabis users have a lower commitment or motivation to work. Support for this conclusion was provided by Hyggen (2012), who also observed lower levels of work commitment among cannabis users and noted that this decreased work commitment was evident from late adolescence (17–20 years) through middle age (early to mid-40s). The finding that frequent cannabis use may be correlated with a lack of motivation to achieve occupational goals may be a developmental continuation of the finding reflecting the relationship between cannabis use and poor educational achievement (Brook et al. 1999).

Prospective longitudinal studies examining associations between cannabis use and subsequent occupational success in young and middle adulthood demonstrate that high levels of cannabis use in adolescence predict higher levels of unemployment and reduced income at age 25 (Brook et al. 2011; Fergusson and Boden 2008), as well as a greater likelihood of being unemployed at age 43 compared with nonusers or light users (Zhang et al. 2016). In a study of urban Black youth who were followed from ages 6 to 42, heavy cannabis use during adolescence was associated with being poor in midlife, and post-adolescent cannabis use also predicted having lower income in midlife (Green et al. 2017). Finally, Capaldi et al. (2022) assessed cannabis use and psychosocial adjustment among males (N=206) across three developmental stages: adolescence (13–20 years), early adulthood (20–30 years), and mid-adulthood (30–38 years). Results revealed that cannabis use in prior developmental periods was linked with lower income levels in adulthood, even after controlling for potential confounds.

The age at which cannabis use was initiated appears to impact future employment success. Green and Ensminger (2006) reported that the use of cannabis on 20 or more occasions prior to age 17 was associated with a greater risk of unemployment at age 32–33 years in their sample of 530 Black Americans. Similar findings were reported by Barry et al. (2022), who analyzed data from the French TEMPO cohort study comparing early cannabis use experimentation (at age 16 or earlier) with late experimentation (after age 16) and found that any cannabis use, but especially use prior to age 17, increased the odds of unemployment in mid–young adulthood.

Trajectories of cannabis use in different developmental periods also may influence the association between cannabis use and occupational functioning. Differences in work commitment and financial stability as a function of varying levels of cannabis use were assessed in a sample of Black and Puerto Rican individuals (N=816) from ages 14 to 29 (Brook et al. 2013). Those classified as chronic users (i.e., did not use cannabis at age 14, used about two and a half times per month at age 19, weekly at age 24, and several times per month at age 29) were more likely to be unemployed or be incapacitated at work (i.e., drunk or high on the job) and less likely to be financially independent. The authors concluded that some negative consequences of cannabis use may include difficulty finding or keeping a job, being financially dependent on others, and financial instability (Brook et al. 2013). Subsequent analysis of the same data with additional assessment at age 36 indicated that chronic cannabis use continued to be associated with a greater risk of being unemployed in middle adulthood (Lee et al. 2015a). Finally, Thompson et al. (2019) reported lower occupational prestige and lower income in young adults who reported early onset and persistent high or increasingly frequent cannabis use during the transition from adolescence to young adulthood. Interestingly, these individuals did not differ in employment status from nonusers or those who had used heavily in adolescence but quit over time.

It is important to note that other factors may exacerbate, or even account for, the effects of cannabis on occupational functioning. For example, Lee et al. (2015a) reported that the use of substances, including alcohol and tobacco but not cannabis, was related to unemployment. Other studies (e.g., Green and Ensminger 2006; Lee et al. 2015b) have found that some of the negative effects of cannabis use on employment status may be heightened among persons from low socioeconomic status or minority backgrounds. Potential mechanisms underlying the link between cannabis use and occupational underperformance might include educational failure, which itself may be associated with cannabis-related impairments in cognitive functioning. Such impairments might limit one's ability to perform work-related tasks (Ringel et al. 2007) and increase the propensity to engage in behaviors that violate social norms, such as choosing substance-using peers (Brook et al. 2016). Finally, Boden et al. (2017) found evidence of a possible reciprocal causal process involving cannabis use and employment status, such that being unemployed for at least 3 months increased the risk of developing cannabis dependence, and cannabis dependence significantly increased the risk of being unemployed.

In summary, correlational and longitudinal evidence supports a link between cannabis use and future employment status. Some data show that the age at cannabis use initiation and patterns of cannabis use may play a role, although it also appears that other factors, such as alcohol and tobacco use, may account for some of these associations. As with other areas of functioning, establishing causality is a problem (Lee et al. 2015a); it is unclear whether cannabis use contributes to unemployment or whether other shared risk factors related to academic or vocational achievement might account for both cannabis use and cannabis-related problems.

Cannabis and Motivation

Motivation refers to the driving force behind a person's actions and plays a pivotal role in shaping their goals, achievements, and overall well-being. An individual's level of motivation can determine their engagement in tasks, persistence in the face of challenges, and goal attainment. *Amotivational syndrome* is a term coined by McGlothlin and West (1968) to describe the passivity and lack of achievement orientation often observed among adult chronic cannabis users. Additional characteristics involve apathy, defined as reduced motivation to complete goal-directed behavior (Marin et al. 1991), as well as a narrowed focus of interest, decreased ability to concentrate, lack of persistence on tasks that require sustained effort, and difficulty accommodating new material. Amotivational syndrome is estimated to occur in approximately 5%–6% of adult cannabis users (Duncan 1987).

Supporting the validity of this somewhat controversial phenotype are findings that amotivational effects related to chronic cannabis use have been linked with deficits in learning and sustained attention, which are thought to be associated with impaired academic function and motivation (Volkow et al. 2016). Decreased motivation, in turn, may be a potential mediator of poorer functional outcomes (Silins et al. 2014). Support for this theory comes from studies showing that college students who use cannabis regularly report lower levels of energy and productivity, increased procrastination, and more school absences than do nonusing classmates (Buckner et al. 2010), as well as a greater likelihood of delaying graduation or dropping out of college (Suerken et al. 2016). Conversely, in a sample of 401 adolescents (ages 14–17) who completed five assessments (every 6 months over a 2-year period) of their cannabis use and motivation, Pacheco-Colón et al. (2021) found that adolescent cannabis use increased significantly over time, as did several aspects of motivation. However, after controlling for sex, age, depression, and use of alcohol and nicotine, these effects did not remain significant, and the authors concluded that cannabis use and motivation were not linked in this sample.

A recent systematic review of 22 studies examining the effects of cannabis on motivation and self-efficacy found that most of the work in this area is cross-sectional, with only 2 longitudinal studies identified (Pacheco-Colón et al. 2018). The studies included various methodologies, including self-report, performance-based methods (i.e., work for reward), PET scans of dopaminergic functioning, and functional neuroimaging using cue reactivity paradigms or a monetary incentive delay task. Of the 20 cross-sectional studies in the review, 9 found a correlation between greater cannabis use and decreased motivation. However, only 6 of these controlled for possible confounding variables (through the use of covariates or matching on these variables), and only 4 studies controlled for other substance use. Few controlled for co-occurring depression or depressive symptoms, which is notable because two studies in the review found that cannabis use and depression contributed additive effects (Musty and Kaback 1995; Wright et al. 2016).

In terms of causal relationships, the two longitudinal studies found similar results, although with differing methodologies. Martz et al. (2016) observed blunted activity in the nucleus accumbens during reward anticipation in chronic cannabis users, even when controlling for baseline nucleus accumbens activation and other potential confounds. Preexisting differences in nucleus accumbens activity did not predict later cannabis use. Similarly, after controlling for confounds, Lac and Luk (2018) reported that cannabis-using college students exhibited lower self-efficacy, although lower self-efficacy did not predict subsequent cannabis use. Pacheco-Colón et al. (2018) interpreted these findings as supporting the theory that chronic cannabis use leads to diminished motivation and reward sensitivity. Overall, studies in this review differed substantially in definition and assessment of motivation and whether and which confounds were addressed. Some studies failed to distinguish between different types of motivation and considered motivation and reward sensitivity equivalent. On the basis of the equivocal cross-sectional study findings, Pacheco-Colón et al. (2018) concluded that only partial support was provided for an amotivational syndrome among cannabis users or a cannabis-specific effect on motivation, although the longitudinal study results support a causal relationship between these factors.

Still other studies provide evidence that chronic cannabis use can disrupt motivation through cognitive, neurobiological, and psychosocial mechanisms (Volkow et al. 2016). For example, memory deficits and reduced attention span can hinder the ability to set and pursue goals and engage in tasks. Tetrahydrocannabinol (THC) has been shown to disrupt reward-based learning (Lane and Cherek 2002), and cannabis users exhibit reduced motivation for reward-related behavior compared with control subjects (Lane et al. 2005). Given the role of dopamine signaling in sustaining motivation (Berridge and Robinson 1998), cannabis-related reductions in striatal dopamine synthesis could theoretically underlie amotivation in cannabis users (Volkow et al. 2016). This hypothesis is supported by imaging data revealing reduced reactivity to dopamine stimulation among cannabis users, which has been linked with negative affect and may lead to decreased engagement in activities unrelated to drug use (Volkow et al. 2014). Finally, over time, cannabis itself can become a more powerful motivator than other activities (e.g., studying, working) in the reward hierarchy. As is the case with other outcomes discussed in this chapter, it is not possible to determine whether cannabis is a cause, correlate, or consequence of impaired motivation (Volkow et al. 2016).

Potential Benefits of Cannabis Use on Psychosocial Functioning

On the basis of the research reviewed in this chapter, it is unlikely that cannabis has any potentially beneficial effects on emotional or social development, academic achievement, or occupational success among youth. Moreover, the potentially negative consequences in these areas of function probably outweigh any potential benefits.

Clinical Significance and Recommendations

Results of the research we have presented in this chapter indicate that the prevention, or at least the delay, of cannabis use by adolescents may have broad health and social benefits. For those who have already initiated cannabis use, treatment is paramount. Mental health professionals who treat adolescents and young adults, particularly those presenting with affective or anxiety symptoms, should assess their patients' current and previous cannabis use to determine whether CaUD is present. If use is found to be chronic or severe, clinicians should explore whether current cannabis use or withdrawal may be contributing to or maintaining depressive or anxiety symptoms. Because early cannabis use appears to relate to later negative outcomes and later negative outcomes likely share underlying risk factors with early marijuana use, treatments aimed solely at reducing teen cannabis use without addressing other psychological or familial issues are unlikely to produce long-term positive gains. Thus, interventions should encompass a fairly broad scope addressing issues such as school performance, peer relationships, and community supports in addition to substance use. Given that familial influences also contribute to cannabis use and other outcomes, involving the family in treatment is encouraged. Interventions that address cannabis use and other at-risk areas simultaneously may be most beneficial for supporting academic achievement, reducing drug use in adulthood, increasing personal and interpersonal functioning, and facilitating a more successful transition to adult roles.

Finally, from a public health perspective, protecting adolescents from the potentially adverse consequences of cannabis use should be an important component of cannabis legislative reforms. Given the rapidly changing political and legislative landscape around cannabis, efforts to reform cannabis legislation should be monitored closely to ensure they limit adolescent access to cannabis and cannabis products to reduce the risk of possible negative effects on psychosocial development.

Conclusion

We are just beginning to understand how cannabis use during adolescence and early adulthood affects subsequent psychosocial functioning during early and mid-adulthood. The types of studies that can be conducted largely limit the conclusions that we can draw. Although most of the studies we discussed use longitudinal methods, they are correlational in nature, so it is difficult to determine the causal direction of cannabis use and outcomes in humans. Rigorous and well-controlled longitudinal and twin/adoption studies may help determine causality, but such studies are few and can be limited by numerous factors.

Many of the earlier studies designed to identify negative effects and attribute them specifically to cannabis often did not adequately address confounding factors, particularly those associated with the concurrent use of multiple substances (a common characteristic of adolescent and young adult cannabis use). Moreover, research in this area often involves diverse samples, encompassing both adolescents and adults, individuals with varying histories of cannabis use (chronic vs. acute), and differing patterns of use (e.g., frequency, dose, and quantity). Other sociodemographic variables, such as sex/gender, family socioeconomic status, and psychological factors, including depression and anxiety, also need to be considered (Macleod et al. 2004). These differences may contribute to the mixed or inconsistent findings on the specific effects of cannabis on particular outcomes. Furthermore, relying solely on correlational analysis or logistic regression models may result in overestimating the association between cannabis use and adverse social, educational, and mental health outcomes. Advanced statistical techniques, such as propensity scoring, can be used to correct for overreliance on correlational and regression methods, mitigate selection bias (Chassin et al. 2010), and reduce confounding by measured factors (McCaffrey et al. 2010).

Despite these limitations of the current literature, the potential for negative impacts of cannabis on emotional, social, academic, vocational, and motivational development cannot be ignored. The landscape of cannabis use is changing rapidly in terms of cannabis legality, the availability of newer ways of using cannabis, and much higher product potencies. THC concentrations have increased significantly since 1995 (ElSohly 2014), and high-potency THC concentrates are readily available at dispensaries. The detrimental effects of these highly potent THC products may be more severe than those of cannabis products used by youth who participated in studies published a decade or more ago. Thus, it is essential that future studies continue to explore both the relationship between cannabis use and developmental challenges and the cannabis-related and psychosocial factors that may mediate or moderate these risks.

Key Points

- Longitudinal research demonstrates that cannabis use during adolescence is associated with difficulties in early and sometimes middle adulthood, including emotional, psychiatric, social, educational, vocational, and motivational functioning.
- Because of the correlational nature of the research, it is difficult to determine whether cannabis use is a direct cause of deficits, and some studies find that these deficits disappear once confounding factors (e.g., tobacco and alcohol use) are controlled for.
- Additional research is needed to determine the extent to which and under what circumstances adolescent cannabis use is harmful (e.g., frequent or heavy use, co-use with other substances).
- Clinically, it is important that providers advise patients that any level of cannabis use during adolescence may be harmful.
- No evidence has shown positive effects of cannabis use on adolescents' psychosocial functioning.

References

Arnett JJ: Emerging adulthood: a theory of development from the late teens through the twenties. Am Psychol 55(5):469–480, 2000 10842426

Arria AM, Caldeira KM, Vincent KB, et al: Discontinuous college enrollment: associations with substance use and mental health. Psychiatr Serv 64(2):165–172, 2013 23474608

Barry KM, Gomajee R, Kousignian I, et al: Adolescent cannabis experimentation and unemployment in young to mid-adulthood: results from the French TEMPO cohort study. Drug Alcohol Depend 230:109–201, 2022 34864566

Bell L, Burtless G, Gornick J, et al: Failure to Launch: Cross-National Trends in the Transition to Economic Independence (LIS Working Paper Series No 456). Luxembourg, Luxembourg Income Study, Cross-National Data Center, 2007

Berridge KC, Robinson TE: What is the role of dopamine in reward: hedonic impact, reward learning, or incentive salience? Brain Res Brain Res Rev 28(3):309–369, 1998 9858756

Boden JM, Lee JO, Horwood LJ, et al: Modelling possible causality in the associations between unemployment, cannabis use, and alcohol misuse. Soc Sci Med 175:127–134, 2017 28088618

Braun BL, Hannan P, Wolfson M, et al: Occupational attainment, smoking, alcohol intake, and marijuana use: ethnic-gender differences in the CARDIA study. Addict Behav 25(3):399–414, 2000 10890293

Brook JS, Balka EB, Whiteman M: The risks for late adolescence of early adolescent marijuana use. Am J Public Health 89(10):1549–1554, 1999 10511838

Brook JS, Adams RE, Balka EB, et al: Early adolescent marijuana use: risks for the transition to young adulthood. Psychol Med 32(1):79–91, 2002 11883732

Brook JS, Zhang C, Brook DW: Antisocial behavior at age 37: developmental trajectories of marijuana use extending from adolescence to adulthood. Am J Addict 20(6):509–515, 2011 21999495

Brook JS, Lee JY, Finch SJ, et al: Adult work commitment, financial stability, and social environment as related to trajectories of marijuana use beginning in adolescence. Subst Abus 34(3):298–305, 2013 23844962

Brook JS, Zhang C, Leukefeld CG, et al: Marijuana use from adolescence to adulthood: developmental trajectories and their outcomes. Soc Psychiatry Psychiatr Epidemiol 51(10):1405–1415, 2016 27168181

Buckner JD, Ecker AH, Cohen AS: Mental health problems and interest in marijuana treatment among marijuana-using college students. Addict Behav 35(9):826–833, 2010 20483200

Butler A, Patte KA, Ferro MA, et al: Interrelationships among depression, anxiety, flourishing, and cannabis use in youth. Addict Behav 89:206–215, 2019 30321693

Capaldi DM, Tiberio SS, Kerr DCR, et al: Associations of cannabis use across adolescence and early adulthood with health and psychosocial adjustment in early adulthood and mid-adulthood in men. Subst Abuse 16:1–13, 2022 35677294

Chassin L, Dmitrieva J, Modecki K, et al: Does adolescent alcohol and marijuana use predict suppressed growth in psychosocial maturity among male juvenile offenders? Psychol Addict Behav 24(1):48–60, 2010 20307112

Degenhardt L, Hall W, Lynskey M: Exploring the association between cannabis use and depression. Addiction 98(11):1493–1504, 2003 14616175

Degenhardt L, Coffey C, Carlin JB, et al: Outcomes of occasional cannabis use in adolescence: 10-year follow-up study in Victoria, Australia. Br J Psychiatry 196(4):290–295, 2010 20357305

Duncan DF: Lifetime prevalence of "amotivational syndrome" among users and nonusers of hashish. Psychol Addict Behav 1(2):114–119, 1987

Edwards KA, Hertel-Fernandez A: The Kids Aren't Alright: A Labor Market Analysis of Young Workers (Briefing Paper 258). Washington, DC, Economic Policy Institute, 2010. Available at: http://www.epi.org/page/-/bp258/bp258.pdf. Accessed September 18, 2023.

ElSohly MA: Potency Monitoring Program Quarterly Report 123. Oxford, National Center for Natural Products Research, University of Mississippi, 2014

Fergusson DM, Boden JM: Cannabis use and later life outcomes. Addiction 103(6):969–976, discussion 977–978, 2008 18482420

Fergusson DM, Horwood LJ: Early onset cannabis use and psychosocial adjustment in young adults. Addiction 92(3):279–296, 1997 9219390

Fergusson DM, Lynskey MT, Horwood LJ: The short-term consequences of early onset cannabis use. J Abnorm Child Psychol 24(4):499–512, 1996 8886945

Fergusson DM, Horwood LJ, Swain-Campbell N: Cannabis use and psychosocial adjustment in adolescence and young adulthood. Addiction 97(9):1123–1135, 2002 12199828

Flory K, Lynam D, Milich R, et al: Early adolescent through young adult alcohol and marijuana use trajectories: early predictors, young adult outcomes, and predictive utility. Dev Psychopathol 16(1):193–213, 2004 15115071

Foster KT, Arterberry BJ, Iacono WG, et al: Psychosocial functioning among regular cannabis users with and without cannabis use disorder. Psychol Med 48(11):1853–1861, 2018 29173210

Giedd JN: The amazing teen brain. Sci Am 312(6):32–37, 2015 26336683

Gobbi G, Atkin T, Zytynski T, et al: Association of cannabis use in adolescence and risk of depression, anxiety, and suicidality in young adulthood: a systematic review and meta-analysis. JAMA Psychiatry 76(4):426–434, 2019 30758486

Gonçalves PD, Duarte CS, Corbeil T, et al: Adverse childhood experiences and risk patterns of alcohol and cannabis co-use: a longitudinal study of Puerto Rican youth. J Adolesc Health 73(3):421–427, 2023 37294259

Green KM, Ensminger ME: Adult social behavioral effects of heavy adolescent marijuana use among African Americans. Dev Psychol 42(6):1168–1178, 2006 17087550

Green KM, Doherty EE, Ensminger ME: Long-term consequences of adolescent cannabis use: examining intermediary processes. Am J Drug Alcohol Abuse 43(5):567–575, 2017 27929672

Griebel G, Stemmelin J, Scatton B: Effects of the cannabinoid CB1 receptor antagonist rimonabant in models of emotional reactivity in rodents. Biol Psychiatry 57(3):261–267, 2005 15691527

Hasan A, von Keller R, Friemel CM, et al: Cannabis use and psychosis: a review of reviews. Eur Arch Psychiatry Clin Neurosci 270(4):403–412, 2020 31563981

Heitzeg MM, Cope LM, Martz ME, et al: Brain activation to negative stimuli mediates a relationship between adolescent marijuana use and later emotional functioning. Dev Cogn Neurosci 16:71–83, 2015 26403581

Horwood LJ, Fergusson DM, Hayatbakhsh MR, et al: Cannabis use and educational achievement: findings from three Australasian cohort studies. Drug Alcohol Depend 110(3):247–253, 2010 20456872

Hungund BL, Vinod KY, Kassir SA, et al: Upregulation of CB1 receptors and agonist-stimulated [35S]GTPgammaS binding in the prefrontal cortex of depressed suicide victims. Mol Psychiatry 9(2):184–190, 2004 14966476

Hyggen C: Does smoking cannabis affect work commitment? Addiction 107(7):1309–1315, 2012 22276981

Jacobus J, Squeglia LM, Infante MA, et al: Neuropsychological performance in adolescent marijuana users with co-occurring alcohol use: a three-year longitudinal study. Neuropsychology 29(6):829–843, 2015 25938918

Khantzian EJ: The self-medication hypothesis of substance use disorders: a reconsideration and recent applications. Harv Rev Psychiatry 4(5):231–244, 1997 9385000

Ksir C, Hart CL: Cannabis and psychosis: a critical overview of the relationship. Curr Psychiatry Rep 18(2):12, 2016 26781550

Lac A, Luk JW: Testing the amotivational syndrome: marijuana use longitudinally predicts lower self-efficacy even after controlling for demographics, personality, and alcohol and cigarette use. Prev Sci 19(2):117–126, 2018 28620722

Lane SD, Cherek DR: Marijuana effects on sensitivity to reinforcement in humans. Neuropsychopharmacology 26(4):520–529, 2002 11927176

Lane SD, Cherek DR, Tcheremissine OV, et al: Acute marijuana effects on human risk taking. Neuropsychopharmacology 30(4):800–809, 2005 15775958

Lebowitz ER: "Failure to launch": shaping intervention for highly dependent adult children. J Am Acad Child Adolesc Psychiatry 55(2):89–90, 2016 26802773

Lee JO, Hill KG, Hartigan LA, et al: Unemployment and substance use problems among young adults: does childhood low socioeconomic status exacerbate the effect? Soc Sci Med 143:36–44, 2015a 26342911

Lee JY, Brook JS, Finch SJ, et al: Trajectories of marijuana use from adolescence to adulthood predicting unemployment in the mid 30s. Am J Addict 24(5):452–459, 2015b 25955962

Lembke A: Time to abandon the self-medication hypothesis in patients with psychiatric disorders. Am J Drug Alcohol Abuse 38(6):524–529, 2012 22924576

Lev-Ran S, Roerecke M, Le Foll B, et al: The association between cannabis use and depression: a systematic review and meta-analysis of longitudinal studies. Psychol Med 44(4):797–810, 2014 23795762

Lubman DI, Cheetham A, Yücel M: Cannabis and adolescent brain development. Pharmacol Ther 148:1–16, 2015 25460036

Macleod J, Oakes R, Copello A, et al: Psychological and social sequelae of cannabis and other illicit drug use by young people: a systematic review of longitudinal, general population studies. Lancet 363(9421):1579–1588, 2004 15145631

Maggs JL, Staff J, Kloska DD, et al: Predicting young adult degree attainment by late adolescent marijuana use. J Adolesc Health 57(2):205–211, 2015 26206441

Marin RS, Biedrzycki RC, Firinciogullari S: Reliability and validity of the Apathy Evaluation Scale. Psychiatry Res 38(2):143–162, 1991 1754629

Martin M, Ledent C, Parmentier M, et al: Involvement of CB1 cannabinoid receptors in emotional behaviour. Psychopharmacology (Berl) 159(4):379–387, 2002 11823890

Martz ME, Trucco EM, Cope LM, et al: Association of marijuana use with blunted nucleus accumbens response to reward anticipation. JAMA Psychiatry 73(8):838–844, 2016 27384542

McCaffrey DF, Pacula RL, Han B, et al: Marijuana use and high school dropout: the influence of unobservables. Health Econ 19(11):1281–1299, 2010 19937639

McGlothlin WH, West LJ: The marihuana problem: an overview. Am J Psychiatry 125(3):126–134, 1968 5667203

McNeely C, Blanchard J: The Teen Years Explained: A Guide to Healthy Adolescent Development. Baltimore, MD, Center for Adolescent Health, Johns Hopkins Bloomberg School of Public Health, 2009. Available at: https://www.jhsph.edu/research/centers-and-institutes/center-for-adolescent-health/_docs/TTYE-Guide.pdf. Accessed August 2024.

Medina KL, Nagel BJ, Park A, et al: Depressive symptoms in adolescents: associations with white matter volume and marijuana use. J Child Psychol Psychiatry 48(6):592–600, 2007 17537075

Meier MH, Caspi A, Ambler A, et al: Persistent cannabis users show neuropsychological decline from childhood to midlife. Proc Natl Acad Sci USA 109(40):E2657–E2664, 2012 22927402

Meier MH, Hill ML, Small PJ, et al: Associations of adolescent cannabis use with academic performance and mental health: a longitudinal study of upper middle class youth. Drug Alcohol Depend 156:207–212, 2015 26409752

Melchior M, Bolze C, Fombonne E, et al: Early cannabis initiation and educational attainment: is the association causal? Data from the French TEMPO study. Int J Epidemiol 46(5):1641–1650, 2017 28520946

Mokrysz C, Landy R, Gage SH, et al: Are IQ and educational outcomes in teenagers related to their cannabis use? A prospective cohort study. J Psychopharmacol 30(2):159–168, 2016 26739345

Moore TH, Zammit S, Lingford-Hughes A, et al: Cannabis use and risk of psychotic or affective mental health outcomes: a systematic review. Lancet 370(9584):319–328, 2007 17662880

Musty RE, Kaback L: Relationships between motivation and depression in chronic marijuana users. Life Sci 56(23–24):2151–2158, 1995 7776845

Pacheco-Colón I, Limia JM, Gonzalez R: Nonacute effects of cannabis use on motivation and reward sensitivity in humans: a systematic review. Psychol Addict Behav 32(5):497–507, 2018 29963875

Pacheco-Colón I, Hawes SW, Duperrouzel JC, et al: Evidence lacking for cannabis users slacking: a longitudinal analysis of escalating cannabis use and motivation among adolescents. J Int Neuropsychol Soc 27(6):637–647, 2021 34261556

Palamar JJ, Fenstermaker M, Kamboukos D, et al: Adverse psychosocial outcomes associated with drug use among US high school seniors: a comparison of alcohol and marijuana. Am J Drug Alcohol Abuse 40(6):438–446, 2014 25169838

Patton GC, Coffey C, Carlin JB, et al: Cannabis use and mental health in young people: cohort study. BMJ 325(7374):1195–1198, 2002 12446533

Ringel JS, Ellickson PL, Collins RL: High school drug use predicts job-related outcomes at age 29. Addict Behav 32(3):576–589, 2007 16822622

Schaefer JD, Hamdi NR, Malone SM, et al: Associations between adolescent cannabis use and young-adult functioning in three longitudinal twin studies. Proc Natl Acad Sci USA 118(14):e2013180118, 2021 33782115

Scholes-Balog KE, Hemphill SA, Evans-Whipp TJ, et al: Developmental trajectories of adolescent cannabis use and their relationship to young adult social and behavioural adjustment: a longitudinal study of Australian youth. Addict Behav 53:11–18, 2016 26414206

Schweinsburg AD, Brown SA, Tapert SF: The influence of marijuana use on neurocognitive functioning in adolescents. Curr Drug Abuse Rev 1(1):99–111, 2008 19630709

Shulman S, Feldman B, Blatt S, et al: Emerging adulthood: age-related tasks and underlying self processes. J Adolesc Res 20(5):577–603, 2005

Silins E, Horwood LJ, Patton GC, et al: Young adult sequelae of adolescent cannabis use: an integrative analysis. Lancet Psychiatry 1(4):286–293, 2014 26360862

Steinberg L, Morris AS: Adolescent development. Annu Rev Psychol 52:83–110, 2001 11148300

Suerken CK, Reboussin BA, Egan KL, et al: Marijuana use trajectories and academic outcomes among college students. Drug Alcohol Depend 162:137–145, 2016 27020322

Thompson K, Leadbeater B, Ames M, et al: Associations between marijuana use trajectories and educational and occupational success in young adulthood. Prev Sci 20(2):257–269, 2019 29704147

Troxel WM, Rodriguez A, Seelam R, et al: Longitudinal associations of sleep problems with alcohol and cannabis use from adolescence to emerging adulthood. Sleep 44(10): 202, 2021 33884430

Vinod KY, Arango V, Xie S, et al: Elevated levels of endocannabinoids and CB1 receptor-mediated G-protein signaling in the prefrontal cortex of alcoholic suicide victims. Biol Psychiatry 57(5):480–486, 2005 15737662

Volkow ND, Baler RD, Compton WM, et al: Adverse health effects of marijuana use. N Engl J Med 370(23):2219–2227, 2014 24897085

Volkow ND, Swanson JM, Evins AE, et al: Effects of cannabis use on human behavior, including cognition, motivation, and psychosis: a review. JAMA Psychiatry 73(3):292–297, 2016 26842658

Womack SR, Shaw DS, Weaver CM, et al: Bidirectional associations between cannabis use and depressive symptoms from adolescence through early adulthood among at-risk young men. J Stud Alcohol Drugs 77(2):287–297, 2016 26997187

Wright NE, Scerpella D, Lisdahl KM: Marijuana use is associated with behavioral approach and depressive symptoms in adolescents and emerging adults. PLoS One 11(11):e0166005, 2016 27835662

Zhang C, Brook JS, Leukefeld CG, et al: Trajectories of marijuana use from adolescence to adulthood as predictors of unemployment status in the early forties. Am J Addict 25(3):203–209, 2016 26991779

5

Cannabis and Psychosis

Lucia Sideli, Ph.D.

Edoardo Spinazzola, Ph.D.

Robin M. Murray, Prof., FRS

Marco Colizzi, M.D., Ph.D.

Twenty years ago, very little was known about any link between cannabis use and psychosis. However, a trickle of papers has now turned into an avalanche, partly because of our increasing understanding of the relationship between the two but also provoked by the worldwide relaxation of laws regarding cannabis use and the consequent rise in consumption. In this chapter, we discuss four important areas of this relationship: 1) epidemiological studies, 2) clinical characteristics of cannabis-induced psychosis, 3) experimental studies, and 4) neurobiological studies. Finally, we consider criticisms of the idea that heavy cannabis use is a contributory cause of psychosis.

Current State of Evidence

Epidemiological Studies

Prospective and retrospective studies have provided robust evidence of the association between cannabis use and psychosis, with increased risk for psychotic disorders among cannabis users compared with non-users, and evidence of a dose-response effect (Murray et al. 2016, 2017; Radua et al. 2018; Sideli et al. 2021; see Table 5–1).

A meta-analysis suggested that, on average across reports, 34% of individuals had smoked cannabis regularly (i.e., at least monthly) at the time of their first episode of psychosis (Myles et al. 2016). Cannabis use disorder (CaUD) is the most frequent substance use disorder in the history of patients with a first episode of schizophrenia (Hunt et al. 2018). As early as 2007, a systematic review suggested that cannabis use is a risk factor for psychotic disorders in terms of lifetime use (pooled adjusted OR [AOR] 1.41; 95% CI 1.20, 1.65) and frequent use (pooled AOR 2.09; 95% CI 1.54, 2.84) (Moore et al. 2007).

The psychosis continuum model suggests that psychosis can be best described as a continuous rather than a categorical construct expressed at different levels in the population, ranging from transitory psychotic-like experiences to full-blown psychotic disorders (Linscott and van Os 2013; van Os et al. 2009). In line with this model, cannabis use is not only associated with clinical psychotic disorders but also with sub-clinical psychotic experiences (Matheson et al. 2011; Ragazzi et al. 2018) and schizotypy traits in the general population (Szoke et al. 2014).

Although the effect of cannabis use on mood, motivation, and energy is well documented (Green et al. 2003), there are fewer studies on affective psychosis (i.e., depressive and bipolar disorders with psychotic features) compared with those on schizophrenia spectrum disorders. Rodriguez et al.'s (2021) meta-analysis found that cannabis use was associated with a threefold risk for affective psychosis. Evidence suggested a stronger risk for bipolar than for depressive outcomes, with an increased odds of 2.97 (95% CI 1.8, 4.9) for manic episodes (Gibbs et al. 2015) compared with odds of 1.49 (95% CI 1.15, 1.94) to 1.62 (95% CI 1.21, 2.16) for depression (Lev-Ran et al. 2014; Moore et al. 2007). Pinto et al. (2019) found that 30% of patients with bipolar disorders had smoked cannabis in their lifetime, 20% had a comorbid CaUD, and cannabis use was significantly associated with psychotic symptoms.

Table 5–1. Meta-analytic findings on the association between cannabis and psychosis

Outcome	Study	Participants	Methods	Main findings	Estimate
Subclinical psychosis	Szoke et al. (2014)	29 studies	Random-effects meta-analysis on schizotypy	Association between lifetime cannabis use and total, positive, negative, and disorganized dimension of schizotypy	Total schizotypy: ES=0.42; 95% CI 0.34, 0.51
	Matheson et al. (2023)	N=31,541 children and adolescents from 11 studies	Random-effects meta-analysis on PLEs	Association between PLEs and lifetime and weekly cannabis use	Lifetime: OR 1.71; 95% CI 1.45, 2.01 Weekly: OR 2.27; 95% CI 1.31, 3.95
UHR/CHR status	Kraan et al. (2016)	N=1,171 UHR patients from 7 studies	Random-effects meta-analysis on transition to psychosis	Association only between transition to psychosis and cannabis use	Lifetime: OR 1.14; 95% CI 0.86, 1.52 Abuse/dependence: OR 1.75; 95% CI 1.15, 2.71

Table 5–1. Meta-analytic findings on the association between cannabis and psychosis (*continued*)

Outcome	Study	Participants	Methods	Main findings	Estimate
UHR/CHR status (*continued*)	Carney et al. (2017)	n=4,205 UHR patients and n=667 control subjects from 30 studies	Random-effects meta-analysis on age at onset of psychosis	Association between UHR status and cannabis use	Lifetime use: OR 2.09; 95% CI 1.04, 4.19 Current use: OR 5.49; 95% CI 1.97, 15.32
	Farris et al. (2020)	N=4,055 CHR participants from 36 studies	Random-effects meta-analysis on transition to psychosis	Nonsignificant association between transition to psychosis and cannabis use	RR=1.11; 95% CI 0.89, 1.37
First-episode psychosis	Large et al. (2011)	N=8,167 substance use patients from 83 studies	Random-effects meta-analysis on age at onset of psychosis	Relationship between earlier onset of psychotic disorder and cannabis use (average 2.70 years earlier)	ES=–2.70; 95% CI –0.53, –0.30

Table 5–1. Meta-analytic findings on the association between cannabis and psychosis (*continued*)

Outcome	Study	Participants	Methods	Main findings	Estimate
First-episode psychosis (*continued*)	Myles et al. (2012)	$n=3,199$ cannabis-using patients and $n=5,715$ non-cannabis-using patients from 38 studies	Random-effects meta-analysis on age at onset of psychosis	Relationship between earlier onset of psychotic disorder and cannabis use (average 32 months earlier)	SMD=−0.40; 95% CI −0.49, −0.31
Psychosis	Moore et al. (2007)	11 samples from 7 cohort studies	Random-effects meta-analysis on psychosis	Relationship between lifetime and most frequent cannabis use and psychosis	Lifetime use: AOR 1.41; 95% CI 1.20, 1.65 Most frequent use: AOR 2.09; 95% CI 1.54, 2.84
	Marconi et al. (2016)	$N=66,816$ individuals from 10 studies	Random-effects meta-analysis on risk of psychosis	High levels of cannabis use increase the risk of psychotic outcomes with a dose-response relationship	OR 3.9; 95% CI 2.84, 5.34

Table 5–1. Meta-analytic findings on the association between cannabis and psychosis (*continued*)

Outcome	Study	Participants	Methods	Main findings	Estimate
Psychosis (*continued*)	Schoeler et al. (2016c)	N=16,565 individuals from 24 studies	Random-effects meta-analysis on clinical outcomes of psychosis	Continued cannabis use after onset of psychosis predicts adverse outcomes than for nonusers	d=0.31; 95% CI 0.04, 0.57
	Kiburi et al. (2021)	18 studies with sample size ranging from 45 to 50,087	Random-effects meta-analysis on psychosis	Relationship between psychotic disorder and cannabis use in adolescence	RR 1.71; 95% CI 1.47, 2.00
	Robinson et al. (2022)	N = 7,390 participants from 10 studies	Random-effects meta-analysis on psychosis	Dose-response relationship between frequency of cannabis use and risk for psychosis	Weekly use: RR 1.35; 95% CI 1.19–1.52 Daily use: RR 1.76; 95% CI 1.47–2.12

Table 5–1. Meta-analytic findings on the association between cannabis and psychosis (*continued*)

Outcome	Study	Participants	Methods	Main findings	Estimate
Bipolar disorders	Gibbs et al. (2015)	$N=5,520$ individuals from 2 studies	Random-effects meta-analysis	Association between cannabis use and (hypo)manic symptoms in the population	OR 2.97; 95% CI 1.8, 4.9
	Pinto et al. (2019)	$N=5,028$ patients with bipolar disorders from 9 studies	Random-effects meta-analysis on onset and clinical outcomes of bipolar disorders	Relationship of cannabis use with earlier onset of bipolar disorder and with psychotic symptoms	Age at onset: SMD −0.46; 95% CI −0.61, −0.31 Psychotic symptoms: OR 1.76; 95% CI 1.20, 2.58
	Rodriguez et al. (2021)	$N=6,427$ patients with bipolar disorders or affective psychosis from 6 studies	Random-effects meta-analysis on risk of affective psychosis	Association between cannabis use and bipolar disorders or affective psychosis	OR 3.03; 95% CI 1.32, 6.96

AOR = adjusted odds ratio; CHR = clinical high risk; PLE = psychotic-like experience; UHR = ultrahigh risk.

Experimental Studies

Experimental studies, henceforth referred to as human laboratory studies, have investigated the association between cannabis and psychosis, addressing some of the limitations of observational research. These studies involved the administration of Δ^9-tetrahydrocannabinol (Δ^9-THC) through different routes (i.e., smoked cannabis, cannabis extract, and oral and intravenous THC) in double-blind, placebo-controlled, randomized trials (Murray et al. 2017). Human laboratory studies have consistently shown that THC can induce transient psychotic states (Ganesh et al. 2020; Hindley et al. 2020). The advantage of such studies is that they allow for causal inferences to be made with confidence because there is a precise temporal relationship between the drug administration and the effect (psychosis), and the dose and administration can be carefully controlled (Murray et al. 2017).

The first modern study was conducted by D'Souza et al. (2004) and showed that the administration of 2.5 mg and 5 mg of intravenous THC induced transient schizophrenia-like positive and negative symptoms, as well as behavioral and cognitive deficits in a group of 22 healthy subjects. A meta-analysis confirmed that a single THC administration—regardless of the route, form, dose, or setting—robustly increased positive, negative, and other psychiatric symptoms in healthy individuals, with large effect sizes (Hindley et al. 2020). Additionally, a mega-analysis that focused specifically on assessing intravenous THC administration indicated that this substance induced consistent positive and negative symptoms (Ganesh et al. 2020).

In individuals with schizophrenia, the administration of THC was associated with a transient exacerbation in core psychotic symptoms and cognitive deficits (D'Souza et al. 2005). These effects were even more pronounced when compared with those experienced by control subjects, and chronic antipsychotic treatment failed to protect these patients from THC-induced symptoms.

Interestingly, when healthy control subjects were pretreated with haloperidol in this study, the psychotomimetic and behavioral effects of THC persisted, which suggests that dopamine receptor 2 (D_2) blockade does not play a major role in mediating the psychotomimetic and perception-altering effects of THC (D'Souza et al. 2008). However, two other human laboratory studies indicated that olanzapine (Kleinloog et al. 2012) and haloperidol (Liem-Moolenaar et al. 2010) may attenuate psychotic symptoms following THC administration.

A few human laboratory studies attempted to identify a link between THC administration and dopamine release, but the findings have been limited. Barkus et al. (2011) administered 2.5 mg of intravenous THC to 11 healthy volunteers, and even though this dose elicited psychotic symptoms, the authors could not find any significant increase in striatal dopamine. Overall, THC seems to release dopamine in the striatum, albeit to a lesser extent than do substances such as amphetamine (Murray et al. 2017).

Another line of research indicated that frequent cannabis users and individuals with higher tobacco use tend to exhibit blunted responses following THC administration, probably due to increased tolerance to the substance (D'Souza et al. 2016; Hindley et al. 2020). This blunted response to THC might be explained by either the evidence of down-regulation of cannabinoid receptors (D'Souza et al. 2016) or the reduced synthesis of dopamine in the striatal and limbic regions (Bloomfield et al. 2014), both of which are observed in chronic cannabis users (Ganesh et al. 2020).

Along with positive psychotic symptoms, THC was also reported to induce negative symptoms, such as blunted affect, emotional withdrawal, psychomotor retardation, lack of spontaneity, and reduced rapport (D'Souza et al. 2004; Radhakrishnan et al. 2014). Although it is difficult to confirm that these symptoms were primary negative symptoms, a human laboratory study has shown that such effects of THC were not attributable merely to sedation, thus suggesting that they may be a direct adverse effect of cannabis exposure (Morrison and Stone 2011). In general, it seems that in experimental settings THC does induce negative symptoms, but to a lesser extent than positive symptoms (Hindley et al. 2020).

In conclusion, human laboratory studies have shown—plausibly inferring causality—that transient psychosis in response to THC intoxication is common and reproducible. However, these studies cannot characterize the effects of chronic, heavy cannabis use because that would be neither feasible nor ethical (Radhakrishnan et al. 2014). The studies were also unable to conclusively confirm a link between THC administration and striatal dopaminergic activity; therefore, the nature of the neurobiological underpinnings of the cannabis-psychosis association is yet to be discovered. What seems most likely is that the cannabinoid system results in complex interactions with various neurotransmitter systems at different levels, and these interactions cannot be teased apart by human laboratory studies alone (Sherif et al. 2016).

Neurobiology

Genetic Vulnerability

Having a family history of psychotic disorders increases sensitivity to the psychotogenic effects of cannabis (Genetic Risk and Outcome in Psychosis [GROUP] Investigators 2011). A number of studies have investigated whether genetic polymorphisms involved in dopamine transmission possibly increase sensitivity to the psychotogenic effects of cannabis. Candidate genes including catechol O-methyltransferase (*COMT*; Vaessen et al. 2018), brain-derived neurotrophic factor (*BDNF*; Decoster et al. 2011), AKT serine/threonine kinase (*AKT1*; Batalla et al. 2018; Bhattacharyya et al. 2012, 2014; Colizzi et al. 2015a; Di Forti et al. 2012; van Winkel et al. 2011), dopamine receptor 2 (*DRD2*; Colizzi et al. 2015c), and FKBP prolyl isomerase 5 (*FKBP5*; Ajnakina et al. 2014) showed promise, but initial findings were not replicated (Misiak et al. 2018; Radhakrishnan et al. 2014). Recently, research has focused on the role of cumulative measures of genetic liability for schizophrenia, defined as polygenic risk score for schizophrenia (PRS-SZ). Large genetic epidemiological studies found that the effect of cannabis use on psychotic symptoms in patients and psychotic-like experiences in community members was over and above the effect of PRS-SZ (Quattrone et al. 2021; Wainberg et al. 2021). Furthermore, in one study, the joint effect of cannabis use and PRS-SZ on risk for psychosis was greater than the sum of their independent effects, suggesting biological interaction (Guloksuz et al. 2019).

In addition to studies examining genetic variation in the dopamine signaling system, there is some evidence that genetically determined variability in the endocannabinoid system may modulate response to the effects of cannabis exposure (Bhattacharyya et al. 2017; Colizzi et al. 2015b; Ruiz-Contreras et al. 2013, 2014; Taurisano et al. 2016). This is of relevance, considering that the cannabinoid 1 (CB_1) receptor is targeted by THC because of its partial agonist properties (Pertwee 2008).

Neuropharmacology

THC, as a partial agonist, competes with the endogenous cannabinoids anandamide and 2-arachidonoylglycerol to activate the CB_1 receptor. The latter is widely expressed in the brain, with implications for the perturbation of endocannabinoid system homeostasis (Pertwee 2008). Because of THC's low intrinsic activity, its effects are highly variable depending on the receptor density, the specific G proteins present, and the level of endocannabinoid tone (Glass and Northup 1999; Savinainen et al. 2001), with all of these being differentially affected by repeated cannabinoid administration (Kelley and Thayer 2004).

With prolonged exposure to cannabinoid agonists, neurons accumulate detrimental changes, such as reduced cell surface receptors, decreased coupling to G proteins, and loss of synaptic modulation (Breivogel and Childers 2000; Kouznetsova et al. 2002; Rubino et al. 1998). Among regular cannabis users, desensitization phenomena may occur, making such individuals less sensitive to the agonist effects of THC and more sensitive to its antagonist effects (Kelley and Thayer 2004), with paradoxically less pronounced psychotomimetic effects and cognitive impairments as a result of partial restoration of the underlying brain function (Colizzi et al. 2018a, 2018b).

Neurotransmitter Abnormalities

The CB_1 receptor modulates the release of multiple neurotransmitters in the brain, governing neuronal activity at a wider level (Pertwee 2008). Therefore, THC ingestion, whether through cannabis consumption or experimental administration, can be expected to result in disrupted neurotransmission. Sustained cannabis use, as in dependence, alters dopamine signaling in the associative striatum (van de Giessen et al. 2017), a crucial brain area for the development of positive symptoms such as delusions and hallucinations (Howes et al. 2009). A direct effect of THC on the dopamine system has been difficult to show in human studies, in contrast with animal studies (Sami et al. 2015). This has pushed researchers into searching for the missing link between the endocannabinoid and dopamine systems.

Thus, it has been hypothesized that the dopaminergic effects of THC are exerted through a CB_1-mediated modulation of glutamate neurotransmission in both cortical and subcortical brain areas (Galanopoulos et al. 2011). More specifically, THC exposure may result in unbalanced, and possibly inhibited, glutamatergic neurotransmission (Matsuda et al. 1993; Pertwee and Ross 2002), which, in turn, would facilitate dopaminergic neurotransmission and consequent psychotic symptoms, suggesting that the effects of THC on glutamate signaling should be easier to detect than those on the dopamine system. This has been corroborated by both animal and human research studies. Preclinical evidence supports a role for THC administration in reducing glutamate uptake via glutamate transporters, with a subsequent increase of the neurotransmitter at the extracellular level. On glutamate accumulation, there

is a reorganization of glutamate receptor subunits with downregulation and internalization. Consequently, neuronal dendritic spines in
the hippocampus rarefy, resulting in long-term impairment of synaptic
plasticity (Chen et al. 2013) and reduced glutamate levels in the synapse
(Galanopoulos et al. 2011).

Preclinical studies have proven the ability of THC to increase cortical glutamate levels both extracellularly (Pistis et al. 2002) and intra-
cellularly (Fan et al. 2010) in several brain regions, such as the dorsal
striatum, nucleus accumbens, hippocampus, and prefrontal cortex
(Galanopoulos et al. 2011). As expected, such an acute THC-induced
increase in glutamate levels is associated with a concomitant rise in
dopamine levels (Pistis et al. 2002). On repeated substance exposure,
there is a progressively greater disruption of the glutamate system, as
reflected by depleted neurotransmitter levels in the striatum in rest
conditions that are followed by striatal glutamatergic firing in the context of acute exposure (Gabriele et al. 2012; Parsegian and See 2014).
Human evidence in this regard is less abundant but sufficiently convincing. In fact, glutamate levels have been found to be disrupted in
both chronically (Chang et al. 2006; Muetzel et al. 2013; Prescot et al.
2011, 2013; Sung et al. 2013) and acutely (Colizzi et al. 2020) exposed
healthy subjects.

Furthermore, for almost two decades it has been known that THC
may directly disrupt GABA neurotransmitter release (Matsuda et al.
1993; Pertwee and Ross 2002). GABAergic interneurons in the medial
temporal cortex express CB_1 receptors, whose activation due to THC
administration has been implicated in impairing cognitive processes,
especially in the domains of memory and learning (Clarke et al. 2008;
Puighermanal et al. 2009; Wise et al. 2009). THC-induced perturbation
of CB_1-expressing interneurons is likely to produce alterations that go
far beyond cognitive function, considering GABA's pivotal role in coor-
dinating neural functions involving various behavioral domains in
health and disease (Freund and Katona 2007; Glickfeld and Scanziani
2006).

Thus, cannabis, mainly through its active component THC, affects
the brain by perturbing different neurotransmitter systems, including
glutamate, GABA, and dopamine. Together, this offers biological plausibility for the psychosis-like effects of cannabis because all of these
neurotransmitter systems have been implicated in schizophrenia spectrum disorders (Lisman et al. 2008). Considering the possibility that
cannabis may accelerate the developmental cascade toward psychosis
through its effects on crucial neurotransmitter systems, researchers

have proposed glutamate alterations as robust biomarkers of psychosis (Davison et al. 2018), even in the prodromal phase (de la Fuente-Sandoval et al. 2013, 2015). It is therefore plausible that among people with any biological (e.g., family history of schizophrenia) or psychosocial (e.g., stressful life events) risk factors for psychosis, cannabis may function as a "second hit" by disrupting neurotransmission at multiple levels. There is thus a need to continue the investigation of the neurobiological underpinnings of cannabis-induced psychosis, starting with the endocannabinoid system itself, which, of course, has been found to be altered in psychosis, independently of cannabis use (Appiah-Kusi et al. 2016; Minichino et al. 2019).

Criticisms of the Causal Hypothesis

Over the years, there have been many criticisms of the hypothesis that heavy cannabis use is a component cause of psychosis. The main ones are as follows:

1. **Reverse causality:** Some researchers have claimed that individuals might have started using cannabis just before the onset of psychosis to get relief from subclinical psychotic experiences (Haney and Evins 2016; Ksir and Hart 2016). However, the evidence suggests that people usually started using cannabis well before the onset of psychosis, and they commonly reported initiating it with friends as opposed to initiating use to "feel better" (Spinazzola et al. 2023). Moreover, the Dunedin birth cohort studies found that the association between adolescent cannabis use and adult schizophreniform disorder (OR 3.12; 95% CI 0.73–13.29) was still evident after controlling for childhood psychotic experiences (Arseneault et al. 2002). Similar results were found by the Christchurch Health and Development birth cohort study, which also reported a negative association between early psychotic symptoms and later cannabis use (Fergusson et al. 2003, 2005). Systematic reviews of longitudinal prospective studies confirmed that the association between early cannabis use and later psychosis is still evident after controlling for personal characteristics and/or other drug use that may foster cannabis consumption (Degenhardt and Hall 2006; Welham et al. 2009). Furthermore, according to a meta-analysis, initiation to regular cannabis use precedes the onset of psychosis by an average of 6 years (Myles et al. 2016).

2. **Genetic confounders:** A more important discussion has taken place concerning the possibility that cannabis use and psychosis may result from shared genetic liability. Some, but not all, Mendelian randomization studies suggested that common genetic variants associated with the risk of schizophrenia might predispose individuals to cannabis use, thus suggesting reverse causality (Gage et al. 2017; Pasman et al. 2018; Vaucher et al. 2018). However, more recent findings have reported that PRS-SZ does not increase the risk for cannabis use (Di Forti et al. 2019b; Guloksuz et al. 2019). A compromise view is that predisposition to schizophrenia may account for a small proportion of the variance in cannabis use, but this is insufficient to explain the association between cannabis use and psychosis (Hjorthøj et al. 2021b; Johnson et al. 2023; Lemvigh et al. 2023).

3. **Use of other drugs and tobacco:** Although cannabis use is often associated with the use of other drugs, prospective (Arseneault et al. 2002) and retrospective (Di Forti et al. 2015) studies found consistent evidence that the cannabis-related risk for psychosis is not confounded by the use of other drugs. Tobacco is often smoked along with cannabis (Hindocha et al. 2016), and this is associated with an increased risk for psychosis (Gurillo et al. 2015). The literature suggests that tobacco use does not fully account for the association between cannabis use and psychosis (Di Forti et al. 2009, 2015) but may interact with cannabis use, conferring a greater risk to individuals using both substances (Jones et al. 2018).

4. **Misclassification of cannabis use:** Compared with biological measures, such as those based on urine or blood samples, self-report measures of cannabis use, such as the Cannabis Experiences Questionnaire (Barkus et al. 2006; Di Forti et al. 2009), used in epidemiological studies have often been criticized as being prone to information bias, including recall bias and social desirability. However, research using both self-report and biological measures has indicated that cannabis questionnaires can be as reliable and complete as laboratory measures regarding the quantity, frequency, and type of cannabis use (Curran et al. 2019; Freeman et al. 2014). Moreover, biological measures provide information only about current cannabis use and not on cumulative cannabis use (e.g., duration or amount of cannabis use).

5. **Insufficient trend studies:** For some time, the findings from epidemiological studies at the individual level (i.e., cohort and case-control) received little confirmation from ecological studies investigating the trends of cannabis use and the incidence of psychosis at the population level. Boydell et al. (2006) were the first to claim that an increase in the incidence of psychosis in South London from the 1960s to the late 1990s could be partly related to increased cannabis consumption. Di Forti et al. (2019a) found that the effect of high-potency cannabis accounted for 12% of new onsets of psychosis in Europe, rising to 30% in London and 50% in Amsterdam, which also have the highest rates of high-potency cannabis consumption. Furthermore, a steady increase in the rate of hospital admissions due to psychotic disorders with comorbid CaUDs was recently observed in Portugal (Gonçalves-Pinho et al. 2020) and Denmark (Hjorthøj et al. 2021a), which was consistent with the greater availability of high-potency cannabis over the same period. Findings from Denmark are particularly interesting because they show that young males seem to be particularly susceptible to the effects of cannabis on schizophrenia (Hjorthøj et al. 2023). Recently, using data from public health resources (i.e., Google Trends and Our World in Data), Di Gennaro and Colizzi (2023) found that trends in cannabis use during the period 2005–2019 strongly correlated with the prevalence of schizophrenia in the United Kingdom.

Deleterious Effects

Impact of Heavy Use

Accumulating evidence has revealed that the impact of regular cannabis use (e.g., weekly or daily) on psychosis is significantly greater compared with the impact of less frequent use (e.g., monthly). The European Network of National Schizophrenia Networks Studying Gene-Environment Interactions (EU-GEI) multicentric incidence study found that daily cannabis use was associated with threefold odds of psychotic onset (AOR 3.2; 95% CI 2.2, 4.1) compared with never-use, whereas weekly cannabis use was associated with only a modest increase (AOR 1.4; 95% CI 1.0, 2.0; Di Forti et al. 2019a). A meta-analysis by Marconi et al. (2016) found that the risk of psychosis associated with the most frequent pattern of cannabis use was significantly higher (OR 3.90; 95% CI 2.84, 5.34) than the risk associated with less frequent use (OR 1.97; 95% CI 1.68, 2.31). The findings were confirmed by a more recent meta-analysis estimating a log-linear association between the frequency of cannabis use and the risk for psychosis, with greater risk associated with daily use (RR 1.76; 95% CI 1.47–2.12) compared with weekly use (RR 1.35; 95% CI 1.19–1.52), and an absence of significant association with monthly use or less (Robinson et al. 2022).

The harmful effect of cannabis use on psychosis has been related to the type of cannabis used, with stronger effects for high-potency types of cannabis (Potter et al. 2018), characterized by higher content of THC, the main psychoactive component of cannabis, and lower content of cannabidiol (CBD), which has no psychotomimetic effects (Freeman et al. 2014; Lafaye et al. 2017). The Genetics and Psychosis case-control study (Di Forti et al. 2009; Murray et al. 2020) was the first to find that, compared with never use, use of high-potency cannabis was associated with threefold odds of having a first episode of psychosis (AOR 2.91; 95% CI 1.52, 3.60), which rose to fivefold odds for daily use of high-potency cannabis (AOR 5.40; 95% CI 2.80, 11.30). By contrast, daily use of low-potency cannabis showed no effect on psychosis (Di Forti et al. 2015). More recently, the EU-GEI study found that, compared with never use, daily use of high-potency cannabis (i.e., with >10% THC) was related to 4.8 increased odds of being diagnosed with first-episode psychosis (95% CI 2.5, 6.3), whereas daily use of low-potency cannabis was related to only 2.2 greater odds of having psychosis (95% CI 1.4, 3.6) (Di Forti et al. 2019a).

Summarizing the literature, Petrilli et al. (2022) stated that high-potency cannabis was consistently linked with an increased risk for psychotic disorders compared with low-potency cannabis. A dose-response relationship between frequency of cannabis use and risk for depressive and manic episodes has also been reported in meta-analyses concerning affective disorders (Gibbs et al. 2015; Moore et al. 2007).

In recent years, with the spread of synthetic cannabinoids (Cohen and Weinstein 2018), cases of long-lasting psychosis following use have been documented in individuals with no previous history of mental disorders (Deng et al. 2018; Orsolini et al. 2019); this effect may turn into a schizophrenia-like psychosis (Papanti et al. 2013). Furthermore, the use of synthetic cannabinoids has been related to an increased risk of relapse in patients affected by schizophrenia (Deng et al. 2018).

Adverse Childhood Events

Some reports indicate that childhood adversity may moderate the effect of cannabis use on psychosis in individuals exposed to both childhood trauma and cannabis (Harley et al. 2010; Houston et al. 2011; Konings et al. 2012), but other studies did not replicate these findings (Kuepper et al. 2011; Morgan et al. 2014; Sideli et al. 2018; Vinkers et al. 2013). This may suggest that the childhood adversities by cannabis interaction may depend on the definition and measure of the exposures. Recently, Trotta et al. (2023) found that cannabis use mediated the effect of household discord, psychological abuse, and sexual abuse, an effect that could result from sensitization of the dopamine system.

Critical Period of Adolescence

Adolescence is a particularly sensitive period for risk of psychosis, especially among substance users (Barkus and Murray 2010; Casadio et al. 2011; Murray et al. 2017; Volkow et al. 2016). The Dunedin birth cohort study first found that, compared with never use, cannabis use before age 15 was associated with a more than fourfold increase in the risk for schizophrenia by age 26 (OR 4.50; 95% CI 1.11–18.21), whereas no significant effect was found for cannabis use after age 18 (OR 1.65; 95% CI 0.65, 4.18) (Arseneault et al. 2002). Meta-analytic findings suggest that children and adolescents who smoke cannabis have a nearly double risk (RR 1.71; 95% CI 1.47, 2.00) for psychotic-like experiences or psychotic symptoms (Kiburi et al. 2021; Matheson et al. 2023). Kiburi et al. (2021) found that the risk for psychosis was particularly high among adolescents with early initiation of cannabis use, heavy cannabis use, and exposure to both cannabis use and childhood adversities.

Cannabis Use and the Prodrome of Psychosis

Consistent findings have shown that heavy cannabis use is associated with clinical conditions predating the onset of psychosis. These syndromes have been referred to as *ultrahigh risk* or *clinical high risk* and are characterized by the presence of one or more of the following criteria during the past year: 1) subclinical psychotic symptoms (i.e., attenuated psychotic symptoms); 2) time-limited, self-remitting, frank psychotic symptoms (i.e., brief limited intermittent psychotic symptoms); and 3) high genetic load combined with functional decline (i.e., trait and state risk factor or trait) (Yung et al. 1996). According to a pooled estimate, about 50% of individuals at ultrahigh risk/clinical high risk have used cannabis in their lifetime, about 25% are current users, and up to 15% are affected by CaUD (Carney et al. 2017; Farris et al. 2020), with ultrahigh risk/clinical high risk being associated with double odds of cannabis use compared with healthy control subjects (Carney et al. 2017). However, the association with the transition to psychosis was not consistent across meta-analyses, suggesting that the impact of cannabis on the transition to psychosis depends on the pattern of use after the development of ultrahigh risk (e.g., ceasing or continuing use), in combination with other biological and environmental risk factors (Dragioti et al. 2022; Farris et al. 2020; Kraan et al. 2016; Oliver et al. 2020).

Beneficial Effects

Recently, there has been increasing interest in the effects of CBD, the second major component of cannabis. This compound acts as a negative allosteric modulator at the CB_1 receptor (Laprairie et al. 2015), which has led to the idea that CBD might reduce THC-induced psychotomimetic effects or even have antipsychotic properties itself (D'Souza et al. 2022; Sherif et al. 2016). Challenge studies reported that high doses of CBD can counteract the psychotomimetic effects of THC, reducing psychotic symptoms in people who were administered THC (Bhattacharyya et al. 2010; Englund et al. 2013). Interestingly, an increased CBD ratio did not seem to alter the pleasurable effects of THC (Haney et al. 2016; Hindocha et al. 2015).

From a public health perspective, this apparent effect of CBD in blunting the psychotomimetic effects of THC was seen as a possible route toward the production of "safer cannabis" (Englund et al. 2017). However, more recent evidence indicates that CBD in doses that mimic the amount in traditional cannabis varieties does not modulate the effects of THC (Hindley et al. 2020). A recent randomized, double-blind crossover study found no proof that such amounts of CBD protect against the acute adverse effects of THC (Englund et al. 2023).

The largest meta-analysis to date on the use of cannabinoids for the treatment of mental disorders reported that although some evidence suggests that the medical use of cannabis might help treat some neurological conditions (e.g., multiple sclerosis), evidence is scarce on the efficacy of cannabinoids (with or without CBD) to treat different mental health conditions, such as anxiety, depressive disorders, ADHD, Tourette's disorder, PTSD, or psychosis (Black et al. 2019). In this meta-analysis, the studies that used only pharmaceutical CBD were separately grouped to specifically assess the effects of this compound. Again, the authors found "little evidence for the effectiveness of pharmaceutical CBD or medicinal cannabis for the treatment of any of these mental disorders" (Black et al. 2019, p. 11).

Clinical Significance and Recommendations

Clinical Presentation and Outcome

Age at Onset

Cannabis use exerts an effect on both the onset and the course of psychotic disorders. Two meta-analyses of prospective studies showed that people who smoke cannabis over their lifetime tend to be diagnosed with psychotic disorders an average of 2–3 years earlier than do nonusers (Large et al. 2011; Myles et al. 2012), and the association is not fully explained by other risk factors associated with early onset of psychosis (Myles et al. 2012), such as male sex and concurrent tobacco use (Gurillo et al. 2015). Di Forti et al. (2014) showed that those who used high-potency cannabis experienced psychosis onset on average 6 years earlier than never users. Cannabis users also show an earlier onset of bipolar disorders compared with nonusers (Pinto et al. 2019).

Symptomatology

Many studies have attempted to identify a clinical picture specific to cannabis-induced psychosis, compared with other psychoses, at both the psychopathological and neurocognitive levels. Most of these studies have been too small to produce reliable results. However, Quattrone et al. (2020) reported convincing findings from an examination of 901 patients experiencing their first episode of psychosis. A linear relationship was seen between positive symptoms and the extent of lifetime exposure to cannabis, with daily users of high-potency cannabis having the highest score. On the other hand, negative symptoms were more common among patients who had never used cannabis.

Cognition

Although cannabis use has generally been shown to impair cognitive functions in otherwise healthy individuals (Grant et al. 2003; Schoeler et al. 2016a), this has not been found in studies of patients with psychosis, in which better cognitive performance has been found in those who used cannabis compared with those who did not. The Genetics and Psychosis study offered a possible explanation by showing that first-episode psychosis patients who had smoked cannabis had not only a higher current IQ but also a higher premorbid IQ than did patients who had never used cannabis (Ferraro et al. 2013); this difference was not found among control subjects. The authors suggested that cannabis plays a role in provoking psychosis in people who are less neurodevelopmentally impaired than is generally the case in psychosis.

Outcome

Although follow-up studies revealed that about 50% of patients with first-episode psychosis subsequently stopped smoking cannabis (Myles et al. 2016), those who continued to use cannabis were at increased risk for relapse, longer duration of hospitalization, and failed response to antipsychotic treatment (Athanassiou et al. 2021; Schoeler et al. 2016b; Wilson and Bhattacharyya 2016), whereas cannabis discontinuation was associated with functional improvement (Schoeler et al. 2016b). Literature suggests that the effect of continued cannabis use on the risk for relapse and the number of relapses is partially mediated by poor medication adherence (Colizzi et al. 2016; Schoeler et al. 2017). The adverse effect of cannabis use on treatment response has been postulated to be related to the impact of regular cannabis use on the dopaminergic and glutamatergic systems (Bloomfield et al. 2014; Egerton 2016). The findings were similar for bipolar disorders, with associations between continued cannabis use and the number of hospitalizations as well as the number of suicide attempts (Pinto et al. 2019).

The use of high-potency cannabis seems to have a stronger effect on the course of the disease (Petrilli et al. 2022), even independent of the frequency of use. According to the Genetics and Psychosis study conducted in London, daily use of high-potency cannabis was associated with a threefold increased risk of relapse at the 2-year follow-up (AOR 3.28; 95% CI 1.22, 9.18), whereas no effect was found for low-potency cannabis use (Schoeler et al. 2016c).

Recommendations for Clinicians

The evidence indicates that mental health clinicians should promote cannabis discontinuation in patients with psychosis because it can lead to significant improvements in hallucinations and levels of functioning (Waterreus et al. 2023). Although psychosocial interventions have shown limited success in addressing continued cannabis use in this population (Hjorthøj et al. 2014), in the future, it might be necessary to explore tailored treatment interventions that consider the heterogeneity of cannabis use in individuals with psychosis, such as variations in frequency and motivations for use (McDonell and Oluwoye 2019).

Regarding pharmacological approaches, only clozapine, among all antipsychotics trialed, has shown some efficacy in reducing cannabis craving in individuals with psychosis (Brunette et al. 2011). However, the current evidence for pharmacological interventions targeting cannabis use in people with psychosis is still scarce, and further research is needed to explore the effectiveness of other medications or combination treatments.

Conclusion

Evidence from epidemiological, clinical, experimental, and neurobiological studies has convinced almost all researchers that heavy cannabis use increases the risk of psychosis; one by one, the arguments of skeptics have been disproved. Consequently, the focus of research has moved from investigating whether cannabis-induced psychosis exists to understanding the mechanisms involved, who is most susceptible, and whether the worldwide trend toward the liberalization of cannabis laws will lead to such an increased consumption (and potency) of cannabis that it will result in an overall increase in the frequency of psychosis (Murray and Hall 2020).

Key Points

- Evidence from multiple types of studies (e.g., epidemiological, experimental, and neurobiological) supports the hypothesis that heavy cannabis use increases the risk of psychosis; longitudinal studies have shown that reverse causality mechanisms are highly unlikely to account for this association.

- Ecological studies have provided evidence of an increase in the incidence of psychosis in regions with higher cannabis consumption, particularly high-potency cannabis.
- Controlled experimental studies have demonstrated that acute administration of cannabis or its primary psychoactive component, Δ^9-tetrahydrocannabinol, can induce transient psychotic-like symptoms in healthy individuals.
- Neurobiological studies have revealed that cannabis can disrupt the endocannabinoid system and alter neurotransmitter systems, particularly dopamine, glutamate, and GABA, which are implicated in the pathophysiology of psychosis.
- The worldwide trend toward cannabis liberalization raises concerns regarding increased consumption and potency potentially leading to an overall increase in the frequency of psychosis.
- Continued research is needed to better understand the mechanisms involved, identify vulnerable populations, and assess the potential impact of cannabis policy changes on mental health outcomes.
- The bulk of evidence suggests that heavy cannabis use is a contributory cause of psychosis, but further research is necessary to fully elucidate the complex relationship between cannabis use and psychosis.

References

Ajnakina O, Borges S, Di Forti M, et al: Role of environmental confounding in the association between FKBP5 and first-episode psychosis. Front Psychiatry 5:84, 2014 25101008

Appiah-Kusi E, Leyden E, Parmar S, et al: Abnormalities in neuroendocrine stress response in psychosis: the role of endocannabinoids. Psychol Med 46(1):27–45, 2016 26370602

Arseneault L, Cannon M, Poulton R, et al: Cannabis use in adolescence and risk for adult psychosis: longitudinal prospective study. BMJ 325(7374):1212–1213, 2002 12446537

Athanassiou M, Dumais A, Gnanhoue G, et al: A systematic review of longitudinal studies investigating the impact of cannabis use in patients with psychotic disorders. Expert Rev Neurother 21(7):779–791, 2021 34120548

Barkus E, Murray RM: Substance use in adolescence and psychosis: clarifying the relationship. Annu Rev Clin Psychol 6:365–389, 2010 20192802

Barkus EJ, Stirling J, Hopkins RS, Lewis S: Cannabis-induced psychosis-like experiences are associated with high schizotypy. Psychopathology 39(4):175–178, 2006 16636640

Barkus E, Morrison PD, Vuletic D, et al: Does intravenous Δ9-tetrahydrocannabinol increase dopamine release? A SPET study. J Psychopharmacol 25(11):1462–1468, 2011 20851843

Batalla A, Lorenzetti V, Chye Y, et al: The influence of DAT1, COMT, and BDNF genetic polymorphisms on total and subregional hippocampal volumes in early onset heavy cannabis users. Cannabis Cannabinoid Res 3(1):1–10, 2018 29404409

Bhattacharyya S, Morrison PD, Fusar-Poli P, et al: Opposite effects of delta-9-tetrahydrocannabinol and cannabidiol on human brain function and psychopathology. Neuropsychopharmacology 35(3):764–774, 2010 19924114

Bhattacharyya S, Atakan Z, Martin-Santos R, et al: Preliminary report of biological basis of sensitivity to the effects of cannabis on psychosis: AKT1 and DAT1 genotype modulates the effects of Δ-9-tetrahydrocannabinol on midbrain and striatal function. Mol Psychiatry 17(12):1152–1155, 2012 22290123

Bhattacharyya S, Iyegbe C, Atakan Z, et al: Protein kinase B (AKT1) genotype mediates sensitivity to cannabis-induced impairments in psychomotor control. Psychol Med 44(15):3315–3328, 2014 25065544

Bhattacharyya S, Egerton A, Kim E, et al: Acute induction of anxiety in humans by delta-9-tetrahydrocannabinol related to amygdalar cannabinoid-1 (CB1) receptors. Sci Rep 7(1):15025, 2017 29101333

Black N, Stockings E, Campbell G, et al: Cannabinoids for the treatment of mental disorders and symptoms of mental disorders: a systematic review and meta-analysis. Lancet Psychiatry 6(12):995–1010, 2019 31672337

Bloomfield MA, Morgan CJ, Egerton A, et al: Dopaminergic function in cannabis users and its relationship to cannabis-induced psychotic symptoms. Biol Psychiatry 75(6):470–478, 2014 23820822

Boydell J, van Os J, Caspi A, et al: Trends in cannabis use prior to first presentation with schizophrenia, in south-east London between 1965 and 1999. Psychol Med 36(10):1441–1446, 2006 16854250

Breivogel CS, Childers SR: Cannabinoid agonist signal transduction in rat brain: comparison of cannabinoid agonists in receptor binding, G-protein activation, and adenylyl cyclase inhibition. J Pharmacol Exp Ther 295(1):328–336, 2000 10991998

Brunette MF, Dawson R, O'Keefe CD, et al: A randomized trial of clozapine vs. other antipsychotics for cannabis use disorder in patients with schizophrenia. J Dual Diagn 7(1–2):50–63, 2011 25914610

Carney R, Cotter J, Firth J, et al: Cannabis use and symptom severity in individuals at ultra high risk for psychosis: a meta-analysis. Acta Psychiatr Scand 136(1):5–15, 2017 28168698

Casadio P, Fernandes C, Murray RM, et al: Cannabis use in young people: the risk for schizophrenia. Neurosci Biobehav Rev 35(8):1779–1787, 2011 21530584

Chang L, Cloak C, Yakupov R, et al: Combined and independent effects of chronic marijuana use and HIV on brain metabolites. J Neuroimmune Pharmacol 1(1):65–76, 2006 18040792

Chen R, Zhang J, Fan N, et al: Δ9-THC-caused synaptic and memory impairments are mediated through COX-2 signaling. Cell 155(5):1154–1165, 2013 24267894

Clarke JR, Rossato JI, Monteiro S, et al: Posttraining activation of CB1 cannabinoid receptors in the CA1 region of the dorsal hippocampus impairs object recognition long-term memory. Neurobiol Learn Mem 90(2):374–381, 2008 18524639

Cohen K, Weinstein AM: Synthetic and non-synthetic cannabinoid drugs and their adverse effects—a review from public health prospective. Front Public Health 6:162, 2018 29930934

Colizzi M, Iyegbe C, Powell J, et al: Interaction between DRD2 and AKT1 genetic variations on risk of psychosis in cannabis users: a case-control study. NPJ Schizophr 1:15025, 2015a 27336035

Colizzi M, Fazio L, Ferranti L, et al: Functional genetic variation of the cannabinoid receptor 1 and cannabis use interact on prefrontal connectivity and related working memory behavior. Neuropsychopharmacology 40(3):640–649, 2015b 25139064

Colizzi M, Iyegbe C, Powell J, et al: Interaction between functional genetic variation of DRD2 and cannabis use on risk of psychosis. Schizophr Bull 41(5):1171–1182, 2015c 25829376

Colizzi M, Carra E, Fraietta S, et al: Substance use, medication adherence and outcome one year following a first episode of psychosis. Schizophr Res 170(2–3):311–317, 2016 26718334

Colizzi M, McGuire P, Giampietro V, et al: Previous cannabis exposure modulates the acute effects of delta-9-tetrahydrocannabinol on attentional salience and fear processing. Exp Clin Psychopharmacol 26(6):582–598, 2018a 30138003

Colizzi M, McGuire P, Giampietro V, et al: Modulation of acute effects of delta-9-tetrahydrocannabinol on psychotomimetic effects, cognition and brain function by previous cannabis exposure. Eur Neuropsychopharmacol 28(7):850–862, 2018b 29935939

Colizzi M, Weltens N, McGuire P, et al: Delta-9-tetrahydrocannabinol increases striatal glutamate levels in healthy individuals: implications for psychosis. Mol Psychiatry 25(12):3231–3240, 2020 30770892

Curran HV, Hindocha C, Morgan CJA, et al: Which biological and self-report measures of cannabis use predict cannabis dependency and acute psychotic-like effects? Psychol Med 49(9):1574–1580, 2019 30176957

Davison J, O'Gorman A, Brennan L, et al: A systematic review of metabolite biomarkers of schizophrenia. Schizophr Res 195:32–50, 2018 28947341

Decoster J, van Os J, Kenis G, et al: Age at onset of psychotic disorder: cannabis, BDNF Val66Met, and sex-specific models of gene-environment interaction. Am J Med Genet B Neuropsychiatr Genet 156B(3):363–369, 2011 21305693

Degenhardt L, Hall W: Is cannabis use a contributory cause of psychosis? Can J Psychiatry 51(9):556–565, 2006 17007222

de la Fuente-Sandoval C, León-Ortiz P, Azcárraga M, et al: Striatal glutamate and the conversion to psychosis: a prospective 1H-MRS imaging study. Int J Neuropsychopharmacol 16(2):471–475, 2013 22717289

de la Fuente-Sandoval C, Reyes-Madrigal F, Mao X, et al: Cortico-striatal GABAergic and glutamatergic dysregulations in subjects at ultra-high risk for psychosis investigated with proton magnetic resonance spectroscopy. Int J Neuropsychopharmacol 19(3):pyv105, 2015 26364273

Deng H, Verrico CD, Kosten TR, et al: Psychosis and synthetic cannabinoids. Psychiatry Res 268:400–412, 2018 30125871

Di Forti M, Morgan C, Dazzan P, et al: High-potency cannabis and the risk of psychosis. Br J Psychiatry 195(6):488–491, 2009 19949195

Di Forti M, Iyegbe C, Sallis H, et al: Confirmation that the AKT1 (rs2494732) genotype influences the risk of psychosis in cannabis users. Biol Psychiatry 72(10):811–816, 2012 22831980

Di Forti M, Sallis H, Allegri F, et al: Daily use, especially of high-potency cannabis, drives the earlier onset of psychosis in cannabis users. Schizophr Bull 40(6):1509–1517, 2014 24345517

Di Forti M, Marconi A, Carra E, et al: Proportion of patients in south London with first-episode psychosis attributable to use of high potency cannabis: a case-control study. Lancet Psychiatry 2(3):233–238, 2015 26359901

Di Forti M, Quattrone D, Freeman TP, et al: The contribution of cannabis use to variation in the incidence of psychotic disorder across Europe (EU-GEI): a multicentre case-control study. Lancet Psychiatry 6(5):427–436, 2019a 30902669

Di Forti M, Wu-Choi B, Quattrone D, et al: The independent and combined influence of schizophrenia polygenic risk score and heavy cannabis use on risk for psychotic disorder: a case-control analysis from the EUGEI study. Laurel Hollow, NY, Cold Spring Harbor Laboratory, 2019b

Di Gennaro G, Colizzi M: Can we interrogate public databases to fill critical gaps in mental health epidemiology? Testing the association between cannabis and psychosis in the UK as an example. Epidemiol Psychiatr Sci 32:e40, 2023 37317558

Dragioti E, Radua J, Solmi M, et al: Global population attributable fraction of potentially modifiable risk factors for mental disorders: a meta-umbrella systematic review. Mol Psychiatry 27(8):3510–3519, 2022 35484237

D'Souza DC, Perry E, MacDougall L, et al: The psychotomimetic effects of intravenous delta-9-tetrahydrocannabinol in healthy individuals: implications for psychosis. Neuropsychopharmacology 29(8):1558–1572, 2004 15173844

D'Souza DC, Abi-Saab WM, Madonick S, et al: Delta-9-tetrahydrocannabinol effects in schizophrenia: implications for cognition, psychosis, and addiction. Biol Psychiatry 57(6):594–608, 2005 15780846

D'Souza DC, Braley G, Blaise R, et al: Effects of haloperidol on the behavioral, subjective, cognitive, motor, and neuroendocrine effects of delta-9-tetrahydrocannabinol in humans. Psychopharmacology (Berl) 198(4):587–603, 2008 18228005

D'Souza DC, Cortes-Briones JA, Ranganathan M, et al: Rapid changes in cannabinoid 1 receptor availability in cannabis-dependent male subjects after abstinence from cannabis. Biol Psychiatry Cogn Neurosci Neuroimaging 1(1):60–67, 2016 29560896

D'Souza DC, DiForti M, Ganesh S, et al: Consensus paper of the WFSBP task force on cannabis, cannabinoids and psychosis. World J Biol Psychiatry 23(10):719–742, 2022 35315315

Egerton A: Brain glutamate levels and antipsychotic response in schizophrenia. Eur Psychiatry 33(S1):S19–S19, 2016

Englund A, Morrison PD, Nottage J, et al: Cannabidiol inhibits THC-elicited paranoid symptoms and hippocampal-dependent memory impairment. J Psychopharmacol 27(1):19–27, 2013 23042808

Englund A, Freeman TP, Murray RM, et al: Can we make cannabis safer? Lancet Psychiatry 4(8):643–648, 2017 28259650

Englund A, Oliver D, Chesney E, et al: Does cannabidiol make cannabis safer? A randomised, double-blind, cross-over trial of cannabis with four different CBD:THC ratios. Neuropsychopharmacology 48(6):869–876, 2023 36380220

Fan N, Yang H, Zhang J, et al: Reduced expression of glutamate receptors and phosphorylation of CREB are responsible for in vivo delta9-THC exposure-impaired hippocampal synaptic plasticity. J Neurochem 112(3):691–702, 2010 19912468

Farris MS, Shakeel MK, Addington J: Cannabis use in individuals at clinical high-risk for psychosis: a comprehensive review. Soc Psychiatry Psychiatr Epidemiol 55(5):527–537, 2020 31796983

Fergusson DM, Horwood LJ, Swain-Campbell NR: Cannabis dependence and psychotic symptoms in young people. Psychol Med 33(1):15–21, 2003 12537032

Fergusson DM, Horwood LJ, Ridder EM: Tests of causal linkages between cannabis use and psychotic symptoms. Addiction 100(3):354–366, 2005 15733249

Ferraro L, Russo M, O'Connor J, et al: Cannabis users have higher premorbid IQ than other patients with first onset psychosis. Schizophr Res 150(1):129–135, 2013 23958486

Freeman TP, Morgan CJ, Hindocha C, et al: Just say 'know': how do cannabinoid concentrations influence users' estimates of cannabis potency and the amount they roll in joints? Addiction 109(10):1686–1694, 2014 24894801

Freund TF, Katona I: Perisomatic inhibition. Neuron 56(1):33–42, 2007 17920013

Gabriele A, Pacchioni AM, See RE: Dopamine and glutamate release in the dorsolateral caudate putamen following withdrawal from cocaine self-administration in rats. Pharmacol Biochem Behav 103(2):373–379, 2012 23026056

Gage SH, Jones HJ, Burgess S, et al: Assessing causality in associations between cannabis use and schizophrenia risk: a two-sample Mendelian randomization study. Psychol Med 47(5):971–980, 2017 27928975

Galanopoulos A, Polissidis A, Papadopoulou-Daifoti Z, et al: Δ(9)-THC and WIN55,212–2 affect brain tissue levels of excitatory amino acids in a phenotype-, compound-, dose-, and region-specific manner. Behav Brain Res 224(1):65–72, 2011 21645556

Ganesh S, Cortes-Briones J, Ranganathan M, et al: Psychosis-relevant effects of intravenous delta-9-tetrahydrocannabinol: a mega analysis of individual participant-data from human laboratory studies. Int J Neuropsychopharmacol 23(9):559–570, 2020 32385508

Genetic Risk and Outcome in Psychosis (GROUP) Investigators: Evidence that familial liability for psychosis is expressed as differential sensitivity to cannabis: an analysis of patient-sibling and sibling-control pairs. Arch Gen Psychiatry 68(2):138–147, 2011 20921112

Gibbs M, Winsper C, Marwaha S, et al: Cannabis use and mania symptoms: a systematic review and meta-analysis. J Affect Disord 171:39–47, 2015 25285897

Glass M, Northup JK: Agonist selective regulation of G proteins by cannabinoid CB(1) and CB(2) receptors. Mol Pharmacol 56(6):1362–1369, 1999 10570066

Glickfeld LL, Scanziani M: Distinct timing in the activity of cannabinoid-sensitive and cannabinoid-insensitive basket cells. Nat Neurosci 9(6):807–815, 2006 16648849

Gonçalves-Pinho M, Bragança M, Freitas A: Psychotic disorders hospitalizations associated with cannabis abuse or dependence: a nationwide big data analysis. Int J Methods Psychiatr Res 29(1):e1813, 2020 31808250

Grant I, Gonzalez R, Carey CL, et al: Non-acute (residual) neurocognitive effects of cannabis use: a meta-analytic study. J Int Neuropsychol Soc 9(5):679–689, 2003 12901774

Green B, Kavanagh D, Young R: Being stoned: a review of self-reported cannabis effects. Drug Alcohol Rev 22(4):453–460, 2003 14660135

Guloksuz S, Pries LK, Delespaul P, et al: Examining the independent and joint effects of molecular genetic liability and environmental exposures in schizophrenia: results from the EUGEI study. World Psychiatry 18(2):173–182, 2019 31059627

Gurillo P, Jauhar S, Murray RM, et al: Does tobacco use cause psychosis? Systematic review and meta-analysis. Lancet Psychiatry 2(8):718–725, 2015 26249303

Haney M, Evins AE: Does cannabis cause, exacerbate or ameliorate psychiatric disorders? An oversimplified debate discussed. Neuropsychopharmacology 41(2):393–401, 2016 26286840

Haney M, Malcolm RJ, Babalonis S, et al: Oral cannabidiol does not alter the subjective, reinforcing or cardiovascular effects of smoked cannabis. Neuropsychopharmacology 41(8):1974–1982, 2016 26708108

Harley M, Kelleher I, Clarke M, et al: Cannabis use and childhood trauma interact additively to increase the risk of psychotic symptoms in adolescence. Psychol Med 40(10):1627–1634, 2010 19995476

Hindley G, Beck K, Borgan F, et al: Psychiatric symptoms caused by cannabis constituents: a systematic review and meta-analysis. Lancet Psychiatry 7(4):344–353, 2020 32197092

Hindocha C, Freeman TP, Schafer G, et al: Acute effects of delta-9-tetrahydrocannabinol, cannabidiol and their combination on facial emotion recognition: a randomised, double-blind, placebo-controlled study in cannabis users. Eur Neuropsychopharmacol 25(3):325–334, 2015 25534187

Hindocha C, Freeman TP, Ferris JA, et al: No smoke without tobacco: a global overview of cannabis and tobacco routes of administration and their association with intention to quit. Front Psychiatry 7:104, 2016 27458388

Hjorthøj C, Baker A, Fohlmann A, et al: Intervention efficacy in trials targeting cannabis use disorders in patients with comorbid psychosis systematic review and meta-analysis. Curr Pharm Des 20(13):2205–2211, 2014 23829367

Hjorthøj C, Larsen MO, Starzer MSK, et al: Annual incidence of cannabis-induced psychosis, other substance-induced psychoses and dually diagnosed schizophrenia and cannabis use disorder in Denmark from 1994 to 2016. Psychol Med 51(4):617–622, 2021a 31839011

Hjorthøj C, Uddin MJ, Wimberley T, et al: No evidence of associations between genetic liability for schizophrenia and development of cannabis use disorder. Psychol Med 51(3):479–484, 2021b 31813396

Hjorthøj C, Compton W, Starzer M, et al: Association between cannabis use disorder and schizophrenia stronger in young males than in females. Psychol Med 53(15):7322–7328, 2023 37140715

Houston JE, Murphy J, Shevlin M, et al: Cannabis use and psychosis: re-visiting the role of childhood trauma. Psychol Med 41(11):2339–2348, 2011 21557896

Howes OD, Montgomery AJ, Asselin MC, et al: Elevated striatal dopamine function linked to prodromal signs of schizophrenia. Arch Gen Psychiatry 66(1):13–20, 2009 19124684

Hunt GE, Large MM, Cleary M, et al: Prevalence of comorbid substance use in schizophrenia spectrum disorders in community and clinical settings, 1990–2017: systematic review and meta-analysis. Drug Alcohol Depend 191:234–258, 2018 30153606

Johnson EC, Colbert SMC, Jeffries PW, et al: Associations between cannabis use, polygenic liability for schizophrenia, and cannabis-related experiences in a sample of cannabis users. Schizophr Bull 49(3):778–787, 2023 36545904

Jones HJ, Gage SH, Heron J, et al: Association of combined patterns of tobacco and cannabis use in adolescence with psychotic experiences. JAMA Psychiatry 75(3):240–246, 2018 29344610

Kelley BG, Thayer SA: Delta 9-tetrahydrocannabinol antagonizes endocannabinoid modulation of synaptic transmission between hippocampal neurons in culture. Neuropharmacology 46(5):709–715, 2004 14996548

Kiburi SK, Molebatsi K, Ntlantsana V, et al: Cannabis use in adolescence and risk of psychosis: are there factors that moderate this relationship? A systematic review and meta-analysis. Subst Abus 42(4):527–542, 2021 33617756

Kleinloog D, Liem-Moolenaar M, Jacobs G, et al: Does olanzapine inhibit the psychomimetic effects of Δ9-tetrahydrocannabinol? J Psychopharmacol 26(10):1307–1316, 2012 22596206

Konings M, Stefanis N, Kuepper R, et al: Replication in two independent population-based samples that childhood maltreatment and cannabis use synergistically impact on psychosis risk. Psychol Med 42(1):149–159, 2012 21676285

Kouznetsova M, Kelley B, Shen M, et al: Desensitization of cannabinoid-mediated presynaptic inhibition of neurotransmission between rat hippocampal neurons in culture. Mol Pharmacol 61(3):477–485, 2002 11854427

Kraan T, Velthorst E, Koenders L, et al: Cannabis use and transition to psychosis in individuals at ultra-high risk: review and meta-analysis. Psychol Med 46(4):673–681, 2016 26568030

Ksir C, Hart CL: Correlation still does not imply causation (comment). Lancet Psychiatry 3(5):401, 2016 27155509

Kuepper R, Henquet C, Lieb R, et al: Non-replication of interaction between cannabis use and trauma in predicting psychosis. Schizophr Res 131(1–3):262–263, 2011 21745727

Lafaye G, Karila L, Blecha L, et al: Cannabis, cannabinoids, and health. Dialogues Clin Neurosci 19(3):309–316, 2017 29302228

Laprairie RB, Bagher AM, Kelly ME, et al: Cannabidiol is a negative allosteric modulator of the cannabinoid CB1 receptor. Br J Pharmacol 172(20):4790–4805, 2015 26218440

Large M, Sharma S, Compton MT, et al: Cannabis use and earlier onset of psychosis: a systematic meta-analysis. Arch Gen Psychiatry 68(6):555–561, 2011 21300939

Lemvigh C, Brouwer R, Hilker R, et al: The relative and interactive impact of multiple risk factors in schizophrenia spectrum disorders: a combined register-based and clinical twin study. Psychol Med 53(4):1266–1276, 2023 35822354

Lev-Ran S, Roerecke M, Le Foll B, et al: The association between cannabis use and depression: a systematic review and meta-analysis of longitudinal studies. Psychol Med 44(4):797–810, 2014 23795762

Liem-Moolenaar M, te Beek ET, de Kam ML, et al: Central nervous system effects of haloperidol on THC in healthy male volunteers. J Psychopharmacol 24(11):1697–1708, 2010 20142302

Linscott RJ, van Os J: An updated and conservative systematic review and meta-analysis of epidemiological evidence on psychotic experiences in children and adults: on the pathway from proneness to persistence to dimensional expression across mental disorders. Psychol Med 43(6):1133–1149, 2013 22850401

Lisman JE, Coyle JT, Green RW, et al: Circuit-based framework for understanding neurotransmitter and risk gene interactions in schizophrenia. Trends Neurosci 31(5):234–242, 2008 18395805

Marconi A, Di Forti M, Lewis CM, et al: Meta-analysis of the association between the level of cannabis use and risk of psychosis. Schizophr Bull 42(5):1262–1269, 2016 26884547

Matheson SL, Shepherd AM, Laurens KR, et al: A systematic meta-review grading the evidence for non-genetic risk factors and putative antecedents of schizophrenia. Schizophr Res 133(1–3):133–142, 2011 21999904

Matheson SL, Laurie M, Laurens KR: Substance use and psychotic-like experiences in young people: a systematic review and meta-analysis. Psychol Med 53(2):305–319, 2023 36377500

Matsuda LA, Bonner TI, Lolait SJ: Localization of cannabinoid receptor mRNA in rat brain. J Comp Neurol 327(4):535–550, 1993 8440779

McDonell MG, Oluwoye O: Cannabis use in first episode psychosis: what we have tried and why it hasn't worked (comment). BMC Med 17(1):194, 2019 31660949

Minichino A, Senior M, Brondino N, et al: Measuring disturbance of the endocannabinoid system in psychosis: a systematic review and meta-analysis. JAMA Psychiatry 76(9):914–923, 2019 31166595

Misiak B, Stramecki F, Gawęda Ł, et al: Interactions between variation in candidate genes and environmental factors in the etiology of schizophrenia and bipolar disorder: a systematic review. Mol Neurobiol 55(6):5075–5100, 2018 28822116

Moore TH, Zammit S, Lingford-Hughes A, et al: Cannabis use and risk of psychotic or affective mental health outcomes: a systematic review. Lancet 370(9584):319–328, 2007 17662880

Morgan C, Reininghaus U, Reichenberg A, et al: Adversity, cannabis use and psychotic experiences: evidence of cumulative and synergistic effects. Br J Psychiatry 204(5):346–353, 2014 24627297

Morrison PD, Stone JM: Synthetic delta-9-tetrahydrocannabinol elicits schizophrenia-like negative symptoms which are distinct from sedation. Hum Psychopharmacol 26(1):77–80, 2011 23055415

Muetzel RL, Marjańska M, Collins PF, et al: In vivo 1H magnetic resonance spectroscopy in young-adult daily marijuana users. Neuroimage Clin 2:581–589, 2013 23956957

Murray RM, Hall W: Will legalization and commercialization of cannabis use increase the incidence and prevalence of psychosis? JAMA Psychiatry 77(8):777–778, 2020 32267480

Murray RM, Quigley H, Quattrone D, et al: Traditional marijuana, high-potency cannabis and synthetic cannabinoids: increasing risk for psychosis. World Psychiatry 15(3):195–204, 2016 27717258

Murray RM, Englund A, Abi-Dargham A, et al: Cannabis-associated psychosis: neural substrate and clinical impact. Neuropharmacology 124:89–104, 2017 28634109

Murray RM, Mondelli V, Stilo SA, et al: The influence of risk factors on the onset and outcome of psychosis: what we learned from the GAP study. Schizophr Res 225:63–68, 2020 32037203

Myles H, Myles N, Large M: Cannabis use in first episode psychosis: meta-analysis of prevalence, and the time course of initiation and continued use. Aust NZ J Psychiatry 50(3):208–219, 2016 26286531

Myles N, Newall H, Nielssen O, et al: The association between cannabis use and earlier age at onset of schizophrenia and other psychoses: meta-analysis of possible confounding factors. Curr Pharm Des 18(32):5055–5069, 2012 22716150

Oliver D, Reilly TJ, Baccaredda Boy O, et al: What causes the onset of psychosis in individuals at clinical high risk? A meta-analysis of risk and protective factors. Schizophr Bull 46(1):110–120, 2020 31219164

Orsolini L, Chiappini S, Papanti D, et al: The bridge between classical and "synthetic"/chemical psychoses: towards a clinical, psychopathological, and therapeutic perspective. Front Psychiatry 10:851, 2019 31849723

Papanti D, Schifano F, Botteon G, et al: "Spiceophrenia": a systematic overview of "spice"-related psychopathological issues and a case report. Hum Psychopharmacol 28(4):379–389, 2013 23881886

Parsegian A, See RE: Dysregulation of dopamine and glutamate release in the prefrontal cortex and nucleus accumbens following methamphetamine self-administration and during reinstatement in rats. Neuropsychopharmacology 39(4):811–822, 2014 23995583

Pasman JA, Verweij KJH, Gerring Z, et al: GWAS of lifetime cannabis use reveals new risk loci, genetic overlap with psychiatric traits, and a causal influence of schizophrenia. Nat Neurosci 21(9):1161–1170, 2018 30150663

Pertwee RG: The diverse CB1 and CB2 receptor pharmacology of three plant cannabinoids: delta9-tetrahydrocannabinol, cannabidiol and delta9-tetrahydrocannabivarin. Br J Pharmacol 153(2):199–215, 2008 17828291

Pertwee RG, Ross RA: Cannabinoid receptors and their ligands. Prostaglandins Leukot Essent Fatty Acids 66(2–3):101–121, 2002 12052030

Petrilli K, Ofori S, Hines L, et al: Association of cannabis potency with mental ill health and addiction: a systematic review. Lancet Psychiatry 9(9):736–750, 2022 35901795

Pinto JV, Medeiros LS, Santana da Rosa G, et al: The prevalence and clinical correlates of cannabis use and cannabis use disorder among patients with bipolar disorder: a systematic review with meta-analysis and meta-regression. Neurosci Biobehav Rev 101:78–84, 2019 30974123

Pistis M, Ferraro L, Pira L, et al: Delta(9)-tetrahydrocannabinol decreases extracellular GABA and increases extracellular glutamate and dopamine levels in the rat prefrontal cortex: an in vivo microdialysis study. Brain Res 948(1–2):155–158, 2002 12383968

Potter DJ, Hammond K, Tuffnell S, et al: Potency of Δ9-tetrahydrocannabinol and other cannabinoids in cannabis in England in 2016: implications for public health and pharmacology. Drug Test Anal 10(4):628–635, 2018 29441730

Prescot AP, Locatelli AE, Renshaw PF, et al: Neurochemical alterations in adolescent chronic marijuana smokers: a proton MRS study. Neuroimage 57(1):69–75, 2011 21349338

Prescot AP, Renshaw PF, Yurgelun-Todd DA: γ-Amino butyric acid and glutamate abnormalities in adolescent chronic marijuana smokers. Drug Alcohol Depend 129(3):232–239, 2013 23522493

Puighermanal E, Marsicano G, Busquets-Garcia A, et al: Cannabinoid modulation of hippocampal long-term memory is mediated by mTOR signaling. Nat Neurosci 12(9):1152–1158, 2009 19648913

Quattrone D, Ferraro L, Tripoli G, et al: Daily use of high-potency cannabis is associated with more positive symptoms in first-episode psychosis patients: the EU-GEI case-control study. Psychol Med 51(8):1329–1337, 2020 32183927

Quattrone D, Reininghaus U, Richards AL, et al: The continuity of effect of schizophrenia polygenic risk score and patterns of cannabis use on transdiagnostic symptom dimensions at first-episode psychosis: findings from the EU-GEI study. Transl Psychiatry 11(1):423, 2021 34376640

Radhakrishnan R, Wilkinson ST, D'Souza DC: Gone to pot: a review of the association between cannabis and psychosis. Front Psychiatry 5:54, 2014 24904437

Radua J, Ramella-Cravaro V, Ioannidis JPA, et al: What causes psychosis? an umbrella review of risk and protective factors. World Psychiatry 17(1):49–66, 2018 29352556

Ragazzi TCC, Shuhama R, Menezes PR, et al: Cannabis use as a risk factor for psychotic-like experiences: a systematic review of non-clinical populations evaluated with the Community Assessment of Psychic Experiences. Early Interv Psychiatry 12(6):1013–1023, 2018 29927066

Robinson T, Ali MU, Easterbrook B, et al: Risk-thresholds for the association between frequency of cannabis use and the development of psychosis: a systematic review and meta-analysis. Psychol Med 53(9):3858–3868, 2022 35321777

Rodriguez V, Alameda L, Trotta G, et al: Environmental risk factors in bipolar disorder and psychotic depression: a systematic review and meta-analysis of prospective studies. Schizophr Bull 47(4):959–974, 2021 33479726

Rubino T, Patrini G, Massi P, et al: Cannabinoid-precipitated withdrawal: a time-course study of the behavioral aspect and its correlation with cannabinoid receptors and G protein expression. J Pharmacol Exp Ther 285(2):813–819, 1998 9580631

Ruiz-Contreras AE, Carrillo-Sánchez K, Gómez-López N, et al: Working memory performance in young adults is associated to the AATn polymorphism of the CNR1 gene. Behav Brain Res 236(1):62–66, 2013 22944513

Ruiz-Contreras AE, Carrillo-Sánchez K, Ortega-Mora I, et al: Performance in working memory and attentional control is associated with the rs2180619 SNP in the CNR1 gene. Genes Brain Behav 13(2):173–178, 2014 24152087

Sami MB, Rabiner EA, Bhattacharyya S: Does cannabis affect dopaminergic signaling in the human brain? A systematic review of evidence to date. Eur Neuropsychopharmacol 25(8):1201–1224, 2015 26068702

Savinainen JR, Järvinen T, Laine K, et al: Despite substantial degradation, 2-arachidonoylglycerol is a potent full efficacy agonist mediating CB(1) receptor-dependent G-protein activation in rat cerebellar membranes. Br J Pharmacol 134(3):664–672, 2001 11588122

Schoeler T, Kambeitz J, Behlke I, et al: The effects of cannabis on memory function in users with and without a psychotic disorder: findings from a combined meta-analysis. Psychol Med 46(1):177–188, 2016a 26353818

Schoeler T, Monk A, Sami MB, et al: Continued versus discontinued cannabis use in patients with psychosis: a systematic review and meta-analysis. Lancet Psychiatry 3(3):215–225, 2016b 26777297

Schoeler T, Petros N, Di Forti M, et al: Effects of continuation, frequency, and type of cannabis use on relapse in the first 2 years after onset of psychosis: an observational study. Lancet Psychiatry 3(10):947–953, 2016c 27567467

Schoeler T, Petros N, Di Forti M, et al: Poor medication adherence and risk of relapse associated with continued cannabis use in patients with first-episode psychosis: a prospective analysis. Lancet Psychiatry 4(8):627–633, 2017 28705600

Sherif M, Radhakrishnan R, D'Souza DC, et al: Human laboratory studies on cannabinoids and psychosis. Biol Psychiatry 79(7):526–538, 2016 26970363

Sideli L, Fisher HL, Murray RM, et al: Interaction between cannabis consumption and childhood abuse in psychotic disorders: preliminary findings on the role of different patterns of cannabis use. Early Interv Psychiatry 12(2):135–142, 2018 26560802

Sideli L, Trotta G, Spinazzola E, et al: Adverse effects of heavy cannabis use: even plants can harm the brain. Pain 162(Suppl 1):S97–S104, 2021 32804835

Spinazzola E, Quattrone D, Rodriguez V, et al: The association between reasons for first using cannabis, later pattern of use, and risk of first-episode psychosis: the EU-GEI case-control study. Psychol Med 53(15):7418–7427, 2023 37129249

Sung YH, Carey PD, Stein DJ, et al: Decreased frontal N-acetylaspartate levels in adolescents concurrently using both methamphetamine and marijuana. Behav Brain Res 246:154–161, 2013 23466689

Szoke A, Galliot AM, Richard JR, et al: Association between cannabis use and schizotypal dimensions: a meta-analysis of cross-sectional studies. Psychiatry Res 219(1):58–66, 2014 24878296

Taurisano P, Antonucci LA, Fazio L, et al: Prefrontal activity during working memory is modulated by the interaction of variation in CB1 and COX2 coding genes and correlates with frequency of cannabis use. Cortex 81:231–238, 2016 27261878

Trotta G, Rodriguez V, Quattrone D, et al: Cannabis use as a potential mediator between childhood adversity and first-episode psychosis: results from the EU-GEI case-control study. Psychol Med 53(15):7375–7384, 2023 38078747

Vaessen TSJ, de Jong L, Schäfer AT, et al: The interaction between cannabis use and the Val158Met polymorphism of the COMT gene in psychosis: a transdiagnostic meta-analysis. PLoS One 13(2):e0192658, 2018 29444152

van de Giessen E, Weinstein JJ, Cassidy CM, et al: Deficits in striatal dopamine release in cannabis dependence. Mol Psychiatry 22(1):68–75, 2017 27001613

van Os J, Linscott RJ, Myin-Germeys I, et al: A systematic review and meta-analysis of the psychosis continuum: evidence for a psychosis proneness-persistence-impairment model of psychotic disorder. Psychol Med 39(2):179–195, 2009 18606047 van Winkel R, van Beveren NJ, Simons C, et al: AKT1 moderation of cannabis-induced cognitive alterations in psychotic disorder. Neuropsychopharmacology 36(12):2529–2537, 2011 21775978

Vaucher J, Keating BJ, Lasserre AM, et al: Cannabis use and risk of schizophrenia: a Mendelian randomization study. Mol Psychiatry 23(5):1287–1292, 2018 28115737

Vinkers CH, Van Gastel WA, Schubart CD, et al: The effect of childhood maltreatment and cannabis use on adult psychotic symptoms is modified by the COMT Val(1)(5)(8)Met polymorphism. Schizophr Res 150(1):303–311, 2013 23954148

Volkow ND, Swanson JM, Evins AE, et al: Effects of cannabis use on human behavior, including cognition, motivation, and psychosis: a review. JAMA Psychiatry 73(3):292–297, 2016 26842658

Wainberg M, Jacobs GR, di Forti M, et al: Cannabis, schizophrenia genetic risk, and psychotic experiences: a cross-sectional study of 109,308 participants from the UK Biobank. Transl Psychiatry 11(1):211, 2021 33837184

Waterreus A, Di Prinzio P, Ambrosi T, et al: Discontinuing cannabis use: symptomatic and functional outcomes in people with an established psychotic disorder. Schizophr Res 254:118–124, 2023 36842223

Welham J, Isohanni M, Jones P, et al: The antecedents of schizophrenia: a review of birth cohort studies. Schizophr Bull 35(3):603–623, 2009 18658128

Wilson RP, Bhattacharyya S: Antipsychotic efficacy in psychosis with co-morbid cannabis misuse: a systematic review. J Psychopharmacol 30(2):99–111, 2016 26510450

Wise LE, Thorpe AJ, Lichtman AH: Hippocampal CB(1) receptors mediate the memory impairing effects of Delta(9)-tetrahydrocannabinol. Neuropsychopharmacology 34(9):2072–2080, 2009 19322169

Yung AR, McGorry PD, McFarlane CA, et al: Monitoring and care of young people at incipient risk of psychosis. Schizophr Bull 22(2):283–303, 1996 8782287

6

Cannabis Use and Cognition

Mary K. Morreale, M.D.
Richard Balon, M.D.

Cognition is described as the mental act of acquiring knowledge and understanding and refers to multiple processes, including learning, attention, memory, processing speed, and executive functioning. The brain might be particularly sensitive to cannabis exposure, because cannabinoid receptors, specifically the cannabinoid 1 (CB_1) receptor that mediates many of the psychoactive effects of cannabis, are abundant throughout, including the cortical areas involved in higher cognition (Burggren et al. 2019). Many individual studies, meta-analyses, and systematic reviews examine how the cannabinoids cannabidiol (CBD) and Δ^9-tetrahydrocannabinol (Δ^9-THC) impact cognition and how this differs during acute intoxication, chronic use, conditions of abstinence, and varying stages of development.

We begin this chapter by providing an overview of the current state of the evidence as it pertains to the impact of cannabis on cognition, followed by a description of the relevant deleterious and beneficial effects. We conclude with a discussion of the clinical relevance of findings and applicable recommendations related to patient care. We have chosen not to address the impact of cannabis on cognition in various mental

illnesses, such as schizophrenia, because of the presence of many confounding variables.

Current State of Evidence

Multiple factors differentially affect the impact of cannabis on cognitive
outcomes in humans, and there are many methodological limitations
to the available literature on this subject. Starting with features specific
to cannabis, low levels of THC metabolites are present in the blood of
users even when they are not using cannabis daily, which makes distinguishing between the effects of residual drug levels, acute intoxication, tolerance, and withdrawal difficult (Mørland and Bramness 2020).
In addition, there is currently no standard unit for cannabis dosing,
standardized measure for history of cannabis exposure, or standardized time of nonuse for someone to be considered abstinent. Depending
on the product and route of administration (i.e., smoking, vaping, edible consumption), blood concentration can vary significantly, as can
ratios of THC versus CBD (Kroon et al. 2021; Volkow and Weiss 2020).

The literature on the impact of cannabis on cognition also varies
widely across the samples examined; some studies separate adolescent
from adult participants, whereas other studies combine data from large
age ranges. Because cognition changes over a lifetime, interpretation of
findings is influenced by these factors. Also, age at onset of use is often
not reported, which can confound analysis given that reports indicate a
larger impact on cognition when use begins at younger ages. Biological
sex differences are not always included, which is problematic because
of reported variance in action and metabolism (Crane et al. 2013). Some
studies examine medical use of cannabis, whereas others recruit recreational users (Ramaekers et al. 2021). Last, genetic variations in human
populations can also affect vulnerability to the neurocognitive effects
of THC (Cosker et al. 2017).

Within meta-analyses and systematic reviews, differing cognitive
processes are assessed using various measures, which makes compa-
rability and interpretation challenging. Additionally, wide variation
exists between inclusion and exclusion criteria, including concurrent
use of other substances. Finally, high-quality longitudinal data and
assessments of baseline cognition prior to cannabis use are lacking,
which makes a causal relationship difficult to infer.

Deleterious Effects

Adolescents

Because of the degree of synaptic pruning and increased myelination, adolescence is known to be a critical period neurodevelopmentally (Spear 2013). Because the endocannabinoid system is involved in regulating certain cognitive processes, the use of exogenous cannabis has the potential to disrupt normal brain development (Volkow et al. 2016). This is concerning given the significant lifetime use among middle school– and high school–age students.

Prefacing that most studies are small and that cognitive measures are heterogeneous and thus difficult to compare, the literature examining potential differences in the acute vulnerability to the cognitive impact of cannabis in adolescents versus adults is mixed. In two separate studies, Lawn et al. (2022, 2023) found similar impairments in adults and adolescents when measuring verbal episodic memory while participants were intoxicated with THC. In contrast, in a study by Murray et al. (2022), younger participants (ages 18–20) intoxicated with THC had a greater dose-dependent decrease in reaction time and response accuracy on several cognitive measures when compared with older participants (ages 30–40). Finally, Mokrysz et al. (2016) demonstrated that intoxicated adolescent users ages 16–17 had less impairment in recall and reaction time compared with adults ages 24–28. Interestingly, the adolescent users in Mokrysz and colleagues' study displayed impaired response inhibition accuracy and increased craving, which was not evident in adult participants.

Although there is broad consensus that acute cannabis intoxication leads to deficits in attention, memory, and executive functioning in adolescents and adults, the residual impact of cannabis on cognition is less clear (Dellazizzo et al. 2022; Zhornitsky et al. 2021). Regarding history of repeated cannabis exposure and cognition, variability also exists in results, which again is likely due to the heterogeneity of exposure to cannabis and cognitive measures used. Meier et al. (2012) examined members of the Dunedin study, a prospective assessment of 1,037 individuals followed from birth to age 38. Looking at individual differences in IQ before and after cannabis use, the authors found that participants with more persistent cannabis dependence demonstrated a greater decline in IQ. Specifically, those individuals who were diagnosed with cannabis dependence at one, two, or three assessments experienced a decline in IQ of −0.11, −0.17, and −0.38 SD units, respectively. Of note, a decline of 0.38 SD units is equivalent to approximately six IQ points. Comparing adolescent with adult onset of cannabis use in this study, the authors noted that only adolescent-onset users experienced a decline in IQ as a function of persistent use.

Scott et al. (2017) examined 4,568 adolescents and young adults between ages 14 and 21, drawn from the prospective Philadelphia Neurodevelopmental Cohort. In this large sample that was separated into nonusers, occasional users (twice per week or less), and frequent users (three times per week or more), adolescents who used cannabis frequently performed slightly worse on measures of executive control (sustained attention and working memory) when compared with nonusers. Although effects were small in magnitude and of unknown clinical significance, for those who used cannabis occasionally, earlier age at use was associated with reduced efficiency of executive control. Surprisingly, occasional users performed better on executive control and memory than nonusers, leading the authors to state that the relationship between cannabis use and cognition in adolescents is clearly complex and to stress the importance of longitudinal assessments.

Specific to adolescent populations, two recent meta-analyses have addressed the residual impact of cannabis on cognition. Scott et al. (2018) evaluated 69 studies of more than 2,100 cannabis users with a mean age of 20.6 years. When they compared cannabis users with a group with minimal cannabis exposure, they found a small overall association (effect sizes all less than one-third of a standard deviation) between the frequency of cannabis use and reduced cognitive functioning in the areas of learning, executive functioning, information processing, delayed memory, and attention. Interestingly, the authors found no difference in effect size for those participants who began use at an earlier age, which contradicts previous studies that revealed an association between younger age at first use and decreased performance on multiple cognitive measures, and they noted that only longitudinal assessments could clarify this discrepancy. Blest-Hopley et al. (2018) conducted a meta-analysis of functional MRI (fMRI) studies that examined the residual effects of cannabis use on the adolescent brain (219 cannabis users to 224 control subjects) and determined that activation was increased in both the inferior parietal gyrus and putamen, which may reflect compensatory cognitive strategies in users.

Twin studies have attempted to disentangle the potential impact of adolescent use of cannabis on cognition from genetic and environmental factors. Jackson et al. (2016) examined changes in IQ subtests in two longitudinal, population-based cohorts of twins. They did not find evidence to support that use of cannabis during adolescence had a direct effect on intellectual decline. Although twin users of cannabis did demonstrate a greater decline in crystallized intelligence, defined as knowledge of vocabulary and general information, the presence of baseline differences before any cannabis use and the lack of a dose-dependent decrease in functioning led the authors to conclude that confounding factors influencing IQ were likely responsible. Similarly, in another sample of adolescent and young adult twins, there was minimal evidence of an association between cannabis use and both intelligence and executive functioning after accounting for other substances and family effects (Ross et al. 2020).

As noted by several authors, longitudinal data related to the impact of chronic cannabis use on cognition in adolescent populations are vital. The currently running longitudinal Adolescent Brain Cognitive Development Study (https://abcdstudy.org), which invited more than 11,000 children to participate, should assist in clarifying discrepancies in the extant data.

Adults

Substantial evidence exists regarding the acute detrimental impact of cannabis on multiple cognitive domains of adult users, even when use is occasional. Studies indicate negative effects on executive functioning, which includes planning, reasoning, and problem-solving, and dose-related impairments in memory and attention (Ameri 1999; Hall and Solowij 1998; Ramaekers et al. 2006). Verbal learning has been found to be particularly sensitive to the acute effects of cannabis (Ranganathan and D'Souza 2006; Solowij and Pesa 2010). Although cognitive changes may be less in those who use cannabis regularly because of tolerance, evidence suggests that cognitive deficits do occur in this population (Broyd et al. 2016).

A lack of consistency in design makes it difficult to compare studies of cognitive impairments resulting from chronic use of cannabis; however, there is evidence for residual impairment that extends beyond intoxication. In a systematic review by Figueiredo et al. (2020), the authors concluded that although effect sizes were small, the association between chronic cannabis use and cognitive impairment existed in multiple domains, including cognitive flexibility and impulsivity, attention, and both short- and long-term memory. In a similar systematic review of meta-analytic studies, Duperrouzel et al. (2020) reported larger effect sizes—between small to medium—across cognitive domains. The available literature demonstrates that cognitive impairments can be attributed to the duration and frequency of use, as well as dose (Pope and Yurgelun-Todd 1996; Pope et al. 2001; Solowij 1998; Solowij et al. 2002). The impact of earlier-onset cannabis use on cognition is unclear, with some studies suggesting an association between early use and worsened cognition and others negating this finding (Duperrouzel et al. 2020; Scott et al. 2018).

Regarding duration of use and degree of exposure, Solowij et al. (2002) assessed 102 near-daily cannabis users (mean duration of use 10.2 years) and found that those who used for a longer period performed significantly worse on tests of attention and memory than did short-term users and control subjects. Specifically, longer-term users had more impairments in learning, retention, and retrieval. Auer et al. (2016) also demonstrated residual cognitive deficits with cumulative lifetime cannabis exposure. Examining data from the Coronary Artery Risk Development in Young Adults study, the authors compared cognitive data on 3,385 participants ages 18–30 with data from a second assessment 25 years later. Cumulative lifetime exposure to cannabis was associated with decreased performance in measures of verbal memory, processing speed, and executive functioning. When the approximately 11% of participants who continued to use up to the time of the second assessment were excluded, cumulative lifetime exposure was associated with worsened verbal memory. Several authors have noted that verbal learning and memory are the cognitive domains that have been most consistently impaired across studies (Solowij and Battisti 2008; Zhornitsky et al. 2021).

Using data related to the deleterious effects of cannabis on adolescent populations from the longitudinal Dunedin study discussed in the previous section, Meier et al. (2012) assessed cognition at age 45. In this sample (N=938), long-term users were defined as those who used cannabis weekly or more frequently over the past year at age 45 or who were diagnosed as cannabis dependent at age 45 and had used cannabis weekly or more frequently at one or more previous assessments. These users demonstrated below-average IQ as adults despite having an average IQ during childhood, and the change in IQ was greater than that seen in long-term alcohol users, although it was not significantly greater than that in midlife recreational users (those who used cannabis between 6 and 51 days per year at ages 32, 38, or 45) and cannabis quitters (those who did not use at 45 but either had been diagnosed with cannabis dependence or had used more than 4 days per week in the past). Study participants who used cannabis more frequently showed a greater reduction in IQ and worse performance on measures of learning, processing speed, verbal memory, and perceptual reasoning when compared with less persistent users. In this sample, the negative associations between the persistence of cannabis use and cognitive functioning could not be explained by recent usage.

Older Adults

The prevalence of cannabis use among adults older than 65 years of age has increased significantly in the recent past, from 0.4% in 2006 to 4.2% in 2018 (Han and Palamar 2020). Despite a lack of evidence to support efficacy, older adults tend to use cannabis to address medical concerns such as pain, anxiety, and insomnia (Abuhasira et al. 2018; Lum et al. 2019; Minerbi et al. 2019; Reynolds et al. 2018). Several age-related factors might affect the cognitive impacts of cannabis in this population, including the propensity of older adults to choose products higher in CBD for their anti-inflammatory effects, a slowing of metabolism leading to extended periods of intoxication, and differences in brain structure and neurotransmitter systems that occur with age (Burstein 2015; Pocuca et al. 2021; Sagar and Gruber 2018).

Regarding cannabis use in healthy older adults, limited data look specifically at the acute impact of intoxication on cognition in this population. Some authors postulate, however, that acute effects could be worse in older adults because of preexisting declines in cognitive function that occur with normal aging, age-related changes in drug metabolism, and neurotransmitter sensitivity (Scott et al. 2019). Sexton et al. (2019) examined survey responses from 2,905 individuals and analyzed data according to age, comparing users ages 50 and older with a younger group ages 18–29. Although some participants subjectively reported detrimental cognitive symptoms such as difficulty concentrating, difficulty finding words, increased forgetfulness, and short-term memory problems, the older cohort was significantly less likely to report these concerns. The authors hypothesized that these older participants may have underreported this change because of perceptions that word-finding difficulties are a consequence of aging rather than potentially associated with cannabis use. In addition, as reported in other literature mentioned previously, older users are more apt to use cannabis products that are higher in CBD (Pocuca et al. 2021). Finally, those older individuals who use cannabis for medicinal purposes may experience decreased symptom burden associated with use (e.g., pain and insomnia) and therefore report fewer negative side effects. Importantly, no cognitive measures were used in the Sexton et al. (2019) study, and all data were self-reported and subjective.

Two studies are available that examined the chronic effects of cannabis on cognition in healthy older adults. Burggren et al. (2018) used MRI and measures of memory, processing speed, and executive function to compare never-using control subjects with subjects between the ages of 57 and 75 who had a history of significant cannabis use during adolescence. Although differences on cognitive measures between the groups were not statistically significant, the average scores of the cannabis-positive group were lower than those of the cannabis-negative group in all cognitive domains. MRI comparisons revealed thinner cortices in several brain regions, including all subregions of the hippocampus. Using MRI and the National Institutes of Health Toolbox Cognition Battery (inhibitory control, attention, memory, vocabulary, processing speed, reading recognition), Thayer et al. (2019) compared adults older than 60 who had consumed cannabis at least once per week for the past year with those who had never consumed it. Although this study found no significant difference in cognitive performance on any of the outcomes and no changes in the structure of the hippocampus, cannabis users did have greater regional volumes in some brain areas. Pocuca et al. (2021) commented on the discrepancies between the studies by Thayer's group and Burggren's group, noting that characteristics of cannabis use were quite varied between the studies (early vs. late onset, long-term vs. short-term, frequent vs. infrequent use).

Although dementia is a qualifying condition in nearly half of the U.S. states with medical cannabis laws, primarily for agitation associated with Alzheimer's disease, limited data are available showing the impact of cannabis on cognition in individuals with dementia (Charernboon et al. 2021; Maust et al. 2016). Two small studies without a control group demonstrated stable Mini Mental State Examination scores after cannabis exposure (Shelef et al. 2016; van den Elsen et al. 2015). In addition, a study examining the use of a synthetic THC analogue in individuals with dementia did not demonstrate a clinically significant impact on cognition, although there was evidence for worsening cognition in those with more severe disease (Herrmann et al. 2019).

Structural Brain Changes

Despite their heterogeneity of design, structural neuroimaging studies have provided consistent evidence of abnormalities in hippocampal volumes and gray matter density in both adolescent and adult cannabis users compared with control subjects (Ashtari et al. 2011; Battistella et al. 2014; Burggren et al. 2018; Rocchetti et al. 2013). Long-term cannabis users showed cognitive deficits and smaller hippocampal volume in midlife (Meier et al. 2022), which may be dose-dependent and related to heavier use, specifically cannabis dependence (Chye et al. 2019; Meier et al. 2022). Although some data show that hippocampal abnormalities persist into adulthood even after abstinence, other data indicate that the hippocampus can recover and that the addition of CBD might protect the hippocampus to some degree (Burggren et al. 2018; Yücel et al. 2016). Interestingly, in adults, larger hippocampal volumes have been associated with better cognitive performance, but smaller volumes did not statistically mediate chronic cannabis use and deficits in cognition (Meier et al. 2022).

Functional Brain Changes

Studies examining the impact of cannabis on cognition have demonstrated alterations to brain function, as measured by fMRI, in adolescents and adults who use cannabis both acutely and chronically (Batalla et al. 2013; Kim et al. 2019; Lorenzetti et al. 2016; Sagar and Gruber 2018; Yanes et al. 2018). Decreased activation, as measured by fMRI, has been observed in several regions, including the anterior cingulate and the dorsolateral prefrontal cortices (Lorenzetti et al. 2016). Conversely, increased activation has been seen in the striatum (Lorenzetti et al. 2016). Finally, structural-functional impairments were noted in the hippocampi and the caudate nuclei of cannabis users (Kim et al. 2019; Yanes et al. 2018). Interestingly, several studies revealed that changes in function occur in the absence of deficits in cognitive performance, which suggests that cannabis users recruit alternative and potentially less efficient neural pathways (Batalla et al. 2013; Lorenzetti et al. 2016; Sagar and Gruber 2018).

Abstinence

Abstinence is an important factor that influences the association between cannabis use and cognitive functioning. Although the accuracy of abstinence is questionable because of the lack of abstinence monitoring in all included studies, in Scott et al.'s (2018) systematic review and analysis, increased time of abstinence led to decreased effect sizes (i.e., decreased cognitive deficits). Specifically, for those participants who abstained for more than 72 hours, the effect size was no longer statistically significant from zero. Although it is difficult to differentiate the cognitive impact of cannabis withdrawal from chronic effects, another meta-analysis reported that a longer period of abstinence—approximately 1 month—was needed for cognitive recovery (Schreiner and Dunn 2012). Interestingly, some studies indicate that subtle cognitive deficits may remain long term in those who quit cannabis, and several studies suggest that adolescent users might be more likely to have persistent cognitive deficits following abstinence (Meier et al. 2022; Zhornitsky et al. 2021). Although the clinical impact on cognition was not studied, PET data revealed that the downregulation of brain cannabinoid receptors that occurs with chronic use recovered after approximately 4 weeks of abstinence (Hirvonen et al. 2012).

Medical Cannabis

In both a systematic review and a scoping review examining the potential cognitive impact of cannabis used for medical purposes, researchers found that the impact was minimal when low to moderate doses of THC were used (Eadie et al. 2021; Wieghorst et al. 2022). Some studies included in the review by Wieghorst et al. (2022) demonstrated a positive effect of cannabis on cognition when it was used for medicinal purposes, which the authors hypothesized might be due to its alleviation of symptoms such as pain, depression, and insomnia and the resultant cognitive benefit. Given the heterogeneity of included studies, neither review was able to specify the amount of THC required to negatively affect cognition. As is the case in many of the studies mentioned thus far, the studies included in both reviews were heterogeneous as far as study design, population, dose and type of cannabis, and cognitive measures, which makes it quite difficult to draw concrete conclusions.

Beneficial Effects

When compared with the literature related to the deleterious impact of cannabis on cognition, far less evidence supports any beneficial effect. Although it is not a concrete beneficial effect, per se, some studies indicate that CBD can counteract the impact of THC on multiple neurocognitive domains. For example, in a between-subjects design by Englund et al. (2013), participants were given either a placebo or 600 mg of oral CBD prior to receiving 1.5 mg of intravenous THC. In those pretreated with CBD, scores on tests of episodic memory were higher compared with baseline than in the control group. Similarly, in a naturalistic study of individuals who were able to use the cannabis product of their choice, which was later analyzed for THC and CBD content, only those participants who smoked cannabis low in CBD showed impairments in immediate and delayed prose recall when intoxicated (Morgan et al. 2010). On the other hand, those using cannabis high in CBD did not demonstrate any acute memory impairments. Finally, in a study of frequent cannabis users who were treated with 10 weeks of CBD and who continued to use other cannabis products as usual, participants displayed statistically significant improvements in attentional switching, verbal learning, and memory posttreatment relative to baseline (Solowij et al. 2018). Importantly, the attenuating effects of CBD might be related to dosing, specifically to the ratio of CBD to THC. This is evident in the results of a randomized, double-blind crossover study by Morgan et al. (2018), which found that THC alone robustly impaired both working and episodic memory but that doses of CBD and THC at a ratio of 2:1 did not attenuate this response.

CBD alone has also been found to enhance cognition. Although the effect size and number of participants ($N=34$) were small in a randomized controlled trial of individuals who vaped a single dose of 12.5 mg of CBD versus placebo prior to learning 15 unrelated nouns, those who received CBD had significantly better recall (Hotz et al. 2021). Frequency of cannabis consumption in the year prior did not have an impact on the results.

Clinical Significance and Recommendations

Although most of the data presented in this chapter suggest a negative association between cannabis use and cognition, it is difficult to understand what these results mean for users' daily functioning. Because those who begin using cannabis during adolescence may be at higher risk for dependency, heavy use may interfere with educational and vocational pursuits (Mokrysz et al. 2016). For young and middle-age adults, cognitive changes could affect career trajectories. Finally, in older adults who are already experiencing age-related cognitive decline, the summative impact of cannabis use on cognition could lead to decreased independence and quality of life. In summary, although results in all examined populations did not reveal severe deficits, it is possible that even minor cognitive changes could translate into impairment of functioning.

Conclusion

Although the research has significant methodological limitations, an abundance of evidence supports that cannabis negatively affects cognition in multiple cognitive domains, during intoxication and with chronic use, and from adolescence to old age. MRI and fMRI studies reveal that chronic use of cannabis leads to both structural and functional changes in the brain. The negative cognitive impact of chronic cannabis use is likely reversible with abstinence, although the duration of time needed for recovery ranges within studies. Finally, the addition of CBD to THC-containing cannabis products may have a beneficial impact on cognitive outcomes.

Key Points

- The significant methodological limitations to the research examining the impact of cannabis on cognition include a lack of a standardized unit for dosing, heterogeneity in the populations studied and cognitive measures used, and trouble differentiating between acute versus chronic effects of use.
- There is broad consensus that acute cannabis intoxication leads to deficits in attention, memory, and executive functioning in both adolescents and adults.
- Results of studies that examine whether adolescents are more vulnerable to the intoxicating impacts of cannabis on cognition are mixed. Some data suggest that adolescents have more cognitive vulnerability, whereas other data support increased resilience.
- Although effect sizes are small, evidence suggests that persistent cannabis use in adolescents and adults leads to a decline in IQ and decreased performance in many cognitive domains.
- Abstinence is an important factor that influences the association between cannabis use and cognitive functioning, although the exact time frame for cognitive recovery is unclear.
- Functional MRI studies show functional impairments within the brain, specifically in the anterior cingulate cortex, dorsolateral

prefrontal cortex, striatum, hippocampus, and caudate nucleus of cannabis users.

- MRI studies reveal structural changes in hippocampal volumes and gray matter density in both adolescent and adult cannabis users.
- The addition of cannabidiol to Δ^9-tetrahydrocannabinol likely leads to less negative cognitive impact of cannabis.

References

Abuhasira R, Schleider LB, Mechoulam R, et al: Epidemiological characteristics, safety and efficacy of medical cannabis in the elderly. Eur J Intern Med 49:44–50, 2018 29398248

Ameri A: The effects of cannabinoids on the brain. Prog Neurobiol 58(4):315–348, 1999 10368032

Ashtari M, Avants B, Cyckowski L, et al: Medial temporal structures and memory functions in adolescents with heavy cannabis use. J Psychiatr Res 45(8):1055–1066, 2011 21296361

Auer R, Vittinghoff E, Yaffe K, et al: Association between lifetime marijuana use and cognitive function in middle age: the Coronary Artery Risk Development in Young Adults (CARDIA) study. JAMA Intern Med 176(3):352–361, 2016 26831916

Batalla A, Bhattacharyya S, Yücel M, et al: Structural and functional imaging studies in chronic cannabis users: a systematic review of adolescent and adult findings. PLoS One 8(2):e55821, 2013 23390554

Battistella G, Fornari E, Annoni JM, et al: Long-term effects of cannabis on brain structure. Neuropsychopharmacology 39(9):2041–2048, 2014 24633558

Blest-Hopley G, Giampietro V, Bhattacharyya S: Residual effects of cannabis use in adolescent and adult brains: a meta-analysis of fMRI studies. Neurosci Biobehav Rev 88:26–41, 2018 29535069

Broyd SJ, van Hell HH, Beale C, et al: Acute and chronic effects of cannabinoids on human cognition-a systematic review. Biol Psychiatry 79(7):557–567, 2016 26858214

Burggren AC, Siddarth P, Mahmood Z, et al: Subregional hippocampal thickness abnormalities in older adults with a history of heavy cannabis use. Cannabis Cannabinoid Res 3(1):242–251, 2018 30547094

Burggren AC, Shirazi A, Ginder N, et al: Cannabis effects on brain structure, function, and cognition: considerations for medical uses of cannabis and its derivatives. Am J Drug Alcohol Abuse 45(6):563–579, 2019 31365275

Burstein S: Cannabidiol (CBD) and its analogs: a review of their effects on inflammation. Bioorg Med Chem 23(7):1377–1385, 2015 25703248

Charernboon T, Lerthattasilp T, Supasitthumrong T: Effectiveness of cannabinoids for treatment of dementia: a systematic review of randomized controlled trials. Clin Gerontol 44(1):16–24, 2021 32186469

Chye Y, Lorenzetti V, Suo C, et al: Alteration to hippocampal volume and shape confined to cannabis dependence: a multi-site study. Addict Biol 24(4):822–834, 2019 30022573

Cosker E, Schwitzer T, Ramoz N, et al: The effect of interactions between genetics and cannabis use on neurocognition: a review. Prog Neuropsychopharmacol Biol Psychiatry 82:95–106, 2017 29191570

Crane NA, Schuster RM, Fusar-Poli P, et al: Effects of cannabis on neurocognitive functioning: recent advances, neurodevelopmental influences, and sex differences. Neuropsychol Rev 23(2):117–137, 2013 23129391

Dellazizzo L, Potvin S, Giguère S, et al: Evidence on the acute and residual neurocognitive effects of cannabis use in adolescents and adults: a systematic meta-review of meta-analyses. Addiction 117(7):1857–1870, 2022 35048456

Duperrouzel JC, Granja K, Pacheco-Colón I, et al: Adverse effects of cannabis use on neurocognitive functioning: a systematic review of meta-analytic studies. J Dual Diagn 16(1):43–57, 2020 31232216

Eadie L, Lo LA, Christiansen A, et al: Duration of neurocognitive impairment with medical cannabis use: a scoping review. Front Psychiatry 12:638962, 2021 33790818

Englund A, Morrison PD, Nottage J, et al: Cannabidiol inhibits THC-elicited paranoid symptoms and hippocampal-dependent memory impairment. J Psychopharmacol 27(1):19–27, 2013 23042808

Figueiredo PR, Tolomeo S, Steele JD, et al: Neurocognitive consequences of chronic cannabis use: a systematic review and meta-analysis. Neurosci Biobehav Rev 108:358–369, 2020 31715191

Hall W, Solowij N: Adverse effects of cannabis. Lancet 352(9140):1611–1616, 1998 9843121

Han BH, Palamar JJ: Trends in cannabis use among older adults in the United States, 2015–2018. JAMA Intern Med 180(4):609–611, 2020 32091531

Herrmann N, Ruthirakuhan M, Gallagher D, et al: Randomized placebo-controlled trial of nabilone for agitation in Alzheimer's disease. Am J Geriatr Psychiatry 27(11):1161–1173, 2019 31182351

Hirvonen J, Goodwin RS, Li CT, et al: Reversible and regionally selective downregulation of brain cannabinoid CB1 receptors in chronic daily cannabis smokers. Mol Psychiatry 17(6):642–649, 2012 21747398

Hotz J, Fehlmann B, Papassotiropoulos A, et al: Cannabidiol enhances verbal episodic memory in healthy young participants: a randomized clinical trial. J Psychiatr Res 143:327–333, 2021 34536664

Jackson NJ, Isen JD, Khoddam R, et al: Impact of adolescent marijuana use on intelligence: results from two longitudinal twin studies. Proc Natl Acad Sci U S A 113(5):E500–E508, 2016 26787878

Kim DJ, Schnakenberg Martin AM, et al: Aberrant structural-functional coupling in adult cannabis users. Hum Brain Mapp 40(1):252–261,2019 30203892

Kroon E, Kuhns L, Cousijn J: The short-term and long-term effects of cannabis on cognition: recent advances in the field. Curr Opin Psychol 38:49–55, 2021

Lawn W, Fernandez-Vinson N, Mokrysz C, et al: The CannTeen study: verbal episodic memory, spatial working memory, and response inhibition in adolescent and adult cannabis users and age-matched controls. Psychopharmacology (Berl) 239(5):1629–1641, 2022 35486121

Lawn W, Trinci K, Mokrysz C, et al: The acute effects of cannabis with and without cannabidiol in adults and adolescents: a randomised, double-blind, placebo-controlled, crossover experiment. Addiction 118(7):1282–1294, 2023 36750134

Lorenzetti V, Alonso-Lana S, Youssef GJ, et al: Adolescent cannabis use: what is the evidence for functional brain alteration? Curr Pharm Des 22(42):6353–6365, 2016 27514709

Lum HD, Arora K, Croker JA, et al: Patterns of marijuana use and health impact: a survey among older Coloradans. Gerontol Geriatr Med 5:2333721419843707, 2019 31065574

Maust DT, Bonar EE, Ilgen MA, et al: Agitation in Alzheimer disease as a qualifying condition for medical marijuana in the United States. Am J Geriatr Psychiatry 24(11):1000–1003, 2016 27389672

Meier MH, Caspi A, Ambler A, et al: Persistent cannabis users show neuropsychological decline from childhood to midlife. Proc Natl Acad Sci U S A 109(40):E2657–E2664, 2012 22927402

Meier MH, Caspi A, Knodt AR, et al: Long-term cannabis use and cognitive reserves and hippocampal volume in midlife. Am J Psychiatry 179(5):362–374, 2022 35255711

Minerbi A, Häuser W, Fitzcharles MA: Medical cannabis for older patients. Drugs Aging 36(1):39–51, 2019 30488174

Mokrysz C, Freeman TP, Korkki S, et al: Are adolescents more vulnerable to the harmful effects of cannabis than adults? A placebo-controlled study in human males. Transl Psychiatry 6(11):e961, 2016 27898071

Morgan CJ, Schafer G, Freeman TP, et al: Impact of cannabidiol on the acute memory and psychotomimetic effects of smoked cannabis: naturalistic study: naturalistic study [corrected]. Br J Psychiatry 197(4):285–290, 2010 20884951

Morgan CJA, Freeman TP, Hindocha C, et al: Individual and combined effects of acute delta-9-tetrahydrocannabinol and cannabidiol on psychotomimetic symptoms and memory function. Transl Psychiatry 8(1):181, 2018 30185793

Mørland J, Bramness JG: Delta-9-tetrahydrocannabinol (THC) is present in the body between smoking sessions in occasional non-daily cannabis users. Forensic Sci Int 309:110188, 2020 32120192

Murray CH, Huang Z, Lee R, et al: Adolescents are more sensitive than adults to acute behavioral and cognitive effects of THC. Neuropsychopharmacology 47(7):1331–1338, 2022 35110688

Pocuca N, Walter TJ, Minassian A, et al: The effects of cannabis use on cognitive function in healthy aging: a systematic scoping review. Arch Clin Neuropsychol 36(5):673–685, 2021 33159510

Pope HG Jr, Yurgelun-Todd D: The residual cognitive effects of heavy marijuana use in college students. JAMA 275(7):521–527, 1996 8606472

Pope HG Jr, Gruber AJ, Hudson JI, et al: Neuropsychological performance in long-term cannabis users. Arch Gen Psychiatry 58(10):909–915, 2001 11576028

Ramaekers JG, Kauert G, van Ruitenbeek P, et al: High-potency marijuana impairs executive function and inhibitory motor control. Neuropsychopharmacology 31(10):2296–2303, 2006 16572123

Ramaekers JG, Mason NL, Kloft L, et al: The why behind the high: determinants of neurocognition during acute cannabis exposure. Nat Rev Neurosci 22(7):439–454, 2021 34045693

Ranganathan M, D'Souza DC: The acute effects of cannabinoids on memory in humans: a review. Psychopharmacology (Berl) 188(4):425–444, 2006 17019571

Reynolds IR, Fixen DR, Parnes BL, et al: Characteristics and patterns of marijuana use in community-dwelling older adults. J Am Geriatr Soc 66(11):2167–2171, 2018 30291748

Rocchetti M, Crescini A, Borgwardt S, et al: Is cannabis neurotoxic for the healthy brain? A meta-analytical review of structural brain alterations in non-psychotic users. Psychiatry Clin Neurosci 67(7):483–492, 2013 24118193

Ross JM, Ellingson JM, Rhee SH, et al: Investigating the causal effect of cannabis use on cognitive function with a quasi-experimental co-twin design. Drug Alcohol Depend 206:107712, 2020 31753729

Sagar KA, Gruber SA: Marijuana matters: reviewing the impact of marijuana on cognition, brain structure and function, and exploring policy implications and barriers to research. Int Rev Psychiatry 30(3):251–267, 2018 29966459

Sagar KA, Gruber SA: Interactions between recreational cannabis use and cognitive function: lessons from functional magnetic resonance imaging. Ann N Y Acad Sci 1451(1):42–70, 2019 30426517

Schreiner AM, Dunn ME: Residual effects of cannabis use on neurocognitive performance after prolonged abstinence: a meta-analysis. Exp Clin Psychopharmacol 20(5):420–429, 2012 22731735

Scott JC, Wolf DH, Calkins ME, et al: Cognitive functioning of adolescent and young adult cannabis users in the Philadelphia Neurodevelopmental Cohort. Psychol Addict Behav 31(4):423–434, 2017 28414475

Scott JC, Slomiak ST, Jones JD, et al: Association of cannabis with cognitive functioning in adolescents and young adults: a systematic review and meta-analysis. JAMA Psychiatry 75(6):585–595, 2018 29710074

Scott EP, Brennan E, Benitez A: A systematic review of the neurocognitive effects of cannabis in older adults. Curr Addict Rep 6(4):443–455, 2019 32477850

Sexton M, Cuttler C, Mischley LK: A survey of cannabis acute effects and withdrawal symptoms: differential responses across user types and age. J Altern Complement Med 25(3):326–335, 2019 30383388

Shelef A, Barak Y, Berger U, et al: Safety and efficacy of medical cannabis oil for behavioral and psychological symptoms of dementia: an open label, add-on, pilot study. J Alzheimers Dis 51(1):15–19, 2016 26757043

Solowij N: Cannabis and Cognitive Functioning. Cambridge, UK, Cambridge University Press, 1998

Solowij N, Battisti R: The chronic effects of cannabis on memory in humans: a review. Curr Drug Abuse Rev 1(1):81–98, 2008 19630708

Solowij N, Pesa N: Cognitive abnormalities and cannabis use. Braz J Psychiatry 32(Suppl 1):S31–S40, 2010 20512268

Solowij N, Stephens RS, Roffman RA, et al: Cognitive functioning of long-term heavy cannabis users seeking treatment. JAMA 287(9):1123–1131, 2002 11879109

Solowij N, Broyd SJ, Beale C, et al: Therapeutic effects of prolonged cannabidiol treatment on psychological symptoms and cognitive function in regular cannabis users: a pragmatic open-label clinical trial. Cannabis Cannabinoid Res 3(1):21–34, 2018 29607408

Spear LP: Adolescent neurodevelopment. J Adolesc Health 52(2 Suppl 2):S7–S13, 2013 23332574

Thayer RE, York Williams SL, Hutchison KE, et al: Preliminary results from a pilot study examining brain structure in older adult cannabis users and nonusers. Psychiatry Res Neuroimaging 285:58–63, 2019 30785022

van den Elsen GA, Ahmed AI, Verkes RJ, et al: Tetrahydrocannabinol for neuropsychiatric symptoms in dementia: a randomized controlled trial. Neurology 84(23):2338–2346, 2015 25972490

Volkow ND, Weiss SRB: Importance of a standard unit dose for cannabis research. Addiction 115(7):1219–1221 2020 32083354

Volkow ND, Swanson JM, Evins AE, et al: Effects of cannabis use on human behavior, including cognition, motivation, and psychosis: a review. JAMA Psychiatry 73(3):292–297, 2016 26842658

Wieghorst A, Roessler KK, Hendricks O, et al: The effect of medical cannabis on cognitive functions: a systematic review. Syst Rev 11(1):210, 2022 36192811

Yanes JA, Riedel MC, Ray KL, et al: Neuroimaging meta-analysis of cannabis use studies reveals convergent functional alterations in brain regions supporting cognitive control and reward processing. J Psychopharmacol 32(3):283–295, 2018 29338547

Yücel M, Lorenzetti V, Suo C, et al: Hippocampal harms, protection and recovery following regular cannabis use. Transl Psychiatry 6(1):e710, 2016 26756903

Zhornitsky S, Pelletier J, Assaf R, et al: Acute effects of partial CB1 receptor agonists on cognition—a meta-analysis of human studies. Prog Neuropsychopharmacol Biol Psychiatry 104:110063, 2021 32791166

7

Cannabis and Depression

An Update on Co-Occurrence and Underlying Mechanisms

Aviv Weinstein, Ph.D.
Daniel Feingold, Ph.D.

Major depressive disorder (MDD) is a common psychiatric disorder characterized by persistent low mood and loss of interest or pleasure in activities normally enjoyed. The global 12-month prevalence rate of MDD is approximately 3.8% in the general population and 5% among adults. This represents approximately 280 million people worldwide (Institute for Health Metrics and Evaluation 2021). The lifetime prevalence of MDD has varied from 2% in China to 6.7% in South Korea, 20.5% in Chile, and 21% in France, and the 12-month prevalence rate varies between 1.1% in China and 10.4% in Brazil. The highest prevalence rates were reported in Europe and the lowest in Asia (Gutiérrez-Rojas et al. 2020). In the United States, of the 36,309 adult participants in the National Epidemiologic Survey on Alcohol and Related Conditions, Third Edition (NESARC-III), 12-month and lifetime prevalences of MDD were 10.4% and 20.6%, respectively (Hasin et al. 2018).

MDD is recurrent and may become a serious health problem that impairs daily functioning at school, at work, and within the family. Depression is associated with suicide, which is the fourth leading cause of death among 15- to 29-year-olds (Institute for Health Metrics and Evaluation 2021). It has therefore become important to identify risk factors for developing MDD, including substance use and substance use disorders (SUDs; Feingold and Weinstein 2021; Moore et al. 2007; Whiteford et al. 2013).

Cannabis is the most extensively used substance worldwide. In 2020, more than 4% of the world population ages 15–64 (209 million people) had used cannabis in the past year (United Nations Office on Drugs and Crime 2022). This past-year prevalence had increased from 3.8% in 2010, while the estimated crude number of annual cannabis users had increased by 23%, from 170 million people, partly because of an increase in the global population. The past-year prevalence of cannabis use was reported to be higher among adolescents (5.8% in those ages 15–16) compared with adults. Scientific evidence has shown that early initiation of substance use may affect the developing brain of adolescents and increase the likelihood of transitioning to regular use and SUD in both late adolescence and young adulthood.

In this chapter we review the current state of the evidence on the co-occurrence of major depression and cannabis use and the evidence for both the deleterious and possible beneficial effects of cannabis on depression, as shown by preclinical and clinical studies. Finally, we review the clinical significance and make recommendations regarding comorbid cannabis use disorder (CaUD) and depression.

Current State of Evidence

Cross-Sectional Evidence

Earlier studies showed evidence of the co-occurrence of heavy or problematic cannabis use (but not infrequent cannabis use) and depression, which was mainly based on cohort and cross-sectional studies in the general population (Degenhardt et al. 2003). There was also a modest association between early-onset, regular cannabis use and later depression, which persisted after controlling for potential confounding variables. Little evidence was found of a higher risk for later cannabis use among depressed individuals and hence little support for the self-medication hypothesis suggesting that drug-dependent individuals use it for dealing with negative emotional states.

Results from the National Comorbidity Survey showed that MDD patients had a lifetime prevalence of cannabis use of 60% (Chen et al. 2002). The U.S. National Survey on Drug Use and Health (NSDUH) indicated that the past-year prevalence of cannabis use among adolescents with depression was about 25%, compared with only 12% among those without depression, which was substantially higher than findings in the adult population (Substance Abuse and Mental Health Services Administration 2007). According to a Dutch survey, the 3-year incidence of MDD among cannabis users was 11.7%, compared with 5% among nonusers (van Laar et al. 2007). de Graaf et al. (2010) reported on the World Mental Health Survey Initiative (2001–2005), a population-based study of 85,088 participants from 17 countries conducted by the World Health Organization. The correlation seen in this study between early-onset cannabis use and later risk of a depressive episode was modest (controlling for sex and age; RR 1.5 and 95% CI 1.4, 1.7), and it showed no sex differences. The association did not change dramatically with statistical adjustment for mental health problems except for childhood conduct problems, which reduced the association to nonsignificance. In a study of European adolescents ages 14–17, the odds for concurrent MDD were higher than in comparison studies in adult populations. Specifically, the prevalence of lifetime MDD was significantly higher among individuals with lifetime cannabis use and lifetime CaUD compared with nonusers (Wittchen et al. 2007).

NESARC data focusing on adults with past-year MDD or dysthymia (n=6,534) showed 10% prevalence of cannabis use over the past year, which was nearly equally distributed between regular users (4.5% for weekly cannabis use) and occasional users (5.4% for less than weekly use) (Aspis et al. 2015). The NESARC also provided evidence that lifetime and past-year CaUD were related to an increased risk for a past-year diagnosis of MDD (past-year use: OR 2.8 and 95% CI 2.33–3.41; lifetime use: OR 2.6 and 95% CI 2.26–2.95) (Hasin et al. 2016).

A more recent study of more than 28,000 cannabis users indicated that a past-year major depressive episode was related to meeting a higher number of DSM-IV CaUD criteria, irrespective of the frequency of using cannabis (American Psychiatric Association 1994; Dierker et al. 2018). In this study by Dierker et al. (2018), depressed participants were prone to use more cannabis than they had intended, and they spent a significant amount of time acquiring, using, or recovering from the effects of cannabis use compared with those without depression. They were also more likely to continue using cannabis despite adverse consequences, repeatedly fail in efforts to stop or reduce cannabis use, have important activities in life superseded by cannabis use, and need progressively larger amounts of cannabis to obtain those same effects.

Recent Evidence

Gukasyan and Strain (2020) analyzed data from the NSDUH, including data from adolescents who used cannabis (n=14,873) and those without a history of cannabis use (*n*=73,079). Adolescents with a history of using cannabis had higher prevalence of past-year and lifetime MDD and past-year suicide attempts. Surprisingly, heavy users had lower prevalence of lifetime and past-year MDD compared with light users and those who had used cannabis more than a year previously. Reece and Hulse (2020) reported results from a cohort study of the NSDUH from 2010 to 2012 and 2014 to 2016 combined with a 5-year American Community Survey of 410,138 NSDUH participants. Cannabis use correlated with any mental illness, major depressive episodes, serious mental illness, and suicidal ideation, and in each case, cannabis alone correlated with adverse effects on mental health. There was an upward trend of serious mental illness that doubled (from 3.62% to 7.06%) as cannabis use increased. Decriminalization of cannabis was associated with increased mental disorder prevalence compared with the rates prior to decriminalization. A study of 281,650 adults ages 18–34 years who participated in the NSDUH found that from 2008 to 2019, suicidal ideation, plans, or attempts increased from 40% to 60%, which was attributed to cannabis use and major depressive episodes (Han et al. 2021). A meta-analysis of Canadian nationally representative epidemiological surveys of CaUD and MDD suggested that MDD was strongly related to CaUD, and this link was stronger with cannabis dependence (pooled OR 4.83) (Onaemo et al. 2021).

Longitudinal Evidence

Longitudinal studies enable us to examine the extent to which cannabis use is related to a future onset of MDD or an increase in depressive symptoms. Whereas earlier studies indicated that baseline cannabis use correlated with an increased risk for future MDD (Bovasso 2001; Fergusson and Horwood 1997), later studies indicated that cannabis users (including heavy users) were not more prone to develop MDD compared with nonusers (Degenhardt et al. 2013; Georgiades and Boyle 2007).

According to a meta-analysis by Moore et al. (2007) based on eight prospective studies, the risk of depression among individuals with the most frequent cannabis use (i.e., those with CaUD or who smoked cannabis at least every week) was slightly greater than that among nonusers (OR 1.49; 95% CI 1.15, 1.94), with evidence of a dose-response relationship between low- and high-frequency users. A subsequent meta-analysis suggested that any cannabis use (adjusted OR [AOR] 1.17; 95% CI 1.05–1.30) and heavy use in particular (AOR 1.62; 95% CI 1.21–2.16) may be related to a moderate increased risk of developing depression. However, there was a lack of consistency between these studies in terms of adjusting for confounders. A subsequent review by Lev-Ran et al. (2013) of 14 studies with 76,058 participants found a marginally significant greater risk of depression in relation to cannabis use (OR 1.17; 95% CI 1.05, 1.30), which was slightly higher for heavy users (OR 1.62; 95% CI 1.21, 2.16).

Two population-based longitudinal studies support the notion that when taking confounders into account, cannabis use does not elevate the risk for depression. In a Swedish population-based study, crude analyses indicated that cannabis use at baseline was associated with greater odds for consequent depression, yet after controlling for baseline confounders, significance was not maintained (Danielsson et al. 2016). Another study applied similar methodology based on waves 1 and 2 of the NESARC and, after controlling for baseline confounders, found that cannabis use, even daily use, was not related to an increased risk of MDD onset at follow-up (Feingold et al. 2015). Reports by the World Health Organization (2016) and the National Academies of Sciences, Engineering, and Medicine (2017) argued that cannabis use does not increase the probability of developing depression and that there is limited evidence that cannabis use and CaUD influence the onset of depression. Recently, Yana et al. (2023) reported on a retrospective longitudinal study of patients who received medical cannabis from 2014 to 2019 in Ontario. A total of 54,006 cannabis-using patients and 161,265 control participants were analyzed. The adjusted hazard ratio for depression was 2.02 (95% CI 1.83–2.22), and it was 2.23 (95% CI 1.95–2.55) among participants without previous mental health disorders.

An inverse relationship focused on the possible contribution of depression to the initiation of or increase in future cannabis use has also been addressed in research. The notion that substance use may be triggered by negative mood was reported in several clinical observations (e.g., Khantzian and Albanese 2008), exploratory studies (e.g.,

Ogborne et al. 2000), and retrospective studies (e.g., Gruber et al. 1997). It was first suggested that individuals experiencing psychological distress self-medicated their negative affect through substance use (Khantzian 1985), but this was not supported by longitudinal studies (Degenhardt et al. 2003). In a large population-based survey, nearly 9% of individuals with MDD reported that they used substances or misused prescription medication to relieve depression (Bolton et al. 2009); however, cannabis use was not specifically addressed. A longitudinal study by Feingold et al. (2015) showed that, among individuals who abstained from cannabis, MDD at baseline predicted cannabis use within a 3-year period (AOR 1.72; 95% CI 1.10, 2.69). However, this was not replicated in a study by Danielsson et al. (2016) in which, after controlling for additional illicit drug use, baseline depression was not related to higher risk for cannabis use onset at follow-up (RR 1.24; 95% CI 0.99–1.54).

In conclusion, some evidence suggests that cannabis use relates to the onset of depression. Evidence is inconsistent on the relationship between depression and the initiation of or increase in cannabis use.

Studies in Adolescents

Cannabis use is highly common among adolescents and may be prevalent as early as age 13 (European Monitoring Centre for Drugs and Drug Addiction 2017). Initial estimates suggest that 13.8 million people ages 15–16 use cannabis every year, equivalent to a rate of 5.6% (World Health Organization 2016). The relatively high availability of cannabis, along with perceptions of a low risk of harm, makes it one of the most common substances used during adolescence. On the basis of U.S. national monitoring data collected in 2012, the prevalence of cannabis use peaks around age 20, with a general decrease in use starting at age 25, suggesting that use may decrease with age as responsibilities (e.g., work, family) increase (Substance Abuse and Mental Health Services Administration 2014). At young ages, there is a strong correlation between cannabis use and depression; for example, adolescents who use cannabis report more symptoms of depression than do nonusers at ages 13–18 (Kaasbøll et al. 2018), and the frequency of past-year cannabis use relates to more symptoms of depression at ages 16–19 (Leadbeater et al. 2019). However, the link between cannabis use and depression may weaken in magnitude over time. For example, among participants age 18 and older, no differences were found between the frequency of cannabis use and the number of depressive symptoms

(Leadbeater et al. 2019). In addition, regular cannabis use at ages 14, 16, and 21 was not related to an increased risk of developing MDD by age 33 (Guttmannova et al. 2017). An Australian longitudinal cohort study revealed that using cannabis prior to age 17, even daily, was not associated with increased odds of depression by age 30 (AOR 1.02; 95% CI 0.52–2.01) (Silins et al. 2014). These findings suggest a gradually decreasing effect of cannabis use on depression over time.

A follow-up study of adolescents over 40 years evaluated the correlation between using cannabis and the likelihood of developing MDD, considering the early onset of cannabis use and the frequency of use (Schoeler et al. 2018). Adjusted analyses revealed that early cannabis use initiation (age <18 years) was related to increased odds for consequent MDD among both frequent users (AOR 8.83; 95% CI 1.29–70.79) and infrequent users (AOR 2.41; 95% CI 1.22–4.76) compared with nonusers. However, late cannabis use initiation (age >27) was not significantly associated with increased odds for MDD at follow-up for both frequent users (AOR 0.68; 95% CI 0.10–2.65) and infrequent users (AOR 2.23; 95% CI 0.26–14.94) compared with nonusers. Additional analyses indicated that early-onset cannabis use predicted a more rapid onset of MDD, regardless of cannabis use frequency, implying that age at first cannabis use plays a major role in modulating the duration to the onset of MDD.

The idea that MDD can facilitate cannabis use in young people has contradictory findings. On the one hand, integrated findings from four Australian cohorts indicated a moderate positive association between baseline frequent cannabis use and depression scores at follow-up (Horwood et al. 2012). The correlation between cannabis use frequency and future depression decreased with age, peaking at age 15 and declining at age 30. In another study, a 1-SD increase in cumulative depression symptom count between ages 12 and 15 was related to 50% increased risk for a DSM-IV CaUD at age 18 (Rhew et al. 2017). However, although an 18-month follow-up of ninth graders in Chile indicated that depression at baseline related to increased cannabis use at follow-up (AOR 1.21; 95% CI 1.09–1.34), this became insignificant after controlling for additional sociodemographic and clinical variables (Stapinski et al. 2016).

A study of male children at risk for behavioral problems indicated that cannabis use during childhood and adolescence was related to increased risk of MDD by age 48, with a fourfold risk in people who smoked cannabis frequently, after controlling for behavioral and mood disorders and other substance use (Schoeler et al. 2018). According to data from the Seattle Social Development Project, regular cannabis use during adulthood but not in adolescence increased the risk for MDD at age 33 more than twofold (Guttmannova et al. 2017). A relationship between problematic cannabis use and depressive symptoms was also observed in a large Swiss prospective study (Baggio et al. 2014), with a stronger effect for early and persistent cannabis use compared with nonuse or late onset. A review by Gobbi et al. (2019) of 11 studies comprising 23,317 individuals from adolescence to young adulthood found that the odds ratio of developing depression for cannabis users in young adulthood compared with nonusers was 1.37 (95% CI 1.16–1.62; I^2=0%). The pooled odds ratio for suicidal ideation was 1.50 (95% CI 1.11–2.03; I^2=0%) and for suicide attempt was 3.46 (95% CI 1.53–7.84, I^2=61.3%). The results indicated low to moderate individual risk for depression and suicidality, which makes this a major public health concern.

An analysis of 1,548 adolescents from the Quebec Longitudinal Study of Child Development supported the finding of a modest link between cannabis and depression in adolescence (London-Nadeau et al. 2021). A further analysis of 1,606 adolescents from the province of Quebec suggested that depressive symptoms in adolescence predicted subsequent weekly use of cannabis (adjusted for comorbid other substance use) that, once initiated, was likely to remain chronic. Weekly use of cannabis increased the risk for suicidal ideation, but not independently from the use of other substances (Bolanis et al. 2020). An analysis of cohorts from the Women and Alcohol in Gothenburg study (N=1,100) from three time periods examined the correlations between cannabis use, anxiety, and depression over time (Rabiee et al. 2020). A higher correlation was found between cannabis use and depression when controlling for time of use rather than cannabis use itself. The youngest cohort demonstrated an increased risk for depression compared with the older cohort. According to a Swiss population-based study of young adults (N=591) that assessed cannabis use in adolescence retrospectively at ages 19 and 20 and depression and suicidality between ages 20 and 50, cannabis use in adolescence was associated with adult depression and suicidality (Hengartner et al. 2020); first use at age 15 or 16 and younger and more frequent use in adolescence were related to higher risk of depression in adult life.

Halladay et al. (2019) reported from the Canadian Community Health Survey's mental health component, which was collected from 2002 to 2012 and included a nationally representative sample of 15- to 60-year-old Canadians. Monthly cannabis use was consistently related to major depressive episodes, and these associations were stronger in 2012 than in 2002. This change over time remained significant when other substance use was controlled. Monthly cannabis use was consistently related to both suicidal ideation and major depressive episode, and these associations were also stronger in 2012 compared with 2002. These findings support the existence of a relationship between cannabis use, depression, and suicide, which should be evaluated in a more robust manner now that recreational cannabis is available in many jurisdictions. Using U.S. National Health and Nutrition Examination Survey data from 2005 to 2018, Diep et al. (2022) conducted a cross-sectional analysis of adults and found that recent cannabis users had experienced suicidal ideation in the past 2 weeks and were more depressed compared with nonusers. Likewise, compared with those who did not report recent use, recent cannabis users were more depressed and experienced an increase in suicidal ideation. This relationship is likely multifactorial, but it highlights the need for specific guidelines and policies for the prescription of medical cannabis for psychiatric therapy. Gorfinkel et al. (2020), using data from the same survey for the period between 2005 and 2016, conducted a cross-sectional study of 16,216 participants between the ages of 20 and 59. Their study revealed that the correlation between cannabis use and depression became greater during this period and that depressed individuals had greater likelihood of having used cannabis in the past month and of using cannabis daily or near daily compared with nondepressed individuals.

Agrawal et al. (2017) performed a logistic regression analysis of cannabis use from retrospective data on same-sex male and female twin pairs drawn from three twin studies of the Australian Twin Registry (1992–1993, 1996–2000, and 2005–2009). They reported that CaUD risk factors may causally influence the risk of developing MDD, but only when the risk for CaUD is high.

Mustonen et al. (2021) analyzed data from 6,325 participants in the Northern Finland Birth Cohort 1986 to assess adolescent cannabis use and depression up to age 33. They found that 352 participants (5.6%) reported using cannabis until age 15–16. At follow-up, 583 participants (9.2%) were diagnosed with unipolar depression. After the authors adjusted for demographics, emotional and behavioral problems, and parental psychiatric disorders, the use of cannabis once or two to four times was related to an increased risk of depression.

In conclusion, longitudinal evidence indicates that cannabis use during childhood and adolescence is related to an increased risk of

MDD. These studies suggest bidirectional pathways between using cannabis use, CaUD, and the onset of depression. Medical cannabis authorization was related to a higher depression risk.

Contributing Factors

Sex as a Possible Moderator

There is some indication for sex differences in the correlation between cannabis use and depression. A stronger link between cannabis use and depressive symptoms was identified in males between ages 18 and 25 compared with females (Leadbeater et al. 2019). This finding may be attributed to heavier use of cannabis, greater impulsivity, sensation seeking, and avoidant coping strategies seen in males at this age. In the same study, at age 25 and older, the correlation between cannabis use and depressive symptoms was higher among females compared with males, suggesting that at these ages females transition from cannabis use to CaUD.

In conclusion, cannabis use is more likely to increase the risk for depression at a younger age. The correlation between cannabis use and mood disorders may be stronger among males in adolescence and emerging adulthood and stronger among females during midlife.

Neurological and Genetic Evidence

Recently, Alcaraz-Silva et al. (2023) reviewed the role of endocannabinoid receptors, as well as enzymes related to the synthesis and degradation of major endocannabinoids, in the development of depressive disorders. They concluded that, with further transitional research, these components of the endocannabinoid system could serve as biomarkers for the diagnosis and treatment of depression.

A major study by Lynskey et al. (2004) linked cannabis use and depression and measured correlations between early cannabis use and lifetime cannabis dependence and MDD, suicidal ideation, and suicide attempts. They investigated 311 same-sex twins who differed in their early start of cannabis use (one started before age 17, the other did not) and 277 same-sex twins discordant for cannabis dependence. They found that cannabis-dependent individuals had higher odds of suicidal ideation and suicide attempts (2.5 and 2.9 times, respectively) compared with their twins who were not cannabis dependent.

Cannabis was also associated with higher risks for MDD in nonidentical twins. Individuals who started using cannabis before age 17 years had higher rates of subsequent suicide attempt (OR 3.5; 95% CI 1.4–8.6) but not of major depression or suicidal ideation. The risk of cannabis dependence was associated with early MDD and suicidal ideation in nonidentical twins who differed in cannabis use but not in identical twins who differed in cannabis use. This evidence supports the notion that comorbidity of cannabis dependence and MDD (but not suicidal ideation) has both genetic and environmental vulnerability factors. Early-onset cannabis use may be a predisposing factor for MDD, or it may share genetic and environmental predisposition.

Otten and Engels (2013) investigated the link between cannabis use, depression, and the short allele of the serotonin-transporter-linked promoter region 5-HTTLPR in 310 adolescents over a period of 4 years. Cannabis use was related to higher depressive symptoms over time but only in those with the short allele of 5-HTTLPR. This is further evidence of the genetic association between cannabis use and depression. Hodgson et al. (2017) studied 1,284 Mexican Americans from 75 large multigenerational families and 57 genetically unrelated spouses. They reported a linkage peak for MDD on chromosome 22 and a peak for cannabis on chromosome 21. Chromosome 11 had a linkage peak and a single nucleotide polymorphism (SNP) related to both MDD and CaUD. Finally, genome-wide association studies identified SNPs that showed an association between schizophrenia, depression, and CaUD (Sherva et al. 2016). Among 14,754 participants, researchers found three SNPs associated with CaUD and genes that affected both MDD and CaUD and risk for schizophrenia. This was the first study to identify specific cannabis addiction risk alleles and potential genetic factors contributing to the comorbidity of cannabis dependence with MDD and schizophrenia.

In conclusion, genetic evidence indicates that early-onset cannabis use may be a predisposing factor for MDD and that genes associated with cannabis use are also shared with MDD, contributing to their comorbidity.

Effect of Cannabis Use on the Outcome of Depression

There is little evidence of the effect of cannabis use on the severity and course of depression. Early evidence suggested that cannabis use was related to elevated dysphoria among individuals with MDD (Ablon and Goodwin 1974), and a later study found that patients with lifetime mood disorders and current CaUD were likely to experience depression and sadness while intoxicated and were reluctant to report experiences of happiness or euphoria (Arendt et al. 2007). In a study focusing on individuals with MDD or dysthymia, women using cannabis regularly (at least weekly) reported reduced quality of life compared with women who were not using cannabis (Aspis et al. 2015).

Several longitudinal studies demonstrated that using cannabis may alter the course of illness in depressed individuals. Otten and Engels (2013) reported that cannabis use was related to an increase in the number of depressive symptoms through adolescence. In another study based on the NESARC sample, individuals who qualified for a baseline diagnosis of MDD ($N=2,300$) were followed throughout a 3-year period (Feingold et al. 2017). Use of cannabis and the presence of CaUD throughout the course of the study correlated with a higher number of symptoms of depression at follow-up, including anhedonia, insomnia or hypersomnia, body weight fluctuations, and psychomotor difficulties. However, for the most part, poorer clinical and functional outcomes of depression among those who used cannabis were attributed not to that use but rather to preliminary differences in psychosocial and clinical factors. Results from this study negated the hypothesis that cannabis use has a positive effect on the development and outcome of depression, suggesting that self-medication is not effective.

Some evidence indicates that cannabis use, particularly frequent use, may reduce the efficiency of pharmacological treatment for mood disorders in a clinical population (Bricker et al. 2007). In a study of 300 psychiatric outpatients receiving treatment for depression, baseline cannabis use predicted more suicidal ideation, less treatment utilization, less improvement in depressive symptoms, and reduced quality of life at 12-month follow-up compared with nonusers (Bahorik et al. 2017).

In recent years, technological and methodological advances have allowed for more sensitive measures of the relationship between cannabis use and depressed mood. For example, Cuttler et al. (2018) analyzed data from the Strainprint application (app), designed to give medical cannabis users a means of tracking changes in their affective symptoms as a function of different doses and cannabis types. Exploring more than 3,000 contacts made by app users, the authors found that participants reported a reduction in depressive symptoms from before to after cannabis use in 89.3% of tracked sessions. Although no sex differences were apparent, individuals using cannabis that was low in Δ^9-tetrahydrocannabinol (Δ^9-THC) and high in cannabidiol (CBD) reported a greater reduction compared with those using cannabis high in THC and low in CBD.

Analyzing session data entered by users over time, the authors reported that participants' rates of baseline depression (right before using cannabis) increased across time and sessions. This may indicate that although cannabis use can diminish depressive symptoms in the short term, longer-term use can lead to an increase in depressive symptoms. This conclusion is supported by findings from a study comparing adolescent nonusers with adolescent cannabis users that revealed a decline in depression in the latter group after 28 days of abstinence (Jacobus et al. 2017).

Deleterious Effects: Conclusions

Cannabis has been thought to induce a sense of euphoria; however, many individuals begin using it during depressive episodes (Feingold et al. 2015). According to NESARC data, both cannabis use and CaUD were related to an earlier onset of MDD, but no effect was found on the course of either MDD (Feingold et al. 2017) or any anxiety disorders (Feingold et al. 2018). In a substance use intervention trial with depressed outpatients, cannabis use was related to increased depression and anxiety (Bahorik et al. 2017). In another medication trial of cannabis cessation in 302 adults (ages 18–50), cannabis reduction predicted decreased anxiety and depressive symptoms (Hser et al. 2017). Additionally, a study of 400 participants older than 40 years showed that using cannabis increased the risk of being diagnosed with MDD and that an early start of cannabis use shortened the time to being diagnosed with MDD (Schoeler et al. 2018). Evidence of an association between cannabis use and MDD is supported by studies showing that chronic use strengthened the association (Hodgson et al. 2017; Rasic et al. 2013). Most studies described weekly cannabis use as being sufficient for developing MDD, and only one study found the association only in those with CaUD and not in occasional users (Baggio et al. 2014; Horwood et al. 2012). Further investigation is needed into whether the frequency and potency of CBD and THC mediate this association. Furthermore, cannabis use can also promote the progression of depressive symptoms and predict MDD (Bahorik et al. 2017; Moitra et al. 2016). There is strong evidence that cannabis use has negative effects on MDD (Lowe et al. 2019); however, there is debate over its role in affecting the outcomes of depression. The findings are limited because these are observational studies that are constrained by selection bias and the inability to regulate the source of the cannabis (Mammen et al. 2018; Sideli et al. 2020). Table 7–1 summarizes studies showing deleterious effects of cannabis on depression.

Beneficial Effects

Preclinical Studies on Cannabinoids As an Antidepressant

Preclinical studies have suggested that MDD can also occur with alterations in the endocannabinoid system (Aso et al. 2011; Gorzalka and Hill 2011; Mechoulam and Parker 2013) and that genetic deletion of cannabinoid 1 (CB_1) receptors has led to depressive-like behaviors in rodents (Aso et al. 2011; Valverde and Torrens 2012). Preclinical studies analyzed by Parolaro et al. (2010) also showed that reduced functionality of the endocannabinoids might be considered a predisposing factor for MDD; therefore, they suggested that boosting endocannabinoid tone might be a useful alternative therapeutic approach for depressive disorders. Rubino et al. (2009) reported that long-lasting impairment of CB_1 receptor function led to the development of a depressive phenotype in female rats, characterized by an anhedonic state, passive coping behavior in the forced swim test, and cognitive deficits.

There is evidence that facilitating endocannabinoid neurotransmission has antidepressant effects in rodent tests or models of depression through mechanisms that resemble the ones triggered by conventional antidepressant treatments. This suggests that enhancers of the cannabinoid system might become new antidepressant medications (Parolaro et al. 2010) and that cannabinoids can play an important role in the diagnosis and treatment of depression (Bright and Akirav 2022). However, the clinical use of the CB_1 antagonist rimonabant in humans was stopped on account of psychiatric side effects, mainly depression.

Table 7–1 Studies showing deleterious effects of cannabis on depression

Study	Type	Sample	Results
Bovasso (2001)	Longitudinal prospective	1,920 participants in the 1980 Baltimore Epidemiologic Catchment Area study reassessed between 1994 and 1996	Participants with no depressive symptoms and diagnosis of cannabis abuse at baseline were four times more likely than those without cannabis abuse to experience depressive symptoms at follow-up, adjusting for age, sex, antisocial symptoms.
Baggio et al. (2014)	Longitudinal prospective	5,084 young Swiss men (mean age 19.98±1.19 years at baseline)	Cannabis disorder symptoms predicted later depression ($B=0.087$; $P<0.001$).
Danielsson et al. (2016)	Longitudinal prospective	8,598 Swedish men and women (ages 20–64) with a 3-year follow-up	Adjusted for participant sex and age, cannabis use at baseline was associated with increased risk ratio for depression at follow-up (RR 1.22; 95% CI 1.06–1.42). After controlling for baseline confounders, significance was not maintained (RR 0.99; 95% CI 0.82–1.17).
Agrawal et al. (2017)	Twin study	13,986 male and female Australian monozygotic and dizygotic twins (mean age 32)	The monozygotic twin who frequently used cannabis was more likely to have MDD (OR 1.98; 95% CI 1.11–3.53) and suicidal ideation (OR 2.47; 95% CI 1.19–5.10) compared with the identical twin who had used cannabis less frequently.

Table 7–1 Studies showing deleterious effects of cannabis on depression (*continued*)

Study	Type	Sample	Results
Guttmannova et al. (2017)	Longitudinal prospective	808 participants from Seattle, WA, tracking regular marijuana use during adolescence and young adulthood	Regular marijuana use in young adulthood was positively related to more symptoms of cannabis use disorder at age 33.
Halladay et al. (2019)	Cross-sectional surveys	43,466 Canadians ages 15–60 from the 2002 and 2012 Canadian Community Health Survey's mental health component	Canadians using cannabis at least once a month in 2012 had 1.59 times (95% CI 1.11–2.27) the likelihood of experiencing suicidal ideation and 1.55 times (95% CI 1.12–2.13) the likelihood of having a major depressive episode compared with reports from 2002.
Gorfinkel et al. (2020)	Cross-sectional survey	16,216 U.S. adults between 2005 and 2016; 7,768 men (mean age 39.12, range 38.23–39.40)	Odds ratio for depression and any past-month cannabis use increased from 1.46 (95% CI 1.07–1.99) in 2005–2006 to 2.30 (95% CI 1.82–2.91) in 2015–2016. Odds ratio for depression and daily or near-daily past-month cannabis use increased from 1.37 (95% CI 0.81–2.32) in 2005–2006 to 3.16 (95% CI 2.23–4.48) in 2015–2016.

Table 7–1 Studies showing deleterious effects of cannabis on depression (*continued*)

Study	Type	Sample	Results
Hengartner et al. (2020)	Longitudinal retrospective	Stratified population-based cohort of young adults (*N*=591) from Zurich, Switzerland, assessed at age 19–20 for cannabis use in adolescence	Cannabis use during adolescence was associated with adult depression (AOR 1.70; 95% CI 1.24–2.32) and suicidality (AOR 1.65; 95% CI 1.11–2.47). First use at age 15–16 and younger and frequent use in adolescence were associated with a higher risk of depression in adult life.
Rabiee et al. (2020)	Cross-sectional prospective	Women and Alcohol in Gothenburg study (*N*=1,100) from three time periods	Cannabis use was associated with depression in the youngest cohort, which was born between 1980 and 1993 and examined from 2000 to 2015 (OR 2.37; 95% CI 1.45–3.86). There was an interaction between cannabis use and depression in the youngest cohort compared with older cohorts (OR 1.68; 95% CI 0.45–2.92).
Mustonen et al. (2021)	Longitudinal prospective	6,325 participants (48.8% male) of Northern Finland Birth Cohort 1986 followed until 2018	Cannabis use until age 15–16 years was reported by 352 participants (5.6%). By the end of the follow-up, 583 participants (9.2%) had been diagnosed with unipolar depression. Cannabis use in adolescence was associated with an increased risk of depression. Using cannabis once (HR 1.93; 95% CI 1.30–2.87) or two to four times (HR 2.02; 95% CI 1.24–3.31) was associated with increased risk of depression.

Table 7–1 Studies showing deleterious effects of cannabis on depression (*continued*)

Study	Type	Sample	Results
Diep et al. (2022)	Cross-sectional prospective	18,599 adults with no recent use and 3,127 recent cannabis users from National Health and Nutrition Examination Survey data, 2005–2018	Compared with those with no recent use, recent users had greater likelihood of having experienced suicidal ideation during the past 2 weeks (AOR 1.54; 95% CI 1.19–2.00; $P<0.001$), being depressed (AOR 1.53; 95% CI 1.29–1.82; $P<0.001$), and having seen a mental health professional in the past 12 months (AOR 1.28; 95% CI 1.04–1.59; $P<0.05$).

AOR = adjusted odds ratio; HR = hazard ratio.

Cross-Sectional Studies of Improved Depressed Mood by Cannabis

Cannabis users often use cannabis to self-medicate depression and manic symptoms (Ashton et al. 2005; Grinspoon and Bakalar 1998). Individuals who used cannabis occasionally or even daily had lower levels of depressive symptoms than those who had never tried it (Denson and Earleywine 2006). Depressed patients also used cannabis to improve their sleep (Babson et al. 2013; Kuhathasan et al. 2022). Despite these reports, a review by Walsh et al. (2017) concluded that the clinical implications of using cannabis for therapeutic purposes among individuals with mood disorders were unclear. More recently, in a longitudinal, cross-sectional study, medicinal cannabis users reported reduced depression and improved quality of life compared with a control group that had considered but had not used medicinal cannabis (Schlienz et al. 2021). Sachedina et al. (2022) conducted a retrospective study of patients using medical cannabis obtained from a Harvest Medicine clinic in Canada. The 7,362 patients in the sample had an average age of 49.8 years, and 53.1% were female. Improvements were noted between baseline and follow-up scores for both anxiety and health, with larger improvements seen for patients who were actively seeking medical cannabis to treat anxiety or depression. Patients reporting depression 18 months after the beginning of the study reported an average decrease in depression scores. This study provides some evidence to support the effectiveness of medical cannabis as treatment for depression. Finally, Mangoo et al. (2022) analyzed a series of 129 uncontrolled cases from the U.K. Medical Cannabis Registry. Medical cannabis treatment correlated with reductions in depression severity at 1, 3, and 6 months. Because of limitations of the study design, a causal relationship cannot be proven, but this analysis provides insight for further study within clinical trial settings.

In conclusion, the evidence so far is anecdotal and relies heavily on single case studies and cross-sectional studies. There are no placebo-controlled clinical trials that show cannabis is useful for treatment of depression.

Clinical Studies on Cannabis as an Antidepressant

Gruber et al. (1996) evaluated the use of cannabis for treatment of MDD. Improvements in depressive symptoms were described in five case reports of individuals with history of cannabis use for whom an anti-depressant effect extended beyond that of acute cannabis intoxication. Four of five patients reported that the efficacy of cannabis superseded the benefits of past treatment trials of antidepressants. However, these findings were limited by retrospective reports, and all cases fulfilled DSM-IV criteria for cannabis or polysubstance abuse. The evidence to date supporting use of cannabis as a psychopharmacological treatment for mood and related disorders appears to comprise a few primarily single-dose studies (Turna et al. 2017). Unfortunately, these studies have small sample sizes and deficits in the overall study designs, which limits the clinical application of the findings. There is limited evidence for the efficacy of cannabis in these disorders, and, together with the risks associated with regular use, it is difficult to objectively place cannabis as a psychopharmacological treatment until further research is conducted and treatment guidelines are developed.

Turna et al. (2019) analyzed the responses to an online survey from 2,032 licensed users of cannabis for medical purpose in Canada. Of the total sample, 25.7% received cannabis to treat MDD. Most responders endorsed daily cannabis use as improving their anxiety and depressive symptoms, and their symptoms positively correlated with the daily amount of cannabis used. Caveats include the possibility of CaUD and the possibility that improvements in nonpsychiatric conditions could be attributed to improvements in anxiety. These results highlight the need to systematically evaluate medical cannabis use for mental illness. Black et al. (2019) evaluated 42 eligible studies on cannabis treatment for depression (23 randomized controlled trials; $N=2,551$). They reported that medical THC (with or without CBD) had no effect on the main outcomes of mental disorders, but it increased the number of individuals reporting adverse events and withdrawal. There is therefore little evidence that cannabinoids improve mood disorders.

Currently, no clinical trials have been conducted on the use of cannabinoids for treating depression. The evidence so far indicates more harm than therapeutic benefits for the treatment of MDD, and prospective, controlled studies are warranted (Chadwick et al. 2020; Lowe et al. 2019; Stanciu et al. 2021). Table 7–2 describes studies showing beneficial effects of cannabis on depression.

Table 7–2 Studies demonstrating beneficial effects of cannabis on depression

Study	Type	Sample	Results
Denson and Earleywine (2006)	Cross-sectional	4,400 U.S. adult internet users who completed the CES-D scale and measures of marijuana use	Participants who used cannabis once per week or less had less depressed mood, more positive affect, and fewer somatic complaints than nonusers. Daily users reported less depressed mood and more positive affect than nonusers.
Turna et al. (2019)	Online survey	888 (43.7%) Canadian participants who used cannabis for treating anxiety symptoms	Respondents endorsed daily cannabis use, and severity of depressive symptoms was positively associated with the amount of cannabis used per day. The vast majority perceived symptom improvement with cannabis use.
Schlienz et al. (2021)	Cross-sectional, longitudinal, Web-based survey	1,276 participants from a convenience sample of 808 patients with a diagnosed health condition and 468 caregivers from the U.S. nonprofit Realm of Caring Foundation	Cannabis users self-reported lower depression (t[1210]=5.77; $P<0.001$) compared with control participants.

Table 7–2 Studies demonstrating beneficial effects of cannabis on depression (*continued*)

Study	Type	Sample	Results
Sachedina et al. (2022)	Retrospective	7,362 patients (53.1% female) using medical cannabis from a Harvest Medicine clinic in Canada (mean age 49.8 years)	Improvements observed in depression symptoms between baseline and follow-up, with larger improvements seen for patients actively seeking medical cannabis to treat depression.
Mangoo et al. (2022)	Prospective case studies	129 patients from the U.K. Medical Cannabis Registry	Patients who used cannabis for medical purposes showed reductions in depression ratings at 1 month (median 8.0; IQR 4.0–14.0; $P < 0.001$), 3 months (median 7.0; IQR 2.3–12.8; $P < 0.001$), and 6 months (median 7.0; IQR 2.0–9.5; $P < 0.001$).

CES-D = Center for Epidemiologic Studies–Depression; IQR = interquartile range.

Clinical Significance and Recommendations

Recent longitudinal evidence indicates that using cannabis during childhood and adolescence is related to an increased risk of MDD. Kuhns et al. (2022) argued that the current evidence is limited and mixed and suggests that cannabis affects the onset of depression and vice versa. The association between cannabis use and depression is shared by genetic and environmental risk factors. Cannabis use by itself may affect the course of depression, and some people start using cannabis to self-medicate. CaUD is linked with worsening symptoms of depression and suicide. Overall, placebo-controlled, prospective, longitudinal clinical studies are needed that include individuals with comorbid CaUD and MDD.

Because the evidence relies on correlations that do not provide any evidence of causality, several mechanisms may explain the occurrence of comorbid CaUD and MDD (Gobbi et al. 2019). First, the biological effects of cannabis affect brain chemistry, particularly the serotonin system, in multiple ways. Another mechanism is the shared vulnerability of genetic and environmental predispositional factors that may impair psychosocial function. Finally, the self-medication hypothesis suggests that individuals self-medicate to alleviate anxiety and depression (Khantzian 1985).

The matter of using medical cannabis as an antidepressant is at an early stage of examination, and little evidence to date supports it. The evidence so far is anecdotal and relies heavily on single case studies and cross-sectional studies. Placebo-controlled clinical trials are needed to determine whether cannabis is useful for treatment of depression. Psychiatric outpatients who used medical cannabis showed worse mental and physical health function compared with nonusers. Recreational cannabis correlated with increased suicidal ideation and mental health problems and fewer psychiatry visits among patients, and cannabis use over time correlated with lower improvement in depression symptoms and suicidal ideation (Bahorik et al. 2017). Cannabis use by medicated patients with depression can also prevent improvement in their depressive symptoms and impair their treatment. The evidence in favor of cannabis treatment for mood disorders relies on a few single-dose studies with small sample sizes and flawed designs (Turna et al. 2017). There is stronger evidence for harm than benefit from cannabis in MDD, and controlled prospective designs are required (Chadwick et al. 2020; Lowe et al. 2019; Stanciu et al. 2021).

An increase in the use of highly potent cannabis (>15% THC content) has been reported in the United Kingdom and the United States, which is raising concern among mental health professionals because of an increased risk for psychosis and mental problems. An analysis of a substance-using sample from the Global Drug Survey from 2015 and 2016 indicated that individuals with lifetime depression and substance abuse were prone to using extremely high-potency forms of cannabis (Chan et al. 2017), which is concerning because it may reduce the efficacy of pharmacological treatments and impair everyday function in individuals with MDD.

Conclusion

Subjective reports indicate that prescribed medical cannabis can improve depression ratings, but the evidence is anecdotal and based on cross-sectional studies. Contrary evidence shows that medical cannabis relates to an increased risk of depression in medicated psychiatric patients. On balance, the deleterious effects of cannabis use on depression outweigh its beneficial effects. When authorizing patients to use cannabis, clinicians should ensure to also assess the risks, particularly for patients using cannabis for depression treatment.

Key Points

- Recent longitudinal evidence indicates that cannabis use during childhood and adolescence is associated with increased risk of major depressive disorder.
- The use of cannabis as an antidepressant is in the early stages of examination, and no placebo-controlled clinical trials have been conducted that indicate whether cannabis is a useful treatment for depression.
- There is some indication that prescribed medical cannabis can improve depression ratings, but there is also contrary evidence that use of medical cannabis can increase the risk of depression among psychiatric patients.

- Overall, the deleterious effects of cannabis use on depression outweigh its benefits. Extra care should be taken when prescribing medical cannabis to patients who self-medicate for depression.

References

Ablon SL, Goodwin FK: High frequency of dysphoric reactions to tetrahydrocannabinol among depressed patients. Am J Psychiatry 131(4):448–453, 1974 4592555

Agrawal A, Nelson EC, Bucholz KK, et al: Major depressive disorder, suicidal thoughts and behaviours, and cannabis involvement in discordant twins: a retrospective cohort study. Lancet Psychiatry 4(9):706–714, 2017 28750823

Alcaraz-Silva J, Feingold D, Viana-Torre G, et al: The endocannabinoid system as a biomarker for diagnostic and therapeutic applications in depression and anxiety. CNS Neurol Disord Drug Targets 22(3):417–430, 2023 35382720

American Psychiatric Association: Diagnostic and Statistical Manual of Mental Disorders, 4th Edition. Washington, DC, American Psychiatric Association, 1994

Arendt M, Rosenberg R, Fjordback L, et al: Testing the self-medication hypothesis of depression and aggression in cannabis-dependent subjects. Psychol Med 37(7):935–945, 2007 17202003

Ashton CH, Moore PB, Gallagher P, et al: Cannabinoids in bipolar affective disorder: a review and discussion of their therapeutic potential. J Psychopharmacol 19(3):293–300, 2005 15888515

Aso E, Ozaita A, Serra MÀ, et al: Genes differentially expressed in CB1 knockout mice: involvement in the depressive-like phenotype. Eur Neuropsychopharmacol 21(1):11–22, 2011 20692131

Aspis I, Feingold D, Weiser M, et al: Cannabis use and mental health-related quality of life among individuals with depressive disorders. Psychiatry Res 230(2): 341–349, 2015

Babson KA, Boden MT, Bonn-Miller MO: Sleep quality moderates the relation between depression symptoms and problematic cannabis use among medical cannabis users. Am J Drug Alcohol Abuse 39(3):211–216, 2013 23721537

Baggio S, N'Goran AA, Deline S, et al: Patterns of cannabis use and prospective associations with health issues among young males. Addiction 109(6):937–945, 2014 24450535

Bahorik AL, Leibowitz A, Sterling SA, et al: Patterns of marijuana use among psychiatry patients with depression and its impact on recovery. J Affect Disord 213:168–171, 2017 28242498

Black N, Stockings E, Campbell G, et al: Cannabinoids for the treatment of mental disorders and symptoms of mental disorders: a systematic review and meta-analysis. Lancet Psychiatry 6(12):995–1010, 2019 31672337

Bolanis D, Orri M, Castellanos-Ryan N, et al: Cannabis use, depression and suicidal ideation in adolescence: direction of associations in a population based cohort. J Affect Disord 274:1076–1083, 2020 32663935

Bolton JM, Robinson J, Sareen J: Self-medication of mood disorders with alcohol and drugs in the National Epidemiologic Survey on Alcohol and Related Conditions. J Affect Disord 115(3):367–375, 2009 19004504

Bovasso GB: Cannabis abuse as a risk factor for depressive symptoms. Am J Psychiatry 158(12):2033–2037, 2001 11729021

Bricker JB, Russo J, Stein MB, et al: Does occasional cannabis use impact anxiety and depression treatment outcomes? Results from a randomized effectiveness trial. Depress Anxiety 24(6):392–398, 2007 17096386

Bright U, Akirav I: Modulation of endocannabinoid system components in depression: pre-clinical and clinical evidence. Int J Mol Sci 23(10):5526, 2022 35628337

Chadwick VL, Rohleder C, Koethe D, et al: Cannabinoids and the endocannabinoid system in anxiety, depression, and dysregulation of emotion in humans. Curr Opin Psychiatry 33(1):20–42, 2020 31714262

Chan GCK, Hall W, Freeman TP, et al: User characteristics and effect profile of butane hash oil: an extremely high-potency cannabis concentrate. Drug Alcohol Depend 178:32–38, 2017 28624604

Chen CY, Wagner FA, Anthony JC: Marijuana use and the risk of major depressive episode. Epidemiological evidence from the United States National Comorbidity Survey. Soc Psychiatry Psychiatr Epidemiol 37(5):199–206, 2002 12107710

Cuttler C, Spradlin A, McLaughlin RJ: A naturalistic examination of the perceived effects of cannabis on negative affect. J Affect Disord 235:198–205, 2018 29656267

Danielsson AK, Lundin A, Agardh E, et al: Cannabis use, depression and anxiety: a 3-year prospective population-based study. J Affect Disord 193:103–108, 2016 26773900

Degenhardt L, Hall W, Lynskey M: Exploring the association between cannabis use and depression. Addiction 98(11):1493–1504, 2003 14616175

Degenhardt L, Coffey C, Romaniuk H, et al: The persistence of the association between adolescent cannabis use and common mental disorders into young adulthood. Addiction 108(1):124–133, 2013 22775447

de Graaf R, Radovanovic M, van Laar M, et al: Early cannabis use and estimated risk of later onset of depression spells: epidemiologic evidence from the population-based World Health Organization World Mental Health Survey Initiative. Am J Epidemiol 172(2):149–159, 2010 20534820

Denson TF, Earleywine M: Decreased depression in marijuana users. Addict Behav 31(4):738–742, 2006 15964704

Diep C, Bhat V, Wijeysundera DN, et al: The association between recent cannabis use and suicidal ideation in adults: a population-based analysis of the NHANES from 2005 to 2018. Can J Psychiatry 67(4):259–267, 2022 33641436

Dierker L, Selya A, Lanza S, et al: Depression and marijuana use disorder symptoms among current marijuana users. Addict Behav 76:161–168, 2018 28843729

European Monitoring Centre for Drugs and Drug Addiction: European Drug Report Luxembourg. Lisbon, Portugal, European Monitoring Centre for Drugs and Drug Addiction, 2017

Feingold D, Weinstein A: Cannabis and depression, in Cannabinoids and Neuropsychiatric Disorders. Edited by Murillo-Rodriguez E, Pandi-Perumal SR, Monti JM. New York, Springer, 2021 pp 67–80

Feingold D, Weiser M, Rehm J, Lev-Ran S: The association between cannabis use and mood disorders: a longitudinal study. J Affect Disord 172:211–218, 2015 25451420

Feingold D, Rehm J, Lev-Ran S: Cannabis use and the course and outcome of major depressive disorder: a population based longitudinal study. Psychiatry Res 251:225–234, 2017 28214781

Feingold D, Rehm J, Factor H, et al: Clinical and functional outcomes of cannabis use among individuals with anxiety disorders: a 3-year population-based longitudinal study. Depress Anxiety 35(6):490–501, 2018 29486095

Fergusson DM, Horwood LJ: Early onset cannabis use and psychosocial adjustment in young adults. Addiction 92(3):279–296, 1997 9219390

Georgiades K, Boyle MH: Adolescent tobacco and cannabis use: young adult outcomes from the Ontario Child Health Study. J Child Psychol Psychiatry 48(7):724–731, 2007 17593153

Gobbi G, Atkin T, Zytynski T, et al: Association of cannabis use in adolescence and risk of depression, anxiety, and suicidality in young adulthood: a systematic review and meta-analysis. JAMA Psychiatry 76(4):426–434, 2019 30758486

Gorfinkel LR, Stohl M, Hasin D: Association of depression with past-month cannabis use among US adults aged 20 to 59 years, 2005 to 2016. JAMA Netw Open 3(8):e2013802, 2020 32809032

Gorzalka BB, Hill MN: Putative role of endocannabinoid signaling in the etiology of depression and actions of antidepressants. Prog Neuropsychopharmacol Biol Psychiatry 35(7):1575–1585, 2011 21111017

Grinspoon L, Bakalar JB: The use of cannabis as a mood stabilizer in bipolar disorder: anecdotal evidence and the need for clinical research. J Psychoactive Drugs 30(2):171–177, 1998 9692379

Gruber AJ, Pope HG Jr, Brown ME: Do patients use marijuana as an antidepressant? Depression 4(2):77–80, 1996 9160645

Gruber AJ, Pope HG Jr, Oliva P: Very long-term users of marijuana in the United States: a pilot study. Subst Use Misuse 32(3):249–264, 1997 9058474

Gukasyan N, Strain EC: Relationship between cannabis use frequency and major depressive disorder in adolescents: findings from the National Survey on Drug Use and Health 2012–2017. Drug Alcohol Depend 208:107867, 2020 31958677

Gutiérrez-Rojas L, Porras-Segovia A, Dunne H, et al: Prevalence and correlates of major depressive disorder: a systematic review. Br J Psychiatry 42(6):657–672, 2020 32756809

Guttmannova K, Kosterman R, White HR, et al: The association between regular marijuana use and adult mental health outcomes. Drug Alcohol Depend 179:109–116, 2017 28763778

Halladay JE, Boyle MH, Munn C, et al: Sex differences in the association between cannabis use and suicidal ideation and attempts, depression, and psychological distress among Canadians. Can J Psychiatry 64(5):345–350, 2019 30260680

Han B, Compton WM, Einstein EB, et al: Associations of suicidality trends with cannabis use as a function of sex and depression status. JAMA Netw Open 4(6):e2113025, 2021 34156452

Hasin DS, Kerridge BT, Saha TD, et al: Prevalence and correlates of DSM-5 cannabis use disorder, 2012–2013: findings from the National Epidemiologic Survey on Alcohol and Related Conditions–III. Am J Psychiatry 173(6):588–599, 2016 26940807

Hasin DS, Sarvet AL, Meyers JL, et al: Epidemiology of adult DSM-5 major depressive disorder and its specifiers in the United States. JAMA Psychiatry 75(4):336–346, 2018 29450462

Hengartner MP, Angst J, Ajdacic-Gross V, et al: Cannabis use during adolescence and the occurrence of depression, suicidality and anxiety disorder across adulthood: findings from a longitudinal cohort study over 30 years. J Affect Disord 272:98–103, 2020 32379627

Hodgson K, Almasy L, Knowles EE, et al: The genetic basis of the comorbidity between cannabis use and major depression. Addiction 112(1):113–123, 2017 27517884

Horwood LJ, Fergusson DM, Coffey C, et al: Cannabis and depression: an integrative data analysis of four Australasian cohorts. Drug Alcohol Depend 126(3):369–378, 2012 22749560

Hser YI, Mooney LJ, Huang D, et al Reductions in cannabis use are associated with improvements in anxiety, depression, and sleep quality, but not quality of life. J Subst Abuse Treat 81:53–58, 2017 28847455

Institute for Health Metrics and Evaluation: Global Health Data Exchange (GHDx). Seattle, WA, Institute for Health Metrics and Evaluation, 2021. Available at: https://ghdx.healthdata.org/gbd-2021. Accessed January 29, 2023.

Jacobus J, Squeglia LM, Escobar S, et al: Changes in marijuana use symptoms and emotional functioning over 28-days of monitored abstinence in adolescent marijuana users. Psychopharmacology (Berl) 234(23–24):3431–3442, 2017 28900686

Kaasbøll C, Hagen R, Gråwe RW: Population-based associations among cannabis use, anxiety, and depression in Norwegian adolescents. J Child Adolesc Subst Abuse 27(4):238–243, 2018

Khantzian EJ: The self-medication hypothesis of addictive disorders: focus on heroin and cocaine dependence. Am J Psychiatry 142(11):1259–1264, 1985 3904487

Khantzian EJ, Albanese MJ: Understanding Addiction as Self Medication: Finding Hope Behind the Pain. New York, Rowman and Littlefield, 2008

Kuhathasan N, Minuzzi L, MacKillop J, et al: An investigation of cannabis use for insomnia in depression and anxiety in a naturalistic sample. BMC Psychiatry 22(1):303, 2022 35484520

Kuhns L, Kroon E, Colyer-Patel K, et al: Associations between cannabis use, cannabis use disorder, and mood disorders: longitudinal, genetic, and neurocognitive evidence. Psychopharmacology (Berl) 239(5):1231–1249, 2022 34741634

Leadbeater BJ, Ames ME, Linden-Carmichael AN: Age-varying effects of cannabis use frequency and disorder on symptoms of psychosis, depression and anxiety in adolescents and adults. Addiction 114(2):278–293, 2019 30276906

Lev-Ran S, Roerecke M, Le Foll B, et al: The association between cannabis use and depression: a systematic review and meta analysis of longitudinal studies. Psychol Med 44(4):1–14, 2013 23795762

London-Nadeau K, Rioux C, Parent S, et al: Longitudinal associations of cannabis, depression, and anxiety in heterosexual and LGB adolescents. J Abnorm Psychol 130(4):333–345, 2021 34180699

Lowe DJE, Sasiadek JD, Coles AS, et al: Cannabis and mental illness: a review. Eur Arch Psychiatry Clin Neurosci 269(1):107–120, 2019 30564886

Lynskey MT, Glowinski AL, Todorov AA, et al: Major depressive disorder, suicidal ideation, and suicide attempt in twins discordant for cannabis dependence and early onset cannabis use. Arch Gen Psychiatry 61(10):1026–1032, 2004 15466676

Mammen G, Rueda S, Roerecke M, et al: Association of cannabis with long-term clinical symptoms in anxiety and mood disorders: a systematic review of prospective studies. J Clin Psychiatry 79(4):17r11839, 2018 29877641

Mangoo S, Erridge S, Holvey C, et al: Assessment of clinical outcomes of medicinal cannabis therapy for depression: analysis from the UK Medical Cannabis Registry. Expert Rev Neurother 22(11–12):995–1008, 2022 36573268

Mechoulam R, Parker LA: The endocannabinoid system and the brain. Annu Rev Psychol 64:21–47, 2013 22804774

Moitra E, Anderson BJ, Stein MD: Reductions in cannabis use are associated with mood improvement in female emerging adults. Depress Anxiety 33(4):332–338, 2016 26636547

Moore THM, Zammit S, Lingford-Hughes A, et al: Cannabis use and risk of psychotic or affective mental health outcomes: a systematic review. Lancet 370(9584):319–328, 2007 17662880

Mustonen A, Hielscher E, Miettunen J, et al: Adolescent cannabis use, depression and anxiety disorders in the Northern Finland Birth Cohort 1986. BJPsych Open 7(4):e137, 2021 36043688

National Academies of Sciences, Engineering, and Medicine: The Health Effects of Cannabis and Cannabinoids: The Current State of Evidence and Recommendations for Research. Washington, DC, National Academies Press, 2017

Ogborne AC, Smart RG, Weber T, et al: Who is using cannabis as a medicine and why: an exploratory study. J Psychoactive Drugs 32(4):435–443, 2000 11210205

Onaemo VN, Fawehinmi TO, D'Arcy C: Comorbid cannabis use disorder with major depression and generalized anxiety disorder: a systematic review with meta-analysis of nationally representative epidemiological surveys. J Affect Disord 281:467–475, 2021 33360749

Otten R, Engels RC: Testing bidirectional effects between cannabis use and depressive symptoms: moderation by the serotonin transporter gene. Addict Biol 18(5):826–835, 2013 21967091

Parolaro D, Realini N, Vigano D, et al: The endocannabinoid system and psychiatric disorders. Exp Neurol 224(1):3–14, 2010 20353783

Rabiee R, Lundin A, Agardh E, et al: Cannabis use and the risk of anxiety and depression in women: a comparison of three Swedish cohorts. Drug Alcohol Depend 216:108332, 2020 33080503

Rasic D, Weerasinghe S, Asbridge M, et al: Longitudinal associations of cannabis and illicit drug use with depression, suicidal ideation and suicidal attempts among Nova Scotia high school students. Drug Alcohol Depend 129(1–2):49–53, 2013 23041136

Reece AS, Hulse GK: Co-occurrence across time and space of drug- and cannabinoid-exposure and adverse mental health outcomes in the National Survey of Drug Use and Health: combined geotemporospatial and causal inference analysis. BMC Public Health 20(1):1655, 2020 33148213

Rhew IC, Fleming CB, Vander Stoep A, et al: Examination of cumulative effects of early adolescent depression on cannabis and alcohol use disorder in late adolescence in a community-based cohort. Addiction 112(11):1952–1960, 2017 28600897

Rubino T, Realini N, Braida D, et al: The depressive phenotype induced in adult female rats by adolescent exposure to THC is associated with

cognitive impairment and altered neuroplasticity in the prefrontal
cortex. Neurotox Res 15(4):291–302, 2009 19384563

Sachedina F, Chan C, Damji RS, et al: Medical cannabis use in Canada and its
impact on anxiety and depression: a retrospective study. Psychiatry Res
313:114573, 2022 35598566

Schlienz NJ, Scalsky R, Martin EL, et al: A cross-sectional and prospective
comparison of medicinal cannabis users and controls on self-reported
health. Cannabis Cannabinoid Res 6(6):548–558, 2021 33998852

Schoeler T, Theobald D, Pingault J-B, et al: Developmental sensitivity to cannabis
use patterns and risk for major depressive disorder in mid-life: findings
from 40 years of follow-up. Psychol Med 48(13):2169–2176, 2018 29607801

Sherva R, Wang Q, Kranzler H, et al: Genome-wide association study of
cannabis dependence severity, novel risk variants, and shared genetic
risks. JAMA Psychiatry 73(5): 472–480, 2016

Sideli L, Quigley H, La Cascia C, et al: Cannabis use and the risk for
psychosis and affective disorders. J Dual Diagn 16(1):22–42, 2020 31647377

Silins E, Horwood LJ, Patton GC, et al: Young adult sequelae of adolescent
cannabis use: an integrative analysis. Lancet Psychiatry 1(4):286–293, 2014
26360862

Stanciu CN, Brunette MF, Teja N, et al: Evidence for use of cannabinoids
in mood disorders, anxiety disorders, and PTSD: a systematic review.
Psychiatr Serv 72(4):429–436, 2021 33530732

Stapinski LA, Montgomery AA, Araya R: Anxiety, depression and risk
of cannabis use: examining the internalising pathway to use among
Chilean adolescents. Drug Alcohol Depend 166:109–115, 2016

Substance Abuse and Mental Health Services Administration: Results
From the 2006 National Survey on Drug Use and Health: National
Findings. Rockville, MD, Substance Abuse and Mental Health Services
Administration, 2007

Substance Abuse and Mental Health Services Administration: Results From
the 2013 National Survey on Drug Use and Health: Summary of National
Findings. Rockville, MD, Substance Abuse and Mental Health Services
Administration, 2014

Turna J, Patterson B, Van Ameringen M: Is cannabis treatment for anxiety,
mood, and related disorders ready for prime time? Depress Anxiety
34(11):1006–1017, 2017 28636769

Turna J, Simpson W, Patterson B, et al: Cannabis use behaviors and
prevalence of anxiety and depressive symptoms in a cohort of Canadian
medicinal cannabis users. J Psychiatr Res 111:134–139, 2019 30738930

United Nations Office on Drugs and Crime: World Drug Report 2022. New
York, United Nations, 2022

Valverde O, Torrens M: CB1 receptor-deficient mice as a model for depression.
Neuroscience 204:193–206, 2012 21964469

van Laar M, van Dorsselaer S, Monshouwer K, et al: Does cannabis use predict the first incidence of mood and anxiety disorders in the adult population? Addiction 102(8):1251–1260, 2007 17624975

Walsh Z, Gonzalez R, Crosby K, et al: Medical cannabis and mental health: a guided systematic review. Clin Psychol Rev 51:15–29, 2017 27816801

Whiteford HA, Degenhardt L, Rehm J, et al: Global burden of disease attributable to mental and substance use disorders: findings from the Global Burden of Disease Study 2010. Lancet 382(9904):1575–1586, 2013 23993280

Wittchen HU, Fröhlich C, Behrendt S, et al: Cannabis use and cannabis use disorders and their relationship to mental disorders: a 10-year prospective-longitudinal community study in adolescents. Drug Alcohol Depend 88(Suppl 1):S60–S70, 2007 17257779

World Health Organization: The Health and Social Effects of Nonmedical Cannabis Use. Geneva, World Health Organization, 2016

Yana JL, Lee C, Eurich DT, et al: Risk of depressive disorders associated with medical cannabis authorization: a propensity score matched cohort study. Psychiatry Res 320:115047, 2023 36638694

8

Cannabis, Posttraumatic Stress Disorder, and Anxiety Disorders

Jeremy Weleff, D.O.

Anahita Bassir Nia, M.D.

Joao P. De Aquino, M.D.

Posttraumatic stress disorder (PTSD) is a psychiatric disorder that develops after someone experiences or witnesses a traumatic event, such as a natural disaster, combat, sexual or physical assault, or life-threatening event (American Psychiatric Association 2022). The lifetime prevalence of PTSD is approximately 6%–8% among the general population in the United States (Kessler et al. 2005; Pietrzak et al. 2011), and the point prevalence is 11% in primary care clinics (Spottswood et al. 2017). The prevalence of PTSD is higher among females (Breslau et al. 1991). Symptoms of PTSD include reexperiencing the trauma through flashbacks, nightmares, and intrusive thoughts; avoiding triggers associated with the trauma; and being in a state of hyperarousal, including hypervigilance, irritability, and difficulty sleeping. Because the symptoms of PTSD are diverse, they may overlap with those of other conditions. Up to 78.5% of people with PTSD have also been diagnosed with other psychiatric disorders—with the most common being major depressive disorder, anxiety disorders, substance use disorders (SUDs), and psychotic disorders (Blanco et al. 2016; Pietrzak et al. 2011; Qassem et al. 2021). PTSD is particularly associated with SUDs and nonmedical substance use (Pietrzak et al. 2011).

PTSD and cannabis use are closely linked in many observational, epidemiological studies. The prevalence of cannabis use is high among individuals who have PTSD, have experienced trauma, or have experienced other forms of childhood maltreatment or abuse. In 2018, the International Cannabis Policy Study of self-reported cannabis use for medical reasons reported that 17% of respondents in North America used cannabis for PTSD symptoms (Leung et al. 2022), and PTSD is often reported as one of the most common reasons for medical cannabis use (Boehnke et al. 2022). In some U.S. states, as many as 70% of people who receive medical cannabis have PTSD as their state-level qualifying condition (Mahabir et al. 2021). These findings have been replicated across multiple health care settings, including academic health centers, primary care clinics, and Veterans Affairs settings (Bassir Nia et al. 2023; Bonn-Miller et al. 2012; Browne et al. 2022; Bryan et al. 2021; De Aquino et al. 2020; Gentes et al. 2016; Padwa et al. 2022). Although there is a strong correlation between the experience of traumatic events or PTSD and cannabis use, most of the data that have established this correlation come from epidemiological studies, which are prone to various sources of bias and confounding factors (Hicks et al. 2022).

The potential implications of cannabis in the treatment of PTSD continue to be a vast and active area of research. Mirroring the often co-occurring mood and anxiety symptoms found in those with PTSD, frequently cited reasons for cannabis use in national samples of U.S. adults are to relieve anxiety, insomnia, low mood, and other symptoms of PTSD (Azcarate et al. 2020). These accounts have led to various self-medication hypotheses of using cannabis to treat the multitude of diverse, transdiagnostic symptoms of PTSD. Still, despite cannabis being available for PTSD from medical cannabis dispensaries in several U.S. states, few high-quality data are available to support its clinical use in PTSD treatment. Many systematic analyses have shown scant evidence with a high risk of bias, concluding generally that there is insufficient evidence to guide clinical decisions for or against cannabis as a treatment for PTSD (O'Neil et al. 2017; Orsolini et al. 2019; Rehman et al. 2021; Stanciu et al. 2021). Furthermore, in some reports, more than 70% of persons with PTSD who receive medical cannabis may not have undergone adequate treatment trials with evidence-based pharmaco-therapies (Elias et al. 2019).

Nonetheless, because traditional treatments for PTSD can fall short (Bradley et al. 2005) and access to cannabis has increased, the search for effective therapies has prompted both patients and researchers to con-sider the therapeutic potential of cannabis and its constituent cannabi-noids. Although this once-controversial plant has gained increasing acceptance in recent years, several questions remain about its safety and efficacy in treating PTSD.

Anxiety disorders, characterized by excessive worry, tension, fear, or nervousness often related to specific situations or events, commonly occur alongside PTSD. It is estimated that more than 33% of adults in the United States experience an anxiety disorder during their lifetime (Kessler et al. 2012). People with anxiety disorders may exhibit symp-toms such as restlessness, irritability, difficulty sleeping or concentrat-ing, and various physical symptoms, such as an increased heart rate, shortness of breath, or sweating.

The relationship between cannabis and anxiety disorders is com-plex (Berger et al. 2022a; Sharpe et al. 2020). The cannabis plant, *Cannabis sativa*, consists of more than 120 active compounds, with cannabidiol (CBD) and Δ^9-tetrahydrocannabinol (Δ^9-THC) being the most abundant phytocannabinoids (i.e., plant-based cannabinoids). When used for rec-reational purposes, cannabis can elicit effects such as relaxation and anxiolysis. However, the impact of cannabis on anxiety disorders has been assessed in limited clinical trials, and the human experimental data that are available mostly stem from acute dosing studies, such that more research is required to evaluate the effects of chronic cannabis/cannabinoid administration on people with anxiety disorders.

It is also important to note that cannabis use can sometimes trigger anxiety symptoms. A growing number of studies have reported that a subset of individuals using medical cannabis experiences anxiety as an adverse effect, particularly when using higher concentrations of THC (Patel et al. 2014). Some have postulated that this increase in the concen-tration of cannabis products has been linked with the rise in emergency department visits related to cannabis (Roehler et al. 2022). There is also a recognized link between chronic cannabis use and anxiety disor-ders, although it is unclear whether chronic cannabis use contributes to anxiety or individuals with anxiety disorders are more inclined to use cannabis regularly (Onaemo et al. 2021; Single et al. 2022). Countering evidence comes from registry studies from Canada and the United Kingdom, which have suggested some positive results for cannabis leading either to no change in Generalized Anxiety Disorder–7 scores or to clinically significant decreases (Ergisi et al. 2022; Lee et al. 2022; Rifkin-Zybutz et al. 2023).

In light of these findings, the role of cannabis in treating anxiety disorders requires careful examination. Like PTSD, anxiety disorders and their treatment are complex and multifaceted, making the inclusion of cannabis and its constituent cannabinoids in the therapeutic repertoire a topic of ongoing debate.

In this chapter, we explore the intricate relationship between cannabis use, PTSD, and anxiety disorders. Our examination encompasses an analysis of the dose- and time-dependent effects of cannabis on mood, anxiety, and sleep, as well as the potential risks and benefits of its use for individuals with PTSD or anxiety disorders. We also critically evaluate the findings of clinical studies that investigate the use of cannabinoids for treating PTSD and anxiety disorders and discuss the implications of these findings for clinical practice. Our aim is to offer a balanced, nuanced, and insightful perspective on this topic, shedding light on the current state of knowledge and providing direction for future research and clinical practice.

Current State of Evidence

Deleterious Effects

Posttraumatic Stress Disorder

The psychiatric consequences of cannabis use in PTSD have been previously reviewed (De Aquino et al. 2018; Patel et al. 2014). Although frequent cannabis use appears to blunt the stress response in humans (Benowitz et al. 1976; D'Souza et al. 2008; Ranganathan et al. 2009), the replication and clinical significance of this finding among people with PTSD remain less clear (Tull et al. 2016). Some lines of evidence indicate deleterious effects of cannabis among people with PTSD. For instance, although a number of individuals who reported having PTSD and using medical cannabis experienced greater reductions in anxiety following cannabis use, they required progressively higher doses over time to maintain these effects (LaFrance et al. 2020). The chronic effects of cannabis in people with PTSD on their anxiety, sleep, and PTSD symptoms are relatively understudied and deserve further attention, given that repeated use can lead to tolerance, physical dependence, and cannabis withdrawal syndrome (CWS).

Moreover, survey results during the first wave of the coronavirus disease 2019 (COVID-19) pandemic from individuals with a self-reported diagnosis of PTSD showed that 72% of those who used more cannabis during the pandemic experienced a worsening of depressive symptoms (as measured by the 16-item Quick Inventory of Depressive Symptomatology Self-Report), while individuals who had no change or maintained their current cannabis use experienced no significant differences (Murkar et al. 2022). Among military personnel, greater cannabis use was associated with more severe suicidal ideation, suicide-related behavior, and suicide attempts (Adkisson et al. 2019; Allan et al. 2019; Hill et al. 2022; Kimbrel et al. 2017, 2018). The results of these studies should be interpreted with caution, however, because other studies have suggested the opposite, finding that cannabis use in PTSD was associated with less severe mood and suicide-related symptoms (Lake et al. 2020).

Considerable research has focused on the impact of cannabis use on treatment engagement and treatment outcomes for individuals with PTSD. Studies suggest that co-occurring or recent cannabis use may increase the likelihood of dropping out from PTSD treatment (Bedard-Gilligan et al. 2018) and that individuals using cannabis during residential PTSD treatment programs experience less improvement in scores on the PTSD Checklist–Military Version and are more likely to continue cannabis use after treatment, particularly if they have experienced less improvement in avoidance and hyperarousal symptoms (Bonn-Miller et al. 2011). Notably, this effect was observed only for cannabis and not for other substances. Other studies show conflicting results. A study examining cognitive-behavioral therapy for co-occurring PTSD and SUD found that baseline cannabis use had no association with end-of-treatment outcomes (Ruglass et al. 2017). Various other studies have also shown no association between cannabis use and PTSD treatment outcomes (e.g., Petersen et al. 2021).

Complex Posttraumatic Stress Disorder

Complex PTSD (cPTSD) is a condition that results from chronic or long-term exposure to emotional trauma over which an individual has little or no control and from which there is little or no hope of escape, such as childhood sexual abuse, domestic violence, or being a prisoner of war. This form of PTSD is phenomenologically distinct from classic PTSD and includes prominent dissociative symptoms. Although there is biological plausibility to the concern that cannabis may worsen the dissociative symptoms of cPTSD (Dagan and Yager 2020), the data regarding the impact of cannabis use in this specific population are notably scarce, making it challenging to draw concrete conclusions.

Anxiety Disorders

Recent review articles have highlighted large inconsistencies regarding the association between cannabis and anxiety and the usefulness of cannabis as a treatment (Van Ameringen et al. 2020). Low-dose cannabis appears to have anxiolytic effects, but there are indications that higher doses may cause panic attacks (Patel et al. 2014) and that longer-term use alters the neuroendocrine response to stress in ways that further complicate this relationship (Cservenka et al. 2018; Fox et al. 2013). Cannabis use has also been prospectively shown to increase the risk of social anxiety disorder, according to data from the National Epidemiologic Survey on Alcohol and Related Conditions (Blanco et al. 2016), and social anxiety has been shown to be a risk factor for cannabis use disorder (CaUD) (Buckner et al. 2008), thus suggesting a bidirectional relationship between cannabis use and anxiety disorders.

Cannabis Withdrawal Syndrome

CWS is a major complicating issue when discussing the impact of cannabis use on symptoms of PTSD and anxiety disorders. It is a common event, with some reports indicating that up to 47% of people who use cannabis experience CWS following cessation of use (Bahji et al. 2020). The characteristic symptoms of CWS, which include irritability, anger, restlessness, sleep disruptions, and depressed mood, overlap with many symptom clusters of PTSD and may contribute to anxiety (Budney et al. 2004). In addition, in clinical trials of the use of cannabis or other cannabinoid products for PTSD, the withdrawal effects became a serious consideration when interpreting the results. Strategies for the clinical management of CWS have been published elsewhere and include psychosocial interventions and short-term use of medications to manage acute anxiety, nausea, and sleep disturbance (Connor et al. 2022).

Beneficial Effects

Posttraumatic Stress Disorder

Cannabis has been reported to be used for coping with different types of trauma (Brammer et al. 2022; Walukevich-Dienst et al. 2019), and greater severity of PTSD symptoms is associated with cannabis use, with specific symptoms, namely avoidance, appearing to be linked with a higher frequency of use (Patel et al. 2021; Rehder and Bowen 2019). Among U.S. veterans, more avoidance and behavioral disengagement are found among those using cannabis who have varying levels of PTSD symptomatology (Hill et al. 2022). Both PTSD symptoms and the expectancy that cannabis may be helpful for symptoms of PTSD appear to be correlated with cannabis use (Earleywine and Bolles 2014).

Prospective studies have shown that severe intrusive symptoms of PTSD are strongly associated with CaUD (Metrik et al. 2022). Both symptom alleviation and avoidance of trauma appear to be closely linked with reasons for cannabis use among trauma-exposed individuals (Elliott et al. 2015). The use of cannabis to manage negative affect is also endorsed among trauma-exposed individuals (Bonn-Miller et al. 2014), and those with more severe PTSD symptoms report using cannabis more often to regulate negative affect (Boden et al. 2013). Qualitative studies in veterans and their partners suggest reasons beyond obtaining euphorigenic effects (i.e., "high") for cannabis use, such as sleep induction (Krediet et al. 2020), with same-day recorded PTSD symptoms increasing the likelihood of cannabis use (Dworkin et al. 2017). Cluster analyses in those with PTSD show similar results, with elevated anxiety states increasing the likelihood of cannabis use (Buckner et al. 2018).

Having higher PTSD symptom scores and reporting using cannabis for sleep symptoms are more common among those with more frequent cannabis use (Bonn-Miller et al. 2014). Among participants using medical cannabis for PTSD, studies using sleep diaries noted that cannabis use closer to bedtime led to lower rates of nightmares, with variable other effects on sleep (e.g., awakenings and early awakenings) (Sznitman et al. 2022). This is thought to be due to smoked cannabis or oral THC causing reductions in rapid eye movement (REM) sleep, and products with higher CBD concentrations may lead to fewer early awakenings (Schierenbeck et al. 2008). Importantly, cannabis withdrawal can cause REM rebound and other issues with sleep-onset latency, which may be problematic for those with PTSD symptoms. Both open-label investigations and small crossover trials have shown signs that nabilone, an orally active synthetic formulation of THC that is used as an antiemetic, may be helpful for PTSD-related nightmares (Fraser 2009; Jetly et al. 2015).

Some studies have also suggested an association between cannabis use and lower severity of PTSD. Data from the Canadian Community

Health Survey provided some evidence that, among participants with PTSD who were using cannabis, there was no association between cannabis use and recent major depressive episodes and suicidal ideation. Those with PTSD who were not using cannabis were found to be at increased odds of experiencing such events (Lake et al. 2020). As limited as the literature currently is, the possibility that cannabis is somehow helpful in managing some symptoms or components of PTSD in a subset of patients deserves attention.

Anxiety Disorders

Multiple studies have sought to understand the relationship between cannabis use and anxiety, each bringing forth a range of results that span both potential benefits and detrimental impacts (Berger et al. 2022a; Sharpe et al. 2020). Similar to the literature on PTSD, the use of cannabis to self-medicate for anxiety symptoms appears to be commonly reported, but the relationship of its use to self-medicate anxiety disorder symptoms appears less clear and more complicated (Davis et al. 2022). Regarding beneficial effects, a study by García-Gutiérrez et al. (2020) underscored oral CBD as a potential alternative for the treatment of anxiety. Their research suggests that this nonhedonic phytocannabinoid might offer a new avenue for therapeutic approaches to anxiety disorders, along with depression and psychotic disorders.

Kuhathasan et al. (2022) investigated cannabis use for insomnia in depression and anxiety. This research points to a potential application of cannabis for mitigating sleep problems associated with these conditions. The specifics of this application, including dose and timing, need further investigation. These study limitations (around dose and timing of doses) are the same as in larger registry studies that suggest reductions in Generalized Anxiety Disorder–7 scores among individuals who use cannabis products (Lee et al. 2022; Rifkin-Zybutz et al. 2023).

To further complicate this relationship, studies have indicated that the ratio of THC to CBD is also an important factor in determining anxiogenic or anxiolytic effects, with greater amounts of CBD possibly being the factor responsible for decreasing anxiety (Hutten et al. 2022), but the influence of lower doses of THC should also be considered (Freeman et al. 2019). Another important complication is that many studies investigating CBD use oral CBD, which may differ from common naturalistic use in herbal hemp extracts or inhalation via electronic delivery devices (e.g., vape pens) (Leas et al. 2021). These findings suggest areas for future research and question the certainty of epidemiological findings for which dosage, frequency, route of administration, and ratios of THC:CBD were not fully controlled.

In summary, although there are potential benefits to cannabis use in terms of managing symptoms of anxiety, it is clear that more research is necessary. Further studies should focus on dose, strain, route of administration, and individual physiological factors to better understand how cannabis can be used effectively and safely in the treatment of anxiety disorders.

Clinical Significance

Treatment Implications for PTSD

Because of the bidirectional relationship between cannabis and PTSD, there are several uncertainties regarding the impact of cannabis on PTSD treatment outcomes. The main limitation of the research on the clinical implications of cannabis use is the challenge in determining whether PTSD symptoms or overall greater psychopathology are the primary contributors to worse outcomes or cannabis use itself is the key contributor to worse treatment outcomes.

The available data on the impact of cannabis use on psychiatric disorders are often limited, particularly with respect to the duration of use, the potency/concentration of THC, and the proportions of other cannabinoid components used by participants in these studies. Therefore, there is a pressing need for longitudinal, well-controlled studies that can provide detailed insights into the impact of cannabis on the clinical course of psychiatric disorders (Botsford et al. 2020; De Aquino et al. 2018). In addition, it is essential to identify the specific aspects of a multidimensional construct such as PTSD that are affected by cannabis use and to develop outcome measures that accurately capture these impacts. Given the numerous unknowns surrounding the impact of cannabis use on PTSD, specific guidance in this area remains limited.

Prospective Cohorts and Clinical Trials

Some prospective cohort studies have compared individuals with PTSD who use cannabis with those who do not, unveiling evidence that those who used cannabis were less likely to meet PTSD criteria by the end of the observation period (Bonn-Miller et al. 2022). Additionally, longitudinal observational data from the United Kingdom have shown cannabis use to be associated with improvements in quality of life, anxiety, and sleep among individuals with PTSD (Pillai et al. 2022).

A growing number of systematic reviews have shed some light on the usefulness of cannabis and its constituent cannabinoids for treatment of PTSD (Orsolini et al. 2019; Rehman et al. 2021; Stanciu et al. 2021). Stanciu et al. (2021) summarized the results of eight studies conducted among persons with various psychiatric disorders, one of which was a small crossover trial including persons with PTSD. Reviews performed by Orsolini et al. (2019) and Rehman et al. (2021) captured additional studies conducted with individuals with PTSD. These efforts to summarize the literature highlight that the evidence base is thus far composed of mostly nonrandomized studies with no comparators. Furthermore, assessments of safety remain limited, thereby precluding a recommendation of cannabis and its constituent cannabinoids as treatments for PTSD.

PTSD Symptoms

In a double-blind crossover trial involving military veterans who met the DSM-5 (American Psychiatric Association 2013) criteria for PTSD, the *ad libitum* use of smoked cannabis with various THC:CBD concentrations demonstrated satisfactory tolerability (Bonn-Miller et al. 2021). However, no significant alleviation in PTSD symptoms was seen, as measured by the primary outcome—the Clinician-Administered PTSD Scale for DSM-5 (CAPS-5) total severity score (Bonn-Miller et al. 2021). Initially, participants were randomly allocated to receive either active treatment or a placebo for 3 weeks during stage 1, which involved 80 participants. Following a 2-week washout period, these participants were randomly reassigned to receive one of the three alternative active treatments in stage 2, involving 74 participants. The authors noted that cannabis withdrawal symptoms could have been a potential confounding factor, which may offer useful guidance for clinical care and future study design. The symptoms of CWS, encompassing sleep disturbances, irritability, and anxiety, bear significant similarity to PTSD symptoms, thereby necessitating careful accounting for cannabis withdrawal symptoms in clinical trials evaluating cannabis-based interventions for PTSD.

In a 3-week open-label study comprising 10 participants, the oral administration of adjunctive THC was associated with lower PTSD-related hyperarousal symptoms as evidenced by CAPS (DSM-IV) arousal scores, along with a decrease in the frequency of nightmares according to the Nightmare Effects Survey (Roitman et al. 2014). Improvements were also observed in sleep quality, which was measured using the Pittsburgh Sleep Quality Index, and participants also had lower scores on the Clinical Global Impression (CGI) Scale for both CGI-Severity and CGI-Improvement following administration of oral THC. However, the total CAPS (DSM-IV) score did not improve substantially during the study period. An important takeaway from this study is the adequate safety and tolerability of oral THC. One notable aspect is that all participants were already receiving other pharmacotherapies (including at least 50% of all participants taking a benzodiazepine, which is a relative contraindication in PTSD), adding a layer of complexity to the interpretation of results compared with other controlled studies.

PTSD-Related Nightmares

In a small double-blind, placebo-controlled crossover trial involving 10 Canadian military personnel with PTSD and treatment-refractory nightmares, nabilone, a synthetic oral formulation of THC, was started at 0.5 mg/day and titrated to the effective dosage (defined as the dosage that provided nightmare suppression) or a maximum of 3 mg/day (Jetly et al. 2015). Participants were followed for 7 weeks, and then, after a 2-week washout period, the other assigned study medication (either nabilone or placebo) was administered for another 7 weeks. Nabilone administration was well tolerated and temporally associated with improvements in CAPS (DSM-IV) recurring distressing dream scores, as well as scores on the CGI-Change and the General Well Being Questionnaire. These findings were preceded by an open-label trial involving individuals whose PTSD-related nightmares persisted despite standard pharmacotherapy, with a minimum of weekly occurrences (Fraser 2009). Although 72% of the patients in this study ($n=34$; $N=47$) reported reduced nightmare severity, the measurement relied on subjective reports of the presence of nightmares and subsequent relief following nabilone use.

In addition to clinical trials, retrospective chart reviews and case series have been published reporting on the potential therapeutic effects of nabilone and CBD in individuals with PTSD. A retrospective chart review of individuals with PTSD receiving nabilone within a correctional setting demonstrated a decrease in scores on the PTSD Checklist–Civilian Version, improvements in sleep duration, and a reduction in nightmares (Cameron et al. 2014). In an open-label case series, 11 participants with PTSD who reported frequent nightmares were administered CBD over an 8-week period, which resulted in a qualitative reduction in scores on the PTSD Checklist for DSM-5 (Elms et al. 2019). It is crucial to note that these reports have significant limitations due to their nonrandomized and retrospective nature, their heterogeneous patient populations with multiple psychiatric comorbidities, and the confounding effects of previously prescribed medications with various mechanisms of action.

Clinical Studies of Cannabis and Anxiety Disorders

Treatment Implications for Anxiety Disorders

Studies examining the relationship between cannabis or cannabinoids and anxiety have limitations similar to those of the literature in PTSD. With dose-dependent biphasic effects on anxiety, cannabis has the potential to be both anxiolytic (at low doses/THC potency) and anxiogenic (at high doses/THC potency). Furthermore, although the acute administration of low-dose cannabis or THC may be anxiolytic, chronic use may produce anxiety—in part due to neuroadaptations in brain cannabinoid receptors, which are responsible for the regulation of affective states (D'Souza et al. 2016). Also, the mixed relationship between social anxiety disorders and cannabis use provides further clues that a complex association exists (Blanco et al. 2016; Buckner et al. 2008). Most systematic analyses of the evidence conclude that not enough high-quality data are available to determine whether cannabis and its constituent cannabinoids are helpful for those with anxiety disorders (Black et al. 2019). Nevertheless, cannabis has been increasingly used among people with generalized anxiety disorder (Ergisi et al. 2022).

In the section that follows, we review the observational and experimental studies investigating the relationship between cannabis and cannabinoids and anxiety disorders.

Prospective Cohorts and Clinical Trials

Nationally representative epidemiological surveys that were primarily conducted in the United States have shown a very high comorbidity and connection between cannabis use and anxiety disorders (Onaemo et al. 2021). Although these studies are limited by their cross-sectional nature, a large systematic review and meta-analysis of longitudinal studies examining the link between cannabis and the later development of anxiety disorders showed an increased odds of anxiety disorders with cannabis use (OR 1.25; 95% CI 1.01–1.54) (Xue et al. 2021). The timing of cannabis use is an important factor to recognize because other large reviews have indicated that recent use was associated with worsened outcomes for anxiety and mood disorders (Mammen et al. 2018). Compelling data from a secondary analysis of a treatment study for CaUD ($N=302$) provided some evidence that reductions in cannabis use led to decreases in anxiety (as measured by Hospital Anxiety and Depression Scale scores) and depression and improved sleep quality, whereas quality of life was not significantly different (Hser et al. 2017). Hence, further work is necessary to clarify whether these findings extend to people diagnosed with anxiety disorders.

Among phytocannabinoids, CBD appears to be the most studied for anxiety disorders in clinical trials. This is likely due to early evidence that CBD was helpful for counteracting the anxiety-inducing effects of THC (Karniol et al. 1974) and other studies that suggested THC had more anxiogenic potential than CBD or placebo in healthy volunteers (Martin-Santos et al. 2012). Despite these insights, direct comparative studies assessing the anxiety-reducing effects of THC—especially at lower doses, which are more likely to alleviate anxiety—and CBD have yet to be conducted.

A 4-week open-label clinical trial assessing a high-CBD sublingual solution in 14 outpatients with moderate to severe anxiety (score >16 on the Beck Anxiety Inventory or >11 on the Overall Anxiety Severity and Impairment Scale [OASIS]) showed significant reductions in anxiety scores (Dahlgren et al. 2022). For many participants, these reductions occurred as early as week 1, and nearly 100% of responders were identified by week 3.

Additionally, in an open-label trial investigating CBD in participants with treatment-resistant anxiety disorders ($N=31$; ages 12–25 years), defined as no clinical improvement despite CBT and/or antidepressant treatment, a significant reduction in OASIS scores was found at week 12 (Berger et al. 2022b). Participants received CBD on a fixed-flexible schedule, with a target dosage of 800 mg/day as add-on treatment. Of note, there was a relatively high rate of rather minor adverse events such as fatigue and hot flashes, among others (80.6% of participants).

A randomized crossover study (*N*=43) of self-administered CBD-free hempseed oil or placebo investigating CBD expectancy showed evidence that the belief that CBD has anxiolytic properties is associated with lower anxiety after administration of non-CBD-containing products (Spinella et al. 2021). Therefore, the impact of expectancy on the results of clinical studies should remain a factor to consider when designing future trials.

Conclusion

The relationship between cannabis, PTSD, and anxiety disorders is intricate and multilayered, requiring a nuanced understanding of the potential therapeutic benefits and adverse effects of cannabis and its various phytocannabinoids. Although some individuals with PTSD or anxiety disorders use cannabis as a coping strategy, its overall impact on their health and well-being can be a delicate balance. Some evidence shows that cannabis may help manage specific symptoms, but it also introduces potential challenges, including withdrawal symptoms and other dose-dependent detrimental effects that can mimic the phenomenology of PTSD and anxiety disorders. The timing, amount, and proportion of THC and CBD use, as well as other characteristics, are important considerations in weighing the evidence for or against their use in these conditions. Furthermore, although some studies suggest that cannabis may not significantly affect PTSD treatment outcomes, its use has also been linked with increased treatment dropout rates. The complexity of these interconnected relationships underscores the need for continued and rigorous research for clinical practice.

Emerging evidence suggests that certain constituents of cannabis, such as THC (administered as nabilone) and CBD, could potentially offer therapeutic benefits when administered orally to relieve PTSD-related nightmares. However, these promising early signals are based on preliminary findings, and more comprehensive, controlled studies are required to validate these results. One area of interest is the capability of THC to suppress REM sleep, which could in turn reduce nightmare severity, although questions persist about the duration of these effects because individuals build tolerance, and about the possibility of REM rebound and vivid dreams upon cessation of cannabis use (Bolla et al. 2010). It is also crucial to thoroughly evaluate the safety and tolerability of these cannabinoid compounds, especially when used alongside common PTSD pharmacotherapies such as selective serotonin reuptake inhibitors.

For anxiety disorders, the evidence remains mixed concerning the possible long-term reduction in anxiety in those using cannabis versus reductions in anxiety in those who reduce their cannabis use. Overall, the body of clinical studies investigating the use of CBD, a nonhedonic cannabinoid, for anxiety appears to be growing. However, thus far, the study samples have had short follow-up periods and included participants with mild forms of anxiety disorder, such that the clinical significance of longer-term anxiolytic effects of CBD remains unclear.

As it stands, the currently available data are insufficient to endorse the use of cannabis or any of its cannabinoid constituents as treatments for PTSD or anxiety disorders. Therefore, comprehensive and longitudinal studies remain necessary to fully ascertain the potential benefits and risks of cannabis and its constituent cannabinoids in individuals with these conditions.

Key Points

- The relationship between PTSD or anxiety disorder and cannabis use is bidirectional and complex. The severity and type of PTSD symptoms may influence the degree and nature of cannabis use, and cannabis withdrawal symptoms may mimic many symptoms of PTSD, further complicating clinical impressions.
- Early research presented mixed results regarding the efficacy of cannabis and its constituents, such as Δ^9-tetrahydrocannabinol/ nabilone and cannabidiol (CBD), in managing PTSD symptoms and related nightmares. The limitations of study designs and confounding factors, such as concurrent pharmacotherapies and withdrawal symptoms, complicate the interpretation of these results.
- Frequent cannabis use may exacerbate certain psychiatric symptoms and negatively affect engagement in PTSD treatment, often resulting in higher dropout rates. More research is needed to determine the nature of this possible relationship.
- A growing body of literature investigating CBD for anxiety disorders and states appears to show some promise, but it is too early to draw any firm conclusions on the state of the evidence concerning cannabis use, PTSD, and anxiety disorders.

- Further controlled research is crucial to fully understand the therapeutic value and safety of cannabis and its constituent cannabinoids for the treatment of PTSD and anxiety.

References

Adkisson K, Cunningham KC, Dedert EA, et al: Cannabis use disorder and post-deployment suicide attempts in Iraq/Afghanistan-era veterans. Arch Suicide Res 23(4):678–687, 2019 29952737

Allan NP, Ashrafioun L, Kolnogorova K, et al: Interactive effects of PTSD and substance use on suicidal ideation and behavior in military personnel: increased risk from marijuana use. Depress Anxiety 36(11):1072–1079, 2019 31475423

American Psychiatric Association: Diagnostic and Statistical Manual of Mental Disorders, 5th Edition. Arlington, VA, American Psychiatric Association, 2013

American Psychiatric Association: Diagnostic and Statistical Manual of Mental Disorders, 5th Edition, Text Revision. Washington, DC, American Psychiatric Association, 2022

Azcarate PM, Zhang AJ, Keyhani S, et al: Medical reasons for marijuana use, forms of use, and patient perception of physician attitudes among the US population. J Gen Intern Med 35(7):1979–1986, 2020 32291715

Bahji A, Stephenson C, Tyo R, et al: Prevalence of cannabis withdrawal symptoms among people with regular or dependent use of cannabinoids: a systematic review and meta-analysis. JAMA Netw Open 3(4):e202370, 2020 32271390

Bassir Nia A, Weleff J, Fogelman N, et al: Regular cannabis use is associated with history of childhood and lifetime trauma in a non-clinical community sample. J Psychiatr Res 159:159–164, 2023 36736285

Bedard-Gilligan M, Garcia N, Zoellner LA, et al: Alcohol, cannabis, and other drug use: engagement and outcome in PTSD treatment. Psychol Addict Behav 32(3):277–288, 2018 29595297

Benowitz NL, Jones RT, Lerner CB: Depression of growth hormone and cortisol response to insulin-induced hypoglycemia after prolonged oral delta-9-tetrahydrocannabinol administration in man. J Clin Endocrinol Metab 42(5):938–941, 1976 1270583

Berger M, Amminger GP, McGregor IS: Medicinal cannabis for the treatment of anxiety disorders. Aust J Gen Pract 51(8):586–592, 2022a 35908759

Berger M, Li E, Rice S, et al: Cannabidiol for treatment-resistant anxiety disorders in young people: an open-label trial. J Clin Psychiatry 83(5):21m14130, 2022b 35921510

Black N, Stockings E, Campbell G, et al: Cannabinoids for the treatment of mental disorders and symptoms of mental disorders: a systematic review and meta-analysis. Lancet Psychiatry 6(12):995–1010, 2019 31672337

Blanco C, Hasin DS, Wall MM, et al: Cannabis use and risk of psychiatric disorders: prospective evidence from a US national longitudinal study. JAMA Psychiatry 73(4):388–395, 2016 26886046

Boden MT, Babson KA, Vujanovic AA, et al: Posttraumatic stress disorder and cannabis use characteristics among military veterans with cannabis dependence. Am J Addict 22(3):277–284, 2013 23617872

Boehnke KF, Dean O, Haffajee RL, et al: U.S. trends in registration for medical cannabis and reasons for use from 2016 to 2020: an observational study. Ann Intern Med 175(7):945–951, 2022 35696691

Bolla KI, Lesage SR, Gamaldo CE, et al: Polysomnogram changes in marijuana users who report sleep disturbances during prior abstinence. Sleep Med 11(9):882–889, 2010 20685163

Bonn-Miller MO, Vujanovic AA, Drescher KD: Cannabis use among military veterans after residential treatment for posttraumatic stress disorder. Psychol Addict Behav 25(3):485–491, 2011 21261407

Bonn-Miller MO, Harris AHS, Trafton JA: Prevalence of cannabis use disorder diagnoses among veterans in 2002, 2008, and 2009. Psychol Serv 9(4):404–416, 2012 22564034

Bonn-Miller MO, Babson KA, Vandrey R: Using cannabis to help you sleep: heightened frequency of medical cannabis use among those with PTSD. Drug Alcohol Depend 136:162–165, 2014 24412475

Bonn-Miller MO, Sisley S, Riggs P, et al: The short-term impact of 3 smoked cannabis preparations versus placebo on PTSD symptoms: a randomized cross-over clinical trial. PLoS One 16(3):e0246990, 2021 33730032

Bonn-Miller MO, Brunstetter M, Simonian A, et al: The long-term, prospective, therapeutic impact of cannabis on post-traumatic stress disorder. Cannabis Cannabinoid Res 7(2):214–223, 2022 33998874

Botsford SL, Yang S, George TP: Cannabis and cannabinoids in mood and anxiety disorders: impact on illness onset and course, and assessment of therapeutic potential. Am J Addict 29(1):9–26, 2020 31577377

Bradley R, Greene J, Russ E, et al: A multidimensional meta-analysis of psychotherapy for PTSD. Am J Psychiatry 162(2):214–227, 2005 15677582

Brammer WA, Conn BM, Iverson E, et al: Coping motives mediate the association of trauma history with problematic cannabis use in young adult medical cannabis patients and non-patient cannabis users. Subst Use Misuse 57(5):684–697, 2022 35193442

Breslau N, Davis GC, Andreski P, et al: Traumatic events and posttraumatic stress disorder in an urban population of young adults. Arch Gen Psychiatry 48(3):216–222, 1991 1996917

Browne K, Leyva Y, Malte CA, et al: Prevalence of medical and nonmedical cannabis use among veterans in primary care. Psychol Addict Behav 36(2):121–130, 2022 34435834

Bryan JL, Hogan J, Lindsay JA, et al: Cannabis use disorder and posttraumatic stress disorder: the prevalence of comorbidity in veterans of recent conflicts. J Subst Abuse Treat 122:108254, 2021 33509412

Buckner JD, Schmidt NB, Lang AR, et al: Specificity of social anxiety disorder as a risk factor for alcohol and cannabis dependence. J Psychiatr Res 42(3):230–239, 2008 17320907

Buckner JD, Jeffries ER, Crosby RD, et al: The impact of PTSD clusters on cannabis use in a racially diverse trauma-exposed sample: an analysis from ecological momentary assessment. Am J Drug Alcohol Abuse 44(5):532–542, 2018 29442522

Budney AJ, Hughes JR, Moore BA, et al: Review of the validity and significance of cannabis withdrawal syndrome. Am J Psychiatry 161(11):1967–1977, 2004 15514394

Cameron C, Watson D, Robinson J: Use of a synthetic cannabinoid in a correctional population for posttraumatic stress disorder-related insomnia and nightmares, chronic pain, harm reduction, and other indications: a retrospective evaluation. J Clin Psychopharmacol 34(5):559–564, 2014 24987795

Connor JP, Stjepanović D, Budney AJ, et al: Clinical management of cannabis withdrawal. Addiction 117(7):2075–2095, 2022 34791767

Cservenka A, Lahanas S, Dotson-Bossert J: Marijuana use and hypothalamic-pituitary-adrenal axis functioning in humans. Front Psychiatry 9:472, 2018 30327619

Dagan Y, Yager J: Cannabis and complex posttraumatic stress disorder: a narrative review with considerations of benefits and harms. J Nerv Ment Dis 208(8):619–627, 2020 32433200

Dahlgren MK, Lambros AM, Smith RT, et al: Clinical and cognitive improvement following full-spectrum, high-cannabidiol treatment for anxiety: open-label data from a two-stage, phase 2 clinical trial. Commun Med (Lond) 2(1):139, 2022 36352103

Davis JP, Pedersen ER, Tucker JS, et al: Directional associations between cannabis use and anxiety symptoms from late adolescence through young adulthood. Drug Alcohol Depend 241:109704, 2022 36434880

De Aquino JP, Sherif M, Radhakrishnan R, et al: The psychiatric consequences of cannabinoids. Clin Ther 40(9):1448–1456, 2018 29678279

De Aquino JP, Sofuoglu M, Stefanovics EA, et al: Impact of cannabis on nonmedical opioid use and symptoms of posttraumatic stress disorder: a nationwide longitudinal VA study. Am J Drug Alcohol Abuse 46(6):812–822, 2020 33035104

D'Souza DC, Ranganathan M, Braley G, et al: Blunted psychotomimetic and amnestic effects of delta-9-tetrahydrocannabinol in frequent users of cannabis. Neuropsychopharmacology 33(10):2505–2516, 2008 18185500

D'Souza DC, Cortes-Briones JA, Ranganathan M, et al: Rapid changes in cannabinoid 1 receptor availability in cannabis-dependent male subjects after abstinence from cannabis. Biol Psychiatry Cogn Neurosci Neuroimaging 1(1):60–67, 2016 29560896

Dworkin ER, Kaysen D, Bedard-Gilligan M, et al: Daily level associations between PTSD and cannabis use among young sexual minority women. Addict Behav 74:118–121, 2017 28618391

Earleywine M, Bolles JR: Marijuana, expectancies, and post-traumatic stress symptoms: a preliminary investigation. J Psychoactive Drugs 46(3):171–177, 2014 25052875

Elias DA, MacLaren VV, Hill-Elias R, et al: Adherence to prescription guidelines for medical cannabis in disability claimants. Can Fam Physician 65(8):e339–e343, 2019 31413039

Elliott L, Golub A, Bennett A, et al: PTSD and cannabis-related coping among recent veterans in New York City. Contemp Drug Probl 42(1):60–76, 2015 28638168

Elms L, Shannon S, Hughes S, et al: Cannabidiol in the treatment of post-traumatic stress disorder: a case series. J Altern Complement Med 25(4):392–397, 2019 30543451

Ergisi M, Erridge S, Harris M, et al: UK Medical Cannabis Registry: an analysis of clinical outcomes of medicinal cannabis therapy for generalized anxiety disorder. Expert Rev Clin Pharmacol 15(4):487–495, 2022 34937473

Fox HC, Tuit KL, Sinha R: Stress system changes associated with marijuana dependence may increase craving for alcohol and cocaine. Hum Psychopharmacol 28(1):40–53, 2013 23280514

Fraser GA: The use of a synthetic cannabinoid in the management of treatment-resistant nightmares in posttraumatic stress disorder (PTSD). CNS Neurosci Ther 15(1):84–88, 2009 19228182

Freeman AM, Petrilli K, Lees R, et al: How does cannabidiol (CBD) influence the acute effects of delta-9-tetrahydrocannabinol (THC) in humans? A systematic review. Neurosci Biobehav Rev 107:696–712, 2019 31580839

García-Gutiérrez MS, Navarrete F, Gasparyan A, et al: Cannabidiol: a potential new alternative for the treatment of anxiety, depression, and psychotic disorders. Biomolecules 10(11):1575, 2020 33228239

Gentes EL, Schry AR, Hicks TA, et al: Prevalence and correlates of cannabis use in an outpatient VA posttraumatic stress disorder clinic. Psychol Addict Behav 30(3):415–421, 2016 27214172

Hicks TA, Zaur AJ, Keeley JW, et al: The association between recreational cannabis use and posttraumatic stress disorder: a systematic review and methodological critique of the literature. Drug Alcohol Depend 240:109623, 2022 36162309

Hill ML, Loflin M, Nichter B, et al: Cannabis use among U.S. military veterans with subthreshold or threshold posttraumatic stress disorder: psychiatric comorbidities, functioning, and strategies for coping with posttraumatic stress symptoms. J Trauma Stress 35(4):1154–1166, 2022 35275431

Hser Y-I, Mooney LJ, Huang D, et al: Reductions in cannabis use are associated with improvements in anxiety, depression, and sleep quality, but not quality of life. J Subst Abuse Treat 81:53–58, 2017 28847455

Hutten NRPW, Arkell TR, Vinckenbosch F, et al: Cannabis containing equivalent concentrations of delta-9-tetrahydrocannabinol (THC) and cannabidiol (CBD) induces less state anxiety than THC-dominant cannabis. Psychopharmacology (Berl) 239(11):3731–3741, 2022 36227352

Jetly R, Heber A, Fraser G, et al: The efficacy of nabilone, a synthetic cannabinoid, in the treatment of PTSD-associated nightmares: a preliminary randomized, double-blind, placebo-controlled cross-over design study. Psychoneuroendocrinology 51:585–588, 2015 25467221

Karniol IG, Shirakawa I, Kasinski N, et al: Cannabidiol interferes with the effects of delta 9-tetrahydrocannabinol in man. Eur J Pharmacol 28(1):172–177, 1974 4609777

Kessler RC, Chiu WT, Demler O, et al: Prevalence, severity, and comorbidity of 12-month DSM-IV disorders in the National Comorbidity Survey Replication. Arch Gen Psychiatry 62(6):617–627, 2005 15939839

Kessler RC, Petukhova M, Sampson NA, et al: Twelve-month and lifetime prevalence and lifetime morbid risk of anxiety and mood disorders in the United States. Int J Methods Psychiatr Res 21(3):169–184, 2012 22865617

Kimbrel NA, Newins AR, Dedert EA, et al: Cannabis use disorder and suicide attempts in Iraq/Afghanistan-era veterans. J Psychiatr Res 89:1–5, 2017 28129565

Kimbrel NA, Meyer EC, DeBeer BB, et al: The impact of cannabis use disorder on suicidal and nonsuicidal self-injury in Iraq/Afghanistan-era veterans with and without mental health disorders. Suicide Life Threat Behav 48(2):140–148, 2018 28295524

Krediet E, Janssen DG, Heerdink ER, et al: Experiences with medical cannabis in the treatment of veterans with PTSD: results from a focus group discussion. Eur Neuropsychopharmacol 36:244–254, 2020 32576481

Kuhathasan N, Minuzzi L, MacKillop J, et al: An investigation of cannabis use for insomnia in depression and anxiety in a naturalistic sample. BMC Psychiatry 22(1):303, 2022 35484520

LaFrance EM, Glodosky NC, Bonn-Miller M, et al: Short and long-term effects of cannabis on symptoms of post-traumatic stress disorder. J Affect Disord 274:298–304, 2020 32469819

Lake S, Kerr T, Buxton J, et al: Does cannabis use modify the effect of post-traumatic stress disorder on severe depression and suicidal ideation? Evidence from a population-based cross-sectional study of Canadians. J Psychopharmacol 34(2):181–188, 2020 31684805

Leas EC, Moy N, McMenamin SB, et al: Availability and promotion of cannabidiol (CBD) products in online vape shops. Int J Environ Res Public Health 18(13):6719, 2021 34206501

Lee C, Round JM, Hanlon JG, et al: Generalized Anxiety Disorder 7-item (GAD-7) scores in medically authorized cannabis patients: Ontario and Alberta, Canada. Can J Psychiatry 67(6):470–480, 2022 34520280

Leung J, Chan G, Stjepanović D, et al: Prevalence and self-reported reasons of cannabis use for medical purposes in USA and Canada. Psychopharmacology (Berl) 239(5):1509–1519, 2022 35020045

Mahabir VK, Smith CS, Vannabouathong C, et al: Comparing medical cannabis use in 5 US states: a retrospective database study. J Cannabis Res 3(1):15, 2021 34044878

Mammen G, Rueda S, Roerecke M, et al: Association of cannabis with long-term clinical symptoms in anxiety and mood disorders: a systematic review of prospective studies. J Clin Psychiatry 79(4):17r11839, 2018 29877641

Martin-Santos R, Crippa JA, Batalla A, et al: Acute effects of a single, oral dose of Δ9-tetrahydrocannabinol (THC) and cannabidiol (CBD) administration in healthy volunteers. Curr Pharm Des 18(32):4966–4979, 2012 22716148

Metrik J, Stevens AK, Gunn RL, et al: Cannabis use and posttraumatic stress disorder: prospective evidence from a longitudinal study of veterans. Psychol Med 52(3):446–456, 2022 32546286

Murkar A, Kendzerska T, Shlik J, et al: Increased cannabis intake during the COVID-19 pandemic is associated with worsening of depression symptoms in people with PTSD. BMC Psychiatry 22(1):554, 2022 35978287

Onaemo VN, Fawehinmi TO, D'Arcy C: Comorbid cannabis use disorder with major depression and generalized anxiety disorder: a systematic review with meta-analysis of nationally representative epidemiological surveys. J Affect Disord 281:467–475, 2021 33360749

O'Neil ME, Nugent SM, Morasco BJ, et al: Benefits and harms of plant-based cannabis for posttraumatic stress disorder: a systematic review. Ann Intern Med 167(5):332–340, 2017 28806794

Orsolini L, Chiappini S, Volpe U, et al: Use of medicinal cannabis and synthetic cannabinoids in post-traumatic stress disorder (PTSD): a systematic review. Medicina (Kaunas) 55(9):525, 2019 31450833

Padwa H, Huang D, Mooney L, et al: Medical conditions of primary care patients with documented cannabis use and cannabis use disorder in electronic health records: a case control study from an academic health system in a medical marijuana state. Subst Abuse Treat Prev Policy 17(1):36, 2022 35527269

Patel H, Holshausen K, Oshri A, et al: Posttraumatic stress disorder symptomatology and substance use in an outpatient concurrent disorders sample. Can J Psychiatry 66(9):788–797, 2021 33878938

Patel S, Hill MN, Hillard CJ: Effects of phytocannabinoids on anxiety, mood, and the endocrine system, in Handbook of Cannabis. Edited by Pertwee R. New York, Oxford University Press, 2014, pp 189–207

Petersen M, Koller K, Straley C, et al: Effect of cannabis use on PTSD treatment outcomes in veterans. Ment Health Clin 11(4):238–242, 2021 34316419

Pietrzak RH, Goldstein RB, Southwick SM, et al: Prevalence and Axis I comorbidity of full and partial posttraumatic stress disorder in the United States: results from Wave 2 of the National Epidemiologic Survey on Alcohol and Related Conditions. J Anxiety Disord 25(3):456–465, 2011 21168991

Pillai M, Erridge S, Bapir L, et al: Assessment of clinical outcomes in patients with post-traumatic stress disorder: analysis from the UK Medical Cannabis Registry. Expert Rev Neurother 22(11–12):1009–1018, 2022 36503404

Qassem T, Aly ElGabry D, Alzarouni A, et al: Psychiatric co-morbidities in post-traumatic stress disorder: detailed findings from the Adult Psychiatric Morbidity Survey in the English Population. Psychiatr Q 92(1):321–330, 2021 32705407

Ranganathan M, Braley G, Pittman B, et al: The effects of cannabinoids on serum cortisol and prolactin in humans. Psychopharmacology (Berl) 203(4):737–744, 2009 19083209

Rehder K, Bowen S: PTSD symptom severity, cannabis, and gender: a zero-inflated negative binomial regression model. Subst Use Misuse 54(8):1309–1318, 2019 30767607

Rehman Y, Saini A, Huang S, et al: Cannabis in the management of PTSD: a systematic review. AIMS Neuroscience 8(3):414–434, 2021

Rifkin-Zybutz R, Erridge S, Holvey C, et al: Clinical outcome data of anxiety patients treated with cannabis-based medicinal products in the United Kingdom: a cohort study from the UK Medical Cannabis Registry. Psychopharmacology (Berl) 240(8):1735–1745, 2023 37314478

Roehler DR, Hoots BE, Holland KM, et al: Trends and characteristics of cannabis-associated emergency department visits in the United States, 2006–2018. Drug Alcohol Depend 232:109288, 2022 35033959

Roitman P, Mechoulam R, Cooper-Kazaz R, et al: Preliminary, open-label, pilot study of add-on oral Δ9-tetrahydrocannabinol in chronic post-traumatic stress disorder. Clin Drug Investig 34(8):587–591, 2014 24935052

Ruglass LM, Shevorykin A, Radoncic V, et al: Impact of cannabis use on treatment outcomes among adults receiving cognitive-behavioral treatment for PTSD and substance use disorders. J Clin Med 6(2):14, 2017 28178207

Schierenbeck T, Riemann D, Berger M, et al: Effect of illicit recreational drugs upon sleep: cocaine, ecstasy and marijuana. Sleep Med Rev 12(5):381–389, 2008 18313952

Sharpe L, Sinclair J, Kramer A, et al: Cannabis, a cause for anxiety? A critical appraisal of the anxiogenic and anxiolytic properties. J Transl Med 18(1):374, 2020 33008420

Single A, Bilevicius E, Ho V, et al: Cannabis use and social anxiety in young adulthood: a meta-analysis. Addict Behav 129:107275, 2022 35184002

Spinella TC, Stewart SH, Naugler J, et al: Evaluating cannabidiol (CBD) expectancy effects on acute stress and anxiety in healthy adults: a randomized crossover study. Psychopharmacology (Berl) 238(7):1965–1977, 2021 33813611

Spottswood M, Davydow DS, Huang H: The prevalence of posttraumatic stress disorder in primary care: a systematic review. Harv Rev Psychiatry 25(4):159–169, 2017 28557811

Stanciu CN, Brunette MF, Teja N, et al: Evidence for use of cannabinoids in mood disorders, anxiety disorders, and PTSD: a systematic review. Psychiatr Serv 72(4):429–436, 2021 33530732

Sznitman SR, Meiri D, Amit BH, et al: Posttraumatic stress disorder, sleep and medical cannabis treatment: a daily diary study. J Anxiety Disord 92:102632, 2022 36182689

Tull MT, McDermott MJ, Gratz KL: Marijuana dependence moderates the effect of posttraumatic stress disorder on trauma cue reactivity in substance dependent patients. Drug Alcohol Depend 159:219–226, 2016 26790822

Van Ameringen M, Zhang J, Patterson B, et al: The role of cannabis in treating anxiety: an update. Curr Opin Psychiatry 33(1):1–7, 2020 31688192

Walukevich-Dienst K, Dylanne Twitty T, Buckner JD: Sexual minority women and cannabis use: the serial impact of PTSD symptom severity and coping motives. Addict Behav 92:1–5, 2019 30553032

Xue S, Husain MI, Zhao H, et al: Cannabis use and prospective long-term association with anxiety: a systematic review and meta-analysis of longitudinal studies [in French]. Can J Psychiatry 66(2):126–138, 2021 32909828

9

Cannabis Use and Aggressive Behaviors Toward Self and Others

Mélissa Beaudoin, M.Sc.

Laura Dellazizzo, M.D., Ph.D.

Sabrina Giguère, M.Sc.

Stéphane Potvin, Ph.D.

Alexandre Dumais, M.D., Ph.D.

Violence represents a significant social burden affecting people of all ages and sexes. In the United States, more than seven people per hour die from violence (National Center for Injury Prevention and Control 2021). Worldwide, there are approximately 475,000 homicides yearly (Butchart et al. 2015). One in three women will be a victim of physical and/or sexual violence at least once in their lifetime after age 15, and as much as 50% of all children between ages 2 and 17 have experienced violence (Hillis et al. 2016; Sardinha et al. 2022). An even more significant problem is violence against oneself (e.g., self-harm, suicidal behaviors), which causes more than 700,000 deaths per year, representing more than 1 in 100 deaths in 2019 (World Health Organization 2021). This burden disproportionately affects youth; in 2019, suicide was the fourth leading cause of death among males and females between ages

15 and 19 (World Health Organization 2021). Overall, many factors may affect the likelihood of a person committing an act of violence directed toward others or oneself. According to a recent meta-analysis, substance use is the most significant factor, with seven times the risk of hetero-aggressive violent behavior, surpassing antisocial behavior, violent victimization in childhood, and severe mental illnesses (Fazel et al. 2018). Substance use is also a significant risk factor for suicidal thoughts, suicide attempts, and fatal acts of self-harm (Favril et al. 2022; Ilgen et al. 2010).

Substance use and abuse are important public health concerns associated with multiple adverse outcomes. The Global Burden of Disease study recently estimated that 494,000 deaths could be attributed to substance use in 2019 alone, representing an increase of more than 15% in the previous 10 years (Global Burden of Disease Collaborative Network 2022). As a result of premature deaths and disability attributable to substance use, 30.9 million quality-adjusted life years were lost. Substance use also affects hospitalizations, which are becoming more frequent and of longer duration (Young and Jesseman 2014). This problem has a substantial financial burden and uses many resources, especially in the health care and justice systems. Moreover, a drop in general productivity can affect all workplaces (Harms Scientific Working Group 2020), and an increase in the risk of violent behaviors affects everyone. Considering the risks associated with substance use overall, it is essential to investigate the effects of each of these substances individually to formulate evidence-based recommendations.

Among substance use disorders (SUDs), cannabis use disorder (CaUD) is the most common after alcohol use disorder, with an age-standardized prevalence of 289.7 cases per 100,000 people worldwide, representing 22.1 million cases (GBD 2016 Alcohol and Drug Use Collaborators 2018). *Cannabis* refers to multiple species of plants (i.e., *Cannabis sativa*, *Cannabis indica*, and *Cannabis ruderalis*) containing various active molecules named cannabinoids. Among them, the most known and studied are Δ^9-tetrahydrocannabinol (Δ^9-THC) and cannabidiol (CBD), with THC being responsible for the psychoactive effects of the drug (Sheikh and Dua 2023). Synthetic cannabinoids, on the other hand, are a chemically diverse group of synthetic substances targeting the endocannabinoid system that produce effects like those of cannabis (National Institute on Drug Abuse 2018; Roque-Bravo et al. 2023). However, these unregulated psychoactive substances seem to be associated with more adverse health effects than regular cannabis. According to the 2016 Global Burden of Disease study, CaUD is especially prevalent in North America, with an age-standardized prevalence of 884.3 per 100,000 (GBD 2016 Alcohol and Drug Use Collaborators 2018). Globally, it was estimated that a loss of 646,500 disability-adjusted life years (8.5 per 100,000 people) was attributable to CaUD in 2016.

Cannabis consumption has steadily increased over the past few years (Hasin et al. 2019; United Nations 2022b). The coronavirus disease 2019 (COVID-19) pandemic and the legalization of cannabis in a few parts of the world (e.g., Canada and some U.S. states) have played a role in the increased prevalence of cannabis use (United Nations 2022a). Notably, the growing popularity of cannabis could be due to greater social acceptance regarding its use (Carliner et al. 2017; Mennis et al. 2023; United Nations 2022a), as well as increased accessibility (Myran et al. 2022; Wadsworth et al. 2022). In addition, the most frequently experienced immediate effects of cannabis are euphoria and relaxation; therefore, the idea that it might be associated with violence can be counterintuitive for consumers (Ashton 2001; Green et al. 2004; Grotenhermen 2003; Morgan et al. 2013). However, the literature shows that it can also be linked with psychosis, irritability, deficits in cognition, and even violence toward others and oneself (Carvalho et al. 2022; Dellazizzo et al. 2019; Escelsior et al. 2021; Hasan et al. 2020; Marconi et al. 2016; Rafiei and Kolla 2022; Schoeler et al. 2016). These aspects have not been thoroughly studied or transferred into clinical practice (Fischer et al. 2019). Although public health measures are in place, and the risks of cannabis use while driving or the risk of developing or exacerbating a psychotic episode with use are commonly discussed in the media, attention to the risks of violence with cannabis use is significantly more limited (Dellazizzo et al. 2020a; Lake et al. 2019). Although some studies have shown a significant relationship between cannabis use and violent behaviors (Carvalho et al. 2022; Escelsior et al. 2021; Rafiei and Kolla 2022; Schoeler et al. 2016), the literature remains scarce.

In this chapter, we summarize current data on the possible relationship between cannabis and violence toward others and oneself. We also address the potential mechanisms underlying this relationship, as well as the limitations of the literature. Our focus is mainly on systematic reviews and meta-analyses, when available. However, we discuss large cohort studies when the literature is scarce on certain topics.

Deleterious Effects

Relationship Between Cannabis and Aggression

Aggression is a broad term describing a wide range of behaviors aimed at physically, psychologically, or emotionally harming others. Common types of violence include physical, sexual, and verbal aggression and cyberaggression (Krug et al. 2002; World Health Organization 2022). For the purposes of this chapter, we emphasize physical violence because it has been more extensively studied in the literature. This includes any physical contact intended to cause pain or injury, such as hitting, kicking, pushing, throwing objects toward someone, or using a weapon. Threatening someone with a potentially lethal weapon (e.g., firearm, knife) is also generally considered to be physically violent.

The relationship between substance abuse and aggression has been described on multiple occasions in the scientific literature (Duke et al. 2017; Grann and Fazel 2004; Kedia et al. 2021; McGinty et al. 2016). For example, a large meta-analysis of meta-analyses concluded that there was a significant relationship between substance use and violence, with a moderate effect size (d=0.45; P<0.001) (Duke et al. 2017). Some patient characteristics increased this association, including male sex, combined alcohol and illicit drug use, and psychotic disorders. Although cannabis is the most widely used substance after alcohol (Centers for Disease Control and Prevention 2021), it is difficult to determine whether it plays a role in this relationship. Indeed, other substances such as alcohol and cocaine have been linked with violent behaviors in previous studies (Czermainski et al. 2020; Miller et al. 1991; Sontate et al. 2021; Witt et al. 2013; Zhong et al. 2020), and therefore their consumption could be responsible for the high incidence of aggressiveness in people with SUDs. However, the impact of each substance specifically on this type of behavior has been very seldom studied, and this is especially true for cannabis. Indeed, a potential link between cannabis and violent behaviors might seem counterintuitive. Nevertheless, such an association has been measured on multiple occasions (Beaudoin et al. 2019, 2020; Dellazizzo et al. 2019, 2020b; Dugré et al. 2017; Johnson et al. 2017; Sorkhou et al. 2022; Zhong et al. 2020). A few potential mechanisms for the cannabis-violence relationship are described later in this chapter.

Violence in the General Population

Among the general adult population, a scoping review of 19 studies concluded that a correlation exists between cannabis use and violence (Rafiei and Kolla 2022). However, despite the increasing body of evidence of this correlation, the current literature is not sufficient to confirm direct causation. Moreover, the strength of the relationship between cannabis use and violence varies according to the study population. For example, the relationship seems to be stronger among individuals with severe and persistent mental illness, offender populations (e.g., prison inmates), individuals with CaUD (indicating more frequent and severe use), and individuals experiencing cannabis withdrawal.

Cannabis Use and Violent Behaviors in Adolescents and Young Adults

Cannabis use may also be associated with subsequent violence in young adults (Dellazizzo et al. 2020b), who are already at higher risk for cannabis-induced psychosis (West and Sharif 2023). A meta-analysis of 30 studies of young individuals (adolescents and adults younger than 30 years) concluded that cannabis users were 2.11 times more at risk of violence (95% CI 1.64–2.72; Dellazizzo et al. 2020b). Moreover, it was found that the risk of violence might be higher for persistent heavy users (OR 2.8; 95% CI 1.7–4.7) compared with past-year users (OR 2.1; 95% CI 1.5–2.8) and lifetime users (OR 1.9; 95% CI 1.3–2.9). However, the reverse relationship between violence and risk of cannabis use has seldom been investigated, and results are highly heterogeneous. Of note, most studies did not consider the role of alcohol and other substances in this relationship. Another systematic review and meta-analysis also concluded that cannabis use alone significantly predicted physical dating violence in people younger than 21 years (OR 1.45; 95% CI 1.20–1.76) (Johnson et al. 2017). It has been suggested that using synthetic cannabinoids during adolescence could lead to even more violent behaviors and injuries (Clayton et al. 2017). However, more studies are needed to investigate the risks associated with synthetic cannabinoids, which have seldom been studied.

Violence and Mental Illness

The association between substance use and violent behaviors has been investigated in patients with psychiatric disorders (Beaudoin et al. 2020; Dellazizzo et al. 2019; Dugré et al. 2017; Sorkhou et al. 2022). In this population, the risk of violence seems to be higher when individuals consume multiple substances (e.g., alcohol, cannabis, or illicit drugs) (Beaudoin et al. 2019; Witt et al. 2013). However, as in the general population, the role of each substance individually has seldom been investigated, particularly the role of cannabis. It has been observed that cumulative cannabis use over 1 year could be an independent risk factor for violence in a psychiatric population (Dugré et al. 2017). Indeed, an analysis performed on participants recruited as part of the MacArthur Violence Risk Assessment Study (data collected between 1992 and 1995 on 1,136 psychiatric patients in the United States) revealed that cumulative cannabis use was associated with an increased risk of violence. In fact, patients who reported having used cannabis at all four follow-up visits, which occurred every 3 months, were 2.44 times more likely to have been violent (95% CI 1.06–5.63; $P<0.05$). The reverse relationship was also tested, but the results were not statistically significant.

Our research team conducted a meta-analysis to review the literature on the association between substance use and violence in individuals with severe mental illnesses (Dellazizzo et al. 2019). The analysis of 12 studies concluded that a moderate association existed between cannabis use and violence in this population, with an odds ratio of 3.02 (95% CI 2.01–4.54; $P=0.0001$). Moreover, this association was much higher when studies specifically considered cannabis misuse (OR 5.8; 95% CI 3.27–10.28) compared with overall cannabis use (OR 2.04; 95% CI 1.36–3.05). However, these studies were highly heterogeneous, notably due to using various definitions for violence. Eight of the studies were cross-sectional, and many were excluded from analysis because they did not distinguish physical violence from overall aggressiveness, which could include verbal violence, violence toward an object, or even irritability. A systematic review by Sorkhou et al. (2022) also concluded that causation could not be established because of methodological limitations.

To address these limitations, our research team replicated these results prospectively in two other psychiatric populations. First, a cross-lagged analysis was conducted in a sample of 965 individuals with schizophrenia recruited as part of the Clinical Antipsychotic Trials of Intervention Effectiveness (CATIE) Schizophrenia Trial, a naturalistically designed clinical trial conducted by the National Institute of Mental Health between 2000 and 2004 in the United States (Beaudoin et al. 2020). It was observed that cumulative cannabis use over a year predicted subsequent violent behaviors and that this association remained significant after controlling for alcohol and stimulant use. Indeed, cumulative cannabis use reported at three follow-up visits occurring every 3 months was a significant predictor of violence during the following 6 months ($P<0.05$). Moreover, cannabis use at baseline predicted subsequent violence even after adjustment for all relevant confounding variables (alcohol and stimulant use, sex, age, education, and childhood antisocial behaviors; $P<0.01$). Conversely, the relationship between violence and subsequent cannabis use was not statistically significant, indicating that this association could be unidirectional. The results of two more case-control studies came to a similar conclusion (Lamsma et al. 2020). Indeed, the analysis of 1,145 individuals with psychotic disorders showed that daily use of cannabis significantly increased the odds of violence compared with nondaily use (OR 1.6; 95% CI 1.2–2.0) or no use (OR 1.7; 95% CI 1.3–2.3). In contrast, nondaily use was not significantly associated with violent behaviors (OR 1.2; 95% CI 0.9–1.7). However, like most of the literature on this association, the temporal relationship was unknown.

Second, our research team conducted a prospective longitudinal study investigating the potential dose-response relationship between cannabis use and violence in individuals with severe mental disorders (Beaudoin et al. 2023). To do so, 98 outpatients with severe mental disorders were recruited at the Institut universitaire en santé mentale de Montréal in Canada. Generalized estimating equations were used to assess the risk of physical hetero-aggression (self-reported and/or assessed using medical, police, or criminal records) based on the frequency profile of cannabis use (self-reported amounts; nonusers vs. occasional vs. regular vs. frequent users). Nonuser status was confirmed through urinary testing. Results were adjusted for the co-occurring effects of time, sex, age, ethnicity, primary diagnosis, personality disorders, impulsivity, alcohol, and stimulant use. It was determined that participants were 1.91 times more likely to engage in violent behaviors for each increase of one profile (95% CI 1.33–2.74; $P<0.001$). The same analysis was conducted to evaluate the association between the severities of cannabis use, measured using the Cannabis Use Problems Identification Test (CUPIT), a self-report scale ranging from 0 to 79 (Bashford et al. 2010). Again, a highly significant dose-response relationship was observed, with an odds ratio of 1.040 for each increase of one unit on that scale (95% CI 1.016–1.064; $P<0.001$) (Beaudoin et al. 2023). Finally, in individuals with newly diagnosed psychosis specifically, earlier use of cannabis was again shown to be a significant risk factor for violent behaviors (OR 4.47; 95% CI 1.13–20.06) (Moulin et al. 2020). These results show that the relationship between cannabis use and violence seems to be stronger in a vulnerable population—that is, in individuals with an underlying mental health disorder. However, once again, multiple confounding factors were not considered (e.g., genetic factors, peer influence). These results need to be replicated, and the mechanism underlying this association must still be elucidated.

Aggressiveness and Delinquent Behaviors

Multiple studies have been conducted on the relationship between cannabis use and aggressiveness. *Aggressivity* is generally described as a broader term than *violence*: whereas *violence* usually refers to physical hetero-violence (e.g., hitting someone) and serious threats (e.g., death threats or threats using a deadly weapon), *aggression* can include verbal violence, delinquency, cyberviolence, and sometimes even self-directed violence (Krug et al. 2002). A recent meta-analysis showed a nonsignificant correlation between cyberaggression and cannabis use (OR 0.13; 95% CI −0.02 to 0.28; κ=3) (Crane et al. 2021). However, this association has not been investigated often, and more studies are needed.

Cannabis use was also a key discriminating factor in increasing the risk of disruptive behaviors in a large sample of adolescents (Dugré et al. 2021). Moreover, multiple studies found significant associations between cannabis use and aggression (physical or verbal, perpetration or victimization) in the context of intimate partner violence (Flanagan et al. 2020; Reingle et al. 2012; Shorey et al. 2014, 2018; Testa et al. 2018). Notably, a study conducted with 9,421 adolescents showed that the use of cannabis between the ages of 15 and 21 was strongly associated with being both a victim and a perpetrator of intimate partner violence at age 26 (consistent cannabis use: OR 2.08; 95% CI 1.53–2.85; $P<0.001$) (Reingle et al. 2012). Some studies on intimate partner violence also suggested that the impact of cannabis use might be more robust and substantial for psychological and verbal aggression than for physical violence (Flanagan et al. 2020; Shorey et al. 2014). However, although cannabis could significantly affect milder forms of aggression, these types of violence have been much less studied than physical violence, probably because they are not as commonly reported and usually do not result in legal charges. Therefore, studying psychological and verbal violence across different contexts may be more challenging. As for overall delinquent behaviors (including violence but also stealing, damaging property, and so on), cannabis use has been shown to be significantly correlated with such acts, particularly in adolescents (Chabrol et al. 2010; Derzon and Lipsey 1999; Rocca et al. 2019).

Early Cannabis Use as a Predictor of Violence

Exposure to cannabis use early in life could also impact the risk of violence later in life. Schoeler et al. (2016) demonstrated this notion by following a cohort of 411 participants throughout their lives using multiwave assessments at ages 8, 10, 14, 16, 18, 21, 32, and 48. By conducting multivariable logistic regression, they found that cannabis use was a significant predictor of subsequent violence, suggesting a possible causal effect. Indeed, the more persistent the cannabis use was over time, the more likely the individual was to commit acts of violence in the future. A more recent longitudinal study investigating health-related outcomes of young males found a significant correlation between adolescent cannabis use and subsequent adult hostility and aggression (Capaldi et al. 2022).

Moreover, early cannabis use could also be associated with other crimes (e.g., drug-related or property crimes) and antisocial behaviors (Brook et al. 2011; Green et al. 2010). These risks were discussed in recent government resources published in Canada and the United States (George and Vaccarino 2015; National Center for Injury Prevention and Control 2021). Finally, it has been suggested that prenatal and immediate postnatal cannabis exposure could influence future aggressive behaviors in animal models (Barthelemy et al. 2016; De Genna et al. 2022). Although these findings are worrisome and provide some evidence against cannabis use during pregnancy and breastfeeding, more research is needed to determine whether this applies to humans. Nevertheless, compared with children not exposed to cannabis in utero, children with prenatal cannabis exposure were found to be more irritable at birth and to display more externalizing behaviors when they grew up, including aggression, impulsivity, and delinquency (El Marroun et al. 2011; Goldschmidt et al. 2000; Murnan et al. 2021).

Relationship Between Cannabis and Violence Toward Oneself

Suicidal behaviors have an extensive range in severity that progresses from the lowest form—suicidal ideation—to the fatal action of completed suicide. Despite numerous studies in this area, information on how to clearly define the phenomenon of suicidality still varies, with countless terms used to describe the same behaviors. Self-directed violence includes fatal and nonfatal suicidal behaviors; nonsuicidal, intentional self-harm; and suicidal ideation (Krug et al. 2002). To better understand self-directed behaviors, it is necessary to distinguish these relevant terms. First, *suicidal ideations* are thoughts of engaging in or planning suicide-related behavior. *Nonsuicidal self-directed violence* includes self-harm, which consists of intentionally injuring oneself with no intention to die by methods such as self-laceration, self-battering, self-burning, taking overdoses, or exhibiting deliberate recklessness. Such acts differ from *suicide attempts* in terms of motivation, which is generally to relieve distress, feel something, induce self-punishment, get attention, or escape a problematic situation. On the other hand, in the case of *suicidal self-directed violence*, there is an intent to die. The person understands the consequences of their actions. A nonfatal self-injurious behavior performed with at least some intent to die is defined as a suicide attempt. When a suicide attempt results in death, the act is defined as a *completed suicide* (Krug et al. 2002).

Preventing suicidal behaviors remains challenging at present because a plethora of complex processes underlying the trigger and development of a suicidal state are not entirely comprehended (Centers for Disease Control and Prevention 2022; Krug et al. 2002; Wordefo et al. 2023). Determining which individuals will go forward with suicidal behaviors and understanding how one person, in comparison with another in a similar context, will partake in such behaviors is very difficult. Therefore, suicidal behaviors tend to be multifaceted, and many risk factors have been reported. Some studies have suggested that variables associated with different forms of suicidal behaviors may be distinct (Chan et al. 2014; Cheek et al. 2016). More specifically, risk factors include but are not limited to stress, impulsivity, exposure to early life adversity (e.g., parental neglect; childhood sexual, physical, and emotional abuse), adverse life events (e.g., loss of employment, familial conflicts, trauma), health-related disorders (e.g., cancer, multiple sclerosis), psychiatric illnesses (e.g., mood disorders, psychotic disorders), and substance use and SUDs (Centers for Disease Control and Prevention 2022; Krug et al. 2002).

Hence, substance use (including alcohol, cannabis, and illicit drugs) remains an important risk factor that has been countlessly investigated (Abdalla et al. 2019; Chau et al. 2019; Kokkevi et al. 2012). Substance use, which may increase impulsivity and negative mood as well as impair judgment and problem-solving skills, could predispose persons to suicidal behaviors (Norström and Rossow 2016); rates as high as 45% have been found in those with SUDs (Ilgen et al. 2010). A meta-analysis by Armoon et al. (2021) aiming to explore variables associated with suicidal behaviors in individuals with SUDs showed that the pooled prevalences of suicidal ideation and attempts among study participants were 35% and 20%, respectively. Specifically, suicidal ideation was associated with smoking, a past history of sexual abuse, alcohol use disorder or CaUD, and depressive disorders. On the other hand, suicide attempts were associated with being female; having a past history of sexual abuse and physical abuse; smoking; using cannabis, alcohol, cocaine, and amphetamine; and being diagnosed with polysubstance disorders and depressive disorders.

Although alcohol has been the most significant substance studied regarding increasing the risk of suicide, research has begun to link cannabis use with suicidal ideation and behaviors (e.g., Carvalho et al. 2022; Gobbi et al. 2019). However, the relationship between cannabis use and these behaviors remains an area that is relatively underinvestigated and associated with conflicting results. The possibility of an association between cannabis use and suicidal behaviors is relevant because cannabis use and CaUD are among the most common forms of substance use and SUDs worldwide (Degenhardt and Hall 2012; Degenhardt et al. 2008). Findings could have implications for improving strategies for suicide prevention.

In the next section, we briefly present data concerning the association between cannabis use and different forms of suicidal behavior.

Suicidal Ideation and Behavior in the General Population

Slight to moderate associations between cannabis use and suicidal ideations were found in meta-analyses. For example, a meta-analysis conducted by Borges et al. (2016) evaluated suicidal ideation in the general population, including adolescents, young adults, and adults. It found that cannabis use significantly increased the odds of suicidal ideations regardless of the amount consumed (OR 1.43; 95% CI 1.13–1.83; κ=6) and that heavy cannabis use moderately increased these odds (OR 2.53; 95% CI 1.00–6.39; κ=5). Additionally, a more recent meta-analysis by Armoon et al. (2021) showed a moderate association between CaUD and the risk of suicidal ideations in the past year (OR 2.01; 95% CI 1.01–4.01; κ=4). However, these results showed high levels of heterogeneity; most studies were cross-sectional, and confounding factors were generally not considered (Armoon et al. 2021; Borges et al. 2016). Cannabis use was linked with self-injurious behaviors: a meta-analysis by Escelsior et al. (2021) showed increased odds of such behaviors in cannabis users (N=12,289; OR 1.569; 95% CI 1.167–2.108) in cross-sectional studies conducted among community samples, psychiatric patients, and healthy populations. Moreover, longitudinal studies showed a greater association between cannabis use and subsequent self-harm (N=258,813; OR 2.569; 95% CI 2.207–3.256), indicating a possible causative link. No heterogeneity was present, and publication bias was noted only for cross-sectional studies. However, confounding factors could not be considered because most studies did not include them in their analyses.

Suicidal ideation and self-injurious behaviors may lead to suicide attempts, which could be linked with cannabis use. The previously mentioned meta-analysis by Borges et al. (2016) showed that cannabis use significantly increased the odds of suicide attempts (OR 2.23; 95% CI 1.24–4.00) and that the risk was higher in cases of cannabis abuse (OR 0.20; 95% CI 1.72–5.94). Regarding completed suicide, it was shown that chronic cannabis use significantly increased the likelihood of suicide (OR 2.56; 95% CI 1.25–5.27; κ=4). High levels of heterogeneity were noted, as well as publication bias; confounding factors were not considered. Additionally, the meta-analysis by Armoon et al. (2021) showed that CaUD was associated with a higher likelihood of attempted suicide in the prior year (OR 1.71; 95% CI 1.37–2.14; κ=5). In that analysis, cannabis was found to be a similar predictor of suicide attempts compared with alcohol use disorder (OR 1.58; 95% CI 1.37–1.81; κ=9), cocaine use disorder (OR 2.01; 95% CI 1.56–2.59; κ=10), and amphetamine use disorder (OR 1.87; 95% CI 1.12–3.12; κ=5). Most of the included studies were cross-sectional.

Cannabis Use in Youth and Increased Risks of Suicidal Ideation and Behavior

A public concern is that cannabis might affect mental health in youth more than in adults. It has been suggested that a younger cannabis initiation age and longer periods of use are associated with worse mental health outcomes, including higher risks of psychosis, other SUDs, depression, and suicidality (Kaur et al. 2022). A recent meta-analysis by Fresán et al. (2022) included a total of 26,937 adolescents and young adults (ages 11–21) and confirmed that the odds of suicidal ideations were higher among cannabis users than nonusers (OR 2.04; 95% CI 1.64–2.53; κ=12). Moreover, an analysis performed on a subsample of 9,054 youth showed a significant association between cannabis use and suicidal plans (OR 1.674; 95% CI 1.554–1.804; κ=3), which seemed to have resulted in higher rates of suicide attempts (OR 2.33; 95% CI

1.78–3.05; κ=16). Moreover, Fresán and colleagues' meta-regression analysis showed that age was a negative predictor, indicating that this relationship was stronger in younger individuals. Of interest, this association varied from one country to another, which could be explained by an earlier age at onset of cannabis use in certain communities. The analyses showed moderate heterogeneity, and all the studies included controlled for several confounding factors.

Another concern is that cannabis use during adolescence could affect an individual's mental health later in life, in particular by altering their brain development (Jacobus and Tapert 2014; Meruelo et al. 2017). Therefore, it could potentially affect one's future risk of suicide as well. On that matter, a meta-analysis conducted by Gobbi et al. (2019) focused on the effects of using cannabis during adolescence on suicidal ideation in adulthood (ages 18–32). Participants who used cannabis before age 18 had slightly higher risks of suicidal ideation in adulthood (OR 1.50; 95% CI 1.11–2.03; κ=3) and a much higher risk of suicide attempts, with an OR of 3.46 (95% CI 1.53–7.84; κ=3) in users compared with nonusers. Although heterogeneity was not assessed, all the included studies controlled for several confounding factors, including age, sex, and depression and/or anxiety at baseline.

Cannabis Use and Suicide in Individuals With Mental Disorders

As previously discussed, cannabis use is associated with a higher likelihood of violent behaviors in individuals with mental health disorders. However, the same was not observed for suicide because risks were comparable with those found in the general population. A meta-analysis by Bartoli et al. (2019) evaluated the relationship between CaUD and suicide attempts from cross-sectional studies in a sample of 6,375 patients diagnosed with bipolar disorder. They found a significant association between CaUD and history of suicide attempts (OR 1.35; 95% CI 1.08–1.70; κ = 11). The authors controlled for age, sex, and the proportion of participants with a diagnosis of bipolar I disorder. The meta-analysis reported no publication bias and moderate heterogeneity.

Additionally, a large cohort study including individuals born in Denmark between 1955 and 2011 assessed the association between cannabis use and suicide attempts in people with various mental health disorders: schizophrenia (*n*=35,625), bipolar disorder (*n*=9,279), unipolar depression (*n*=72,530), and personality disorders (*n*=63,958) (Østergaard et al. 2017). In this analysis, cannabis use was found to slightly increase the risk of suicide attempts in those with schizophrenia (hazard ratio 1.11; 95% CI 1.03–1.19) and was associated with an increased risk of completed suicide only in those with bipolar disorder (hazard ratio 1.86; 95% CI 1.15–2.99). All analyses were adjusted for sex, calendar year (continuous variable), and age at first diagnosis of mental illness.

Another population especially vulnerable to suicide is individuals with a first episode of psychosis. This population has a lifetime suicide death risk of 5.6%, and around 15% of them have already attempted suicide before presenting to mental health services (Addington et al. 2004; Nordentoft et al. 2015). Again, a longitudinal study of 397 individuals followed over 3 years identified cannabis use as a predominant risk factor for suicide attempts across time in this specific population (Ayesa-Arriola et al. 2015). However, to the best of our knowledge, no other studies to date have found a significant difference in suicidal risk between substance users and nonusers (Sánchez-Gutiérrez et al. 2022). Notably, two cohort studies that included people with first-episode psychosis showed no significant difference in cannabis use when comparing individuals with suicidal behaviors with those with no history of such behaviors (Canal-Rivero et al. 2018; Lopez-Morinigo et al. 2019).

Suicidal Risk in Military Veterans

Military veterans are at high risk of suicide, possibly because of their high risk of multiple mental health disorders (e.g., PTSD, depression) (Turna and MacKillop 2021). These individuals are at a higher risk of suicide than the general population, and they generally tend to self-medicate using cannabis. For this reason, health outcomes related to cannabis use, including suicidal thoughts and behaviors, have been investigated in a few cohort studies. Unsurprisingly, a diagnosis of CaUD was found to be associated with suicidal ideations, self-harm, suicidal behaviors, suicide attempts, and completed suicide in this vulnerable population (Adkisson et al. 2019; Bohnert et al. 2017; Kimbrel et al. 2017, 2018). However, the direction of the association was not assessed, and therefore, further studies with longitudinal designs will be needed.

Mechanisms Underlying the Association Between Cannabis and Violence

The association between substance use and violence toward self and others is complex and could be explained by multiple mechanisms.

First, from a neurobiological perspective, it is known that cannabis use may dysregulate the endocannabinoid system located in regions such as limbic structures and the frontal cortex (Maldonado et al. 2020). Several studies have shown that this system is important in regulating mood, impulsivity, and reward responses (Huang et al. 2016; Wrege et al. 2014). Therefore, disruption to the endocannabinoid system may increase the risk of negative mood, cognitive issues, and violent behaviors toward self and others (Agrawal and Lynskey 2014; Leite et al. 2015; Mannekote Thippaiah et al. 2021; Volkow et al. 2017; Wilson et al. 2019). Cannabis use may also promote violent tendencies by inhibiting prefrontal response and downregulating cannabinoid 1 receptors (Broyd et al. 2016; Crean et al. 2011; Rodríguez-Arias et al. 2016; Volkow et al. 2017). The psychopharmacological effects of cannabis intoxication or withdrawal may lower the threshold for violence (Kuhns et al. 2009).

Second, acute cannabis intoxication may place some individuals at greater risk of committing violent acts (Dellazizzo et al. 2020a; Moore and Stuart 2005). Although the use of cannabis has been mostly known to cause relaxation and euphoria, it can also lead to anxiety, paranoia, and panic attacks, which are often accompanied by increased heart rate and blood pressure (Moore and Stuart 2005; Zuardi et al. 1982). Moreover, cannabis intoxication has been shown to possibly impair neurocognitive domains and impair the ability to suppress aggressiveness (Dellazizzo et al. 2020a; Moore and Stuart 2005). The type of cannabis may also matter; it has been suggested that strains with a higher THC:CBD ratio are more likely to induce depression, anxiety, dysphoria, psychosis, impulsivity, and negative affect regulation (Borges et al. 2016; Childs et al. 2017; Gobbi et al. 2019). Cannabis intoxication has also been shown to exacerbate underlying psychiatric symptomatology (e.g., psychosis, depressive symptoms) (Crocker et al. 2021), which may further heighten the propensity for forms of violence (Miller et al. 2020; Moulin et al. 2018). Nevertheless, the hypothesis that cannabis intoxication could directly cause violent behaviors is highly controversial and difficult to confirm (Berenson 2019). Studies from the 1970s and 1980s investigating the effects of controlled THC doses in healthy individuals suggested that moderate to high doses of cannabis could slightly lower the risk of aggression toward others, whereas small doses could increase aggressivity (Myerscough and Taylor 1985; Taylor et al. 1976). However, those studies had many limitations, including small sample sizes. Moreover, the results have never been replicated, likely owing to ethical issues. Now that cannabis is legal in multiple countries and states, this type of experimental study could potentially be reproduced.

Third, it has been proposed that early cannabis use is a possible predictor of violent behaviors later in life. Notably, the impacts of prenatal cannabis exposure on future delinquent and aggressive behaviors have been suggested to be partially attributable to alterations in the glutamate, dopamine, endorphin, and serotonin systems, all of which could be associated with emotional dysregulation and behavioral problems (Murnan et al. 2022; Saez et al. 2014). Moreover, research has suggested that cannabis use during adolescence may alter neural connectivity in the hippocampus and the prefrontal cortex, potentially resulting in reduced inhibition of inappropriate behaviors (Barthelemy et al. 2016; Filbey and Yezhuvath 2013; Volkow et al. 2014).

Fourth, in addition to the effects of acute intoxication, cessation of cannabis use may lead to withdrawal, which is characterized by insomnia, anxiety, and aggression (Budney et al. 2004; Rafiei and Kolla 2022; Ramesh et al. 2011). Irritability or aggression is now considered a cannabis withdrawal symptom in DSM-5 (American Psychiatric Association 2013), and a possible link with violent behaviors has been supported by the results of multiple studies (Mills et al. 2017; Smith et al. 2013). However, the time required between the last dose of cannabis and the increase in aggressiveness remains a matter of debate. An early study on the matter measured aggressivity in 19 subjects with a DSM-IV (American Psychiatric Association 1994) diagnosis of CaUD on days 0 (still smoking), 1, 3, 7, and 28 of a cannabis detoxification period (Kouri et al. 1999). According to the results of this study, aggressiveness was significantly higher than that of a control group composed of 20 former or infrequent cannabis users on days 3 and 7 following withdrawal, and aggressiveness went back to baseline by day 28 (Kouri et al. 1999).

However, recent studies investigating cannabis withdrawal in the general population have shown that symptoms such as irritability, anger, anxiety, and aggression may already begin to increase between days 0 and 3 of abstinence (Budney et al. 2003; Lee et al. 2014). The pharmacokinetic properties of THC, including its long half-life, may be responsible for the delayed expression of these withdrawal symptoms in some individuals (Ramesh et al. 2011). In addition to the delay necessary for such symptoms to appear, the exact prevalence of withdrawal symptoms also remains unclear. In a study of 469 adults who smoked cannabis and attempted to quit on their own, 24.1% reported "feeling aggressive," 28.8% reported having been verbally violent (i.e., insulted, yelled, or swore at a person), 14.7% threw or broke something, and at least 3.6% had been physically violent toward someone else (i.e., pushed, grabbed, or slapped a person) (Levin et al. 2010). The most prevalent mood symptoms included anxiety (50%) and boredom (50%), followed by irritability (45%) and anger (34%). Although these results are interesting and suggest that aggressiveness could be quite common among cannabis quitters, more studies are needed to evaluate how prevalent these symptoms and emotions are and whether they are also experienced by chronic users (e.g., in between doses).

Finally, the cannabis-violence relationship could be mediated by confounding factors. For instance, previous victimization could precede substance use as well as violence (Afifi et al. 2012; Dardis et al. 2015; Duke et al. 2010; Mills et al. 2017). Individuals with antisocial traits could also be predisposed to consuming substances such as cannabis and to committing violence, accounting for part of the association. Notably, a combination of predisposing traits such as impulsivity and the disinhibiting effects of cannabis use may lead to violence (Dumais et al. 2011; Joyal et al. 2004). The association may likewise be environmental or situational. For instance, particularly in relation to violence toward others, criminality (e.g., involvement in organized crime groups) is associated with both substance use and violent behaviors (Calderoni et al. 2022; Spidel et al. 2010). The same could be true for the relationship between cannabis and suicide because some social factors could predispose a person to both (e.g., poverty and involvement with the justice system) (Boch et al. 2021). Cannabis use has also been proposed to act as a gateway substance leading to other addictive behaviors; this could be explained by the influence of the individual's social network, and cannabis could also decrease the reactivity of dopamine neurons modulating the brain's reward regions (Hall and Lynskey 2005; Pistis et al. 2004; Volkow et al. 2014; Williams 2020). Therefore, these substances could potentially be responsible for the increased risk of violence. However, in multiple studies, the association between cannabis use and violence remained significant after adjustments were made regarding the use of other substances (e.g., Beaudoin et al. 2020, 2023; Moulin et al. 2020).

Limitations of Current Data

Reviews and meta-analyses studying this association largely agree that the current literature has many limitations, the first being the considerable heterogeneity in designs and methodologies. Indeed, the definition of violence varied greatly (e.g., physical vs. verbal violence, violence toward others vs. toward objects, violent act vs. overall aggressiveness), as did the measurement tools used (e.g., self-reported vs. convictions). We also noted a great deal of inconsistency in the literature regarding the reporting of cannabis use; for example, whereas some studies only considered heavy cannabis users or individuals with CaUD, others included all users without distinctions. Additionally, the different routes of administration (e.g., smoking, eating, vaping) were generally not considered, and neither was the THC:CBD ratio or the purity of the cannabis. Synthetic cannabinoid users were included in a few studies, but in most studies, cannabis users were included without precisely specifying what the participants were consuming.

This lack of consistency is problematic because these factors could all influence the magnitude of the cannabis-violence relationship, and this should be considered in interpreting these results. For example, THC could cause psychotic symptoms and be linked with impulsivity or even aggressivity (Little and D'Mello 2022; McDonald et al. 2003; Ortiz-Peregrina et al. 2021). Conversely, CBD could benefit individuals with mental disorders, notably by reducing anxiety symptoms (Black et al. 2019; Hartmann et al. 2019; Lowe et al. 2019). Because cannabis is now legal in multiple states and countries, it should become progressively easier to assess precisely what participants are consuming in future studies. Finally, although some longitudinal studies found that cannabis use seems to predispose people to violent behaviors more than the opposite, most of the current literature is based on cross-sectional studies. Therefore, it remains challenging to assess the direction of this association, and consequently, it is impossible to determine whether cannabis use is directly causing violent behaviors. These limitations are difficult to overcome, however, because experimental studies in a controlled setting involving cannabis use and aggressiveness would include several ethical challenges, especially if these were to include individuals with mental illnesses.

Beneficial Effects

Although cannabis use appears to be linked with a higher incidence of violent behaviors, some studies focus on the opposite by using cannabis to reduce agitation and aggressive behaviors in a few specific populations. More specifically, oral cannabis and cannabis extracts containing various concentrations of THC and CBD have been shown to reduce agitation, irritability, and aggressive behaviors in small samples of participants with dementia (Mueller and Fixen 2020; Palmieri and Vadalà 2023), autism spectrum disorder (Bar-Lev Schleider et al. 2019; Fusar-Poli et al. 2020; Silva et al. 2022), and fetal alcohol spectrum disorders (Koren et al. 2021). However, some side effects have been reported, including sleep concerns, irritability, and restlessness (Fusar-Poli et al. 2020). Regarding suicidal behaviors, it has been suggested that cannabis intoxication could reduce the risk of suicide attempts. A cohort study of 363 individuals who recently attempted suicide showed that recent cannabis use alone decreased suicidal behaviors (Bagge and Borges 2017). However, the authors noted that withdrawal symptoms could precipitate these behaviors, making cannabis a poor therapeutic option for suicidal individuals.

CBD oil alone has also been found to reduce the risk of behavioral disturbances in populations with dementia and autism spectrum disorder (Barchel et al. 2019; Hermush et al. 2022). This reduction in aggressive behaviors following the administration of CBD oil has been observed in preclinical studies on mice, rats, and dogs (Andaloussi et al. 2021; Corsetti et al. 2021; Hartmann et al. 2019). Moreover, it has been suggested that CBD might have antipsychotic, antidepressant, and anxiolytic properties, making it a potential therapeutic option for individuals with mental disorders who are at increased risk of violent and suicidal behaviors (Black et al. 2019; Davies and Bhattacharyya 2019; Pajević et al. 2021). However, the evidence remains scarce, and further studies will be needed to assess its efficacy. Additionally, no study to date has assessed the direct effects of CBD on aggressive behaviors toward self and others in this vulnerable population. Finally, using CBD as an anticonvulsant could be beneficial in some cases of epilepsy (White 2019). However, White (2019) noted that suicidal ideation is a possible rare adverse effect of many anticonvulsant drugs, and therefore the FDA is concerned that CBD could cause this adverse effect as well. Nevertheless, this hypothesis remains to be investigated.

In conclusion, these results suggest that cannabis, especially CBD oil, could potentially be beneficial in reducing the risk of physical violence in carefully selected populations. Nevertheless, the level of evidence remains weak. Given that THC and CBD generally have opposing effects, and CBD alone appears to be beneficial, it is possible to hypothesize that this molecule is responsible for the reduction in aggressivity that is sometimes observed in cannabis use. Randomized controlled trials with larger sample sizes will be needed to evaluate the risk-benefit ratio and to determine whether specific types of medical cannabis should be recommended to decrease aggressiveness in certain situations.

Clinical Significance and Recommendations

We have summarized here the available evidence regarding the association between cannabis use and violence. Although the direction of the association and the causality remain to be confirmed, it would be prudent to consider the following recommendations in clinical settings. First, it is important to assess substance use, including cannabis, in patients presenting with aggressive tendencies. Indeed, addressing SUDs could be a critical component of effective treatment. In this situation, clinicians should educate patients about the potential risks of cannabis use and encourage open communication about their substance use habits. Providing evidence-based interventions, such as cognitive-behavioral therapy, family-based therapy, motivational enhancement therapy, and contingency management, has been shown to induce changes in cannabis users (Adams et al. 2023). Moreover, approaches using novel technologies such as mobile health applications and virtual reality are emerging (Giguère et al. 2023; Tatar et al. 2022).

Collaborative care involving substance abuse specialists, mental health professionals, and social support networks can also be crucial in providing comprehensive treatment and support for individuals struggling with CaUD. The collaborative care model has already been shown to be effective for alcohol and opioid use disorders (Watkins et al. 2017); further studies need to be conducted to validate its effectiveness for CaUD. It is also important to screen for aggressive ideation and behaviors directed toward self and others in all patients presenting with an SUD. Indeed, although cannabis is often perceived as less harmful than other substances (Nguyen et al. 2023), it appears to significantly contribute to the well-known relationship between substance use and violence. Clinicians should also be mindful that no specific amount of cannabis has been shown to be safe and that the quantity of cannabis consumed might be just as good a predictor as the severity of the CaUD (Beaudoin et al. 2023). Moreover, considering the THC:CBD ratio might be relevant to harm reduction approaches because THC appears to be the component of cannabis with the most adverse effects on cognition and mental health (Crean et al. 2011), although CBD could oppose the cognitive impairments associated with THC (Wright et al. 2013).

Conclusion

Substance use has consistently been associated with self- and other-directed violence, yet it is essential to investigate the role played by each substance separately in order to formulate comprehensive and relevant recommendations. Understanding this link is crucial for health care professionals working with vulnerable individuals. We have provided an overview of the current evidence regarding the association between cannabis use and violence, which has been described in multiple populations. Several potential mechanisms that could explain this association have been discussed. Notably, acute cannabis intoxication could lead to increased levels of impulsivity and aggression in some cases. Individuals with mental disorders could be at higher risk, possibly through exacerbation of symptoms. Cannabis withdrawal could also play a role, especially in heavy users. Finally, the association between cannabis use and violence could be mediated by psychosocial factors. Although the direction of the association remains uncertain, multiple recommendations could be considered in the clinical setting. For example, health care professionals are encouraged to ensure the accessibility of evidence-based interventions for CaUD and to screen individuals for their risk of aggression.

As for future research, studies need to be conducted to elucidate the mechanisms underlying the associations between cannabis use and violence or suicide. Moreover, more studies are needed to clarify the direction of this association and a potential dose-response relationship. To confirm a potential causal link, participants and collateral individuals (e.g., relatives, witnesses) will have to be questioned to determine the timing of the aggression in relation to the use of cannabis. If possible, the impact of acute cannabis use and withdrawal on neuropsychological components such as impulsivity and aggressivity could be measured in vitro, thereby providing a better understanding of this potential cause-and-effect relationship. Furthermore, there is a critical need to harmonize methodologies so that definitions of violence are consistent across studies. Finally, future studies should try to more precisely assess the quantity as well as the type of cannabis used, especially to control for influential factors such as the THC:CBD ratio.

Key Points

- Self- and other-directed violence is a complex social issue influenced by many factors, including substance use.
- Cannabis has recently been legalized in multiple U.S. states and countries, which may impact its social acceptance and prevalence of use.
- Cannabis use and abuse have been moderately associated with increased risks of interpersonal violence and suicidal thoughts and behaviors. These associations have been seen with varying levels of evidence in multiple populations, including the general population, youth, and individuals with mental disorders.
- Despite multiple studies on the subject, methods remain heterogeneous, and the direction of the associations remains to be clarified.
- The mechanisms underlying the associations between cannabis use and violence remain unknown. Potential explanations include the direct effects of cannabis intoxication, withdrawal syndrome, and social and cultural factors.

References

Abdalla RR, Miguel AC, Brietzke E, et al: Suicidal behavior among substance users: data from the Second Brazilian National Alcohol and Drug Survey (II BNADS). Br J Psychiatry 41(5):437–440, 2019 30785535

Adams ZW, Marriott BR, Hulvershorn LA, et al: Treatment of adolescent cannabis use disorders. Child Adolesc Psychiatr Clin N Am 32(1):141–155, 2023 36410901

Addington J, Williams J, Young J, et al: Suicidal behaviour in early psychosis. Acta Psychiatr Scand 109(2):116–120, 2004 14725592

Adkisson K, Cunningham KC, Dedert EA, et al: Cannabis use disorder and post-deployment suicide attempts in Iraq/Afghanistan-era veterans. Arch Suicide Res 23(4):678–687, 2019 29952737

Afifi TO, Henriksen CA, Asmundson GJ, et al: Childhood maltreatment and substance use disorders among men and women in a nationally representative sample. Can J Psychiatry 57(11):677–686, 2012 23149283

Agrawal A, Lynskey MT: Have the genetics of cannabis involvement gone to pot? Nebr Symp Motiv 61:71–108, 2014 25306780

American Psychiatric Association: Diagnostic and Statistical Manual of Mental Disorders, 4th Edition. Washington, DC, American Psychiatric Association, 1994

American Psychiatric Association: Diagnostic and Statistical Manual of Mental Disorders, 5th Edition. Arlington, VA, American Psychiatric Association, 2013

Andaloussi ZL, Lauer W, Zulu SS, et al: Acute cannabidiol treatment attenuates ethanol-induced place preference and reduces aggressivity in group-housed male rats. Pharmacol Biochem Behav 211:173290, 2021 34662589

Armoon B, SoleimanvandiAzar N, Fleury MJ, et al: Prevalence, sociodemographic variables, mental health condition, and type of drug use associated with suicide behaviors among people with substance use disorders: a systematic review and meta-analysis. J Addict Dis 39(4):550–569, 2021 33896407

Ashton CH: Pharmacology and effects of cannabis: a brief review. Br J Psychiatry 178:101–106, 2001 11157422

Ayesa-Arriola R, Alcaraz EG, Hernández BV, et al: Suicidal behaviour in first-episode non-affective psychosis: specific risk periods and stage-related factors. Eur Neuropsychopharmacol 25(12):2278–2288, 2015 26475577

Bagge CL, Borges G: Acute substance use as a warning sign for suicide attempts: a case-crossover examination of the 48 hours prior to a recent suicide attempt. J Clin Psychiatry 78(6):691–696, 2017 28682530

Barchel D, Stolar O, De-Haan T, et al: Oral cannabidiol use in children with autism spectrum disorder to treat related symptoms and co-morbidities. Front Pharmacol 9:1521, 2019 30687090

Bar-Lev Schleider L, Mechoulam R, Saban N, et al: Real life experience of medical cannabis treatment in autism: analysis of safety and efficacy. Sci Rep 9(1):200, 2019 30655581

Barthelemy OJ, Richardson MA, Cabral HJ, et al: Prenatal, perinatal, and adolescent exposure to marijuana: relationships with aggressive behavior. Neurotoxicol Teratol 58:60–77, 2016 27345271

Bartoli F, Crocamo C, Carrà G: Cannabis use disorder and suicide attempts in bipolar disorder: a meta-analysis. Neurosci Biobehav Rev 103:14–20, 2019 31121199

Bashford J, Flett R, Copeland J: The Cannabis Use Problems Identification Test (CUPIT): development, reliability, concurrent and predictive validity among adolescents and adults. Addiction 105(4):615–625, 2010 20403014

Beaudoin M, Potvin S, Dellazizzo L, et al: Trajectories of dynamic risk factors as predictors of violence and criminality in patients discharged from mental health services: a longitudinal study using growth mixture modeling. Front Psychiatry 10:301, 2019 31139099

Beaudoin M, Potvin S, Giguère CE, et al: Persistent cannabis use as an independent risk factor for violent behaviors in patients with schizophrenia. NPJ Schizophr 6(1):14, 2020 32393793

Beaudoin M, Dellazizzo L, Giguère S, et al: Is there a dose-response relationship between cannabis use and violence? A longitudinal study in individuals with severe mental disorders. Cannabis Cannabinoid Res 9(1):241–251, 2023 36787482

Berenson A: Marijuana is more dangerous than you think. Mo Med 116(2):88–89, 2019 31040486

Black N, Stockings E, Campbell G, et al: Cannabinoids for the treatment of mental disorders and symptoms of mental disorders: a systematic review and meta-analysis. Lancet Psychiatry 6(12):995–1010, 2019 31672337

Boch S, Sezgin E, Ruch D, et al: Unjust: the health records of youth with personal/family justice involvement in a large pediatric health system. Health Justice 9(1):20, 2021 34337696

Bohnert KM, Ilgen MA, Louzon S, et al: Substance use disorders and the risk of suicide mortality among men and women in the US Veterans Health Administration. Addiction 112(7):1193–1201, 2017

Borges G, Bagge CL, Orozco R: A literature review and meta-analyses of cannabis use and suicidality. J Affect Disord 195:63–74, 2016 26872332

Brook JS, Zhang C, Brook DW: Antisocial behavior at age 37: developmental trajectories of marijuana use extending from adolescence to adulthood. Am J Addict 20(6):509–515, 2011 21999495

Broyd SJ, van Hell HH, Beale C, et al: Acute and chronic effects of cannabinoids on human cognition: a systematic review. Biol Psychiatry 79(7):557–567, 2016 26858214

Budney AJ, Moore BA, Vandrey RG, et al: The time course and significance of cannabis withdrawal. J Abnorm Psychol 112(3):393–402, 2003 12943018

Budney AJ, Hughes JR, Moore BA, et al: Review of the validity and significance of cannabis withdrawal syndrome. Am J Psychiatry 161(11):1967–1977, 2004 15514394

Butchart A, Mikton C, Dahlberg LL, et al: Global status report on violence prevention 2014. Inj Prev 21(3):213, 2015 25995201

Calderoni F, Comunale T, Campedelli GM, et al: Organized crime groups: a systematic review of individual-level risk factors related to recruitment. Campbell Syst Rev 18(1):e1218, 2022 36913220

Canal-Rivero M, López-Moríñigo JD, Setién-Suero E, et al: Predicting suicidal behaviour after first episode of non-affective psychosis: the role of neurocognitive functioning. Eur Psychiatry 53:52–57, 2018 29929113

Capaldi DM, Tiberio SS, Kerr DC, et al: Associations of cannabis use across adolescence and early adulthood with health and psychosocial adjustment in early adulthood and midadulthood in men. Subst Abuse 16:11782218221096154, 2022 35677294

Carliner H, Brown QL, Sarvet AL, et al: Cannabis use, attitudes, and legal status in the U.S.: a review. Prev Med 104:13–23, 2017 28705601

Carvalho JV, Souza LS, Moreira EC: Association between cannabis use and suicidal behavior: a systematic review of cohort studies. Psychiatry Res 312:114555, 2022 35461121

Centers for Disease Control and Prevention: Data and Statistics. Atlanta, GA, Centers for Disease Control and Prevention, 2021. Available at: https://www.cdc.gov/cannabis/data-research/facts-stats/. Accessed June 26, 2023.

Centers for Disease Control and Prevention: Risk and Protective Factors. Atlanta, GA, Centers for Disease Control and Prevention, 2022. Available at: https://www.cdc.gov/suicide/factors/index.html. Accessed June 26, 2023.

Chabrol H, Rodgers RF, Sobolewski G, et al: Cannabis use and delinquent behaviors in a non-clinical sample of adolescents. Addict Behav 35(3):263–265, 2010 19896278

Chan LF, Shamsul AS, Maniam T: Are predictors of future suicide attempts and the transition from suicidal ideation to suicide attempts shared or distinct: a 12-month prospective study among patients with depressive disorders. Psychiatry Res 220(3):867–873, 2014 25240940

Chau K, Mayet A, Legleye S, et al: Association between cumulating substances use and cumulating several school, violence and mental health difficulties in early adolescents. Psychiatry Res 280:112480, 2019 31377662

Cheek SM, Nestor BA, Liu RT: Substance use and suicidality: specificity of substance use by injection to suicide attempts in a nationally representative sample of adults with major depression. Depress Anxiety 33(6):541–548, 2016 26393336

Childs E, Lutz JA, de Wit H: Dose-related effects of delta-9-THC on emotional responses to acute psychosocial stress. Drug Alcohol Depend 177:136–144, 2017 28599212

Clayton HB, Lowry R, Ashley C, et al: Health risk behaviors with synthetic cannabinoids versus marijuana. Pediatrics 139(4):e20162675, 2017 28289138

Corsetti S, Borruso S, Malandrucco L, et al: Cannabis sativa L. may reduce aggressive behaviour towards humans in shelter dogs. Sci Rep 11(1):2773, 2021 33531559

Crane CA, Wiernik BM, Berbary CM, et al: A meta-analytic review of the relationship between cyber aggression and substance use. Drug Alcohol Depend 221:108510, 2021 33610092

Crean RD, Crane NA, Mason BJ: An evidence based review of acute and long-term effects of cannabis use on executive cognitive functions. J Addict Med 5(1):1–8, 2011 21321675

Crocker CE, Carter AJE, Emsley JG, et al: When cannabis use goes wrong: mental health side effects of cannabis use that present to emergency services. Front Psychiatry 12:640222, 2021 33658953

Czermainski FR, Lopes FM, Ornell F, et al: Concurrent use of alcohol and crack cocaine is associated with high levels of anger and liability to aggression. Subst Use Misuse 55(10):1660–1666, 2020 32519554

Dardis CM, Dixon KJ, Edwards KM, et al: An examination of the factors related to dating violence perpetration among young men and women and associated theoretical explanations: a review of the literature. Trauma Violence Abuse 16(2):136–152, 2015 24415138

Davies C, Bhattacharyya S: Cannabidiol as a potential treatment for psychosis. Ther Adv Psychopharmacol 9:2045125319881916, 2019 31741731

Degenhardt L, Hall W: Extent of illicit drug use and dependence, and their contribution to the global burden of disease. Lancet 379(9810):55–70, 2012 22225671

Degenhardt L, Chiu WT, Sampson N, et al: Toward a global view of alcohol, tobacco, cannabis, and cocaine use: findings from the WHO World Mental Health Surveys. PLoS Med 5(7):e141, 2008 18597549

De Genna NM, Willford JA, Richardson GA: Long-term effects of prenatal cannabis exposure: pathways to adolescent and adult outcomes. Pharmacol Biochem Behav 214:173358, 2022 35216971

Dellazizzo L, Potvin S, Beaudoin M, et al: Cannabis use and violence in patients with severe mental illnesses: a meta-analytical investigation. Psychiatry Res 274:42–48, 2019 30780061

Dellazizzo L, Potvin S, Athanassiou M, et al: Violence and cannabis use: a focused review of a forgotten aspect in the era of liberalizing cannabis. Front Psychiatry 11:567887, 2020a 33192691

Dellazizzo L, Potvin S, Dou BY, et al: Association between the use of cannabis and physical violence in youths: a meta-analytical investigation. Am J Psychiatry 177(7):619–626, 2020b 32456503

Derzon JH, Lipsey MW: A synthesis of the relationship of marijuana use with delinquent and problem behaviors. Sch Psychol Int 20(1): 57–68, 1999

Dugré JR, Dellazizzo L, Giguère CÉ, et al: Persistency of cannabis use predicts violence following acute psychiatric discharge. Front Psychiatry 8:176, 2017 28983261

Dugré JR, Potvin S, Dellazizzo L, et al: Aggression and delinquent behavior in a large representative sample of high school students: cannabis use and victimization as key discriminating factors. Psychiatry Res 296:113640, 2021 33340870

Duke AA, Smith KMZ, Oberleitner LMS, et al: Alcohol, drugs, and violence: a meta-meta-analysis. Psychol Violence 8:238–249, 2017

Duke NN, Pettingell SL, McMorris BJ, et al: Adolescent violence perpetration: associations with multiple types of adverse childhood experiences. Pediatrics 125(4):e778–e786, 2010 20231180

Dumais A, Potvin S, Joyal C, et al: Schizophrenia and serious violence: a clinical-profile analysis incorporating impulsivity and substance-use disorders. Schizophr Res 130(1–3):234–237, 2011 21441016

El Marroun H, Hudziak JJ, Tiemeier H, et al: Intrauterine cannabis exposure leads to more aggressive behavior and attention problems in 18-month-old girls. Drug Alcohol Depend 118(2–3):470–474, 2011 21470799

Escelsior A, Belvederi Murri M, Corsini GP, et al: Cannabinoid use and self-injurious behaviours: a systematic review and meta-analysis. J Affect Disord 278:85–98, 2021 32956965

Favril L, Yu R, Uyar A, et al: Risk factors for suicide in adults: systematic review and meta-analysis of psychological autopsy studies. Evid Based Ment Health 25(4):148–155, 2022 36162975

Fazel S, Smith EN, Chang Z, et al: Risk factors for interpersonal violence: an umbrella review of meta-analyses. Br J Psychiatry 213(4):609–614, 2018 30058516

Filbey F, Yezhuvath U: Functional connectivity in inhibitory control networks and severity of cannabis use disorder. Am J Drug Alcohol Abuse 39(6):382–391, 2013 24200208

Fischer B, Russell C, Rehm J, et al: Assessing the public health impact of cannabis legalization in Canada: core outcome indicators towards an "index" for monitoring and evaluation. J Public Health (Oxf) 41(2):412–421, 2019 29860521

Flanagan JC, Leone RM, Gilmore AK, et al: Association of cannabis use with intimate partner violence among couples with substance misuse. Am J Addict 29(4):323–330, 2020 32219903

Fresán A, Dionisio-García DM, González-Castro TB, et al: Cannabis smoking increases the risk of suicide ideation and suicide attempt in young individuals of 11–21 years: a systematic review and meta-analysis. J Psychiatr Res 153:90–98, 2022 35810604

Fusar-Poli L, Cavone V, Tinacci S, et al: Cannabinoids for people with ASD: a systematic review of published and ongoing studies. Brain Sci 10(9):572, 2020 32825313

GBD 2016 Alcohol and Drug Use Collaborators: The global burden of disease attributable to alcohol and drug use in 195 countries and territories, 1990–2016: a systematic analysis for the Global Burden of Disease Study 2016. Lancet Psychiatry 5(12):987–1012, 2018 30392731

George T, Vaccarino F (eds): Substance Abuse in Canada: The Effects of Cannabis Use During Adolescence. Ottawa, ON, Canadian Centre on Substance Abuse, 2015

Giguère S, Potvin S, Beaudoin M, et al: Avatar intervention for cannabis use disorder in individuals with severe mental disorders: a pilot study. J Pers Med 13(5):766, 2023 37240936

Global Burden of Disease Collaborative Network: Global Burden of Disease Study 2019 (GBD 2019) Healthcare Access and Quality Index 1990–2019. Seattle, WA, Institute for Health Metrics and Evaluation, 2022

Gobbi G, Atkin T, Zytynski T, et al: Association of cannabis use in adolescence and risk of depression, anxiety, and suicidality in young adulthood: a systematic review and meta-analysis. JAMA Psychiatry 76(4):426–434, 2019 30758486

Goldschmidt L, Day NL, Richardson GA: Effects of prenatal marijuana exposure on child behavior problems at age 10. Neurotoxicol Teratol 22(3):325–336, 2000 10840176

Grann M, Fazel S: Substance misuse and violent crime: Swedish population study. BMJ 328(7450):1233–1234, 2004 15155501

Green B, Kavanagh DJ, Young RM: Reasons for cannabis use in men with and without psychosis. Drug Alcohol Rev 23(4):445–453, 2004 15763749

Green KM, Doherty EE, Stuart EA, et al: Does heavy adolescent marijuana use lead to criminal involvement in adulthood? Evidence from a multiwave longitudinal study of urban African Americans. Drug Alcohol Depend 112(1–2):117–125, 2010 20598815

Grotenhermen F: Pharmacokinetics and pharmacodynamics of cannabinoids. Clin Pharmacokinet 42(4):327–360, 2003 12648025

Hall WD, Lynskey M: Is cannabis a gateway drug? Testing hypotheses about the relationship between cannabis use and the use of other illicit drugs. Drug Alcohol Rev 24(1):39–48, 2005 16191720

Harms Scientific Working Group: Canadian Substance Use Costs and Harms, 2015–2017. Victoria, BC, Canadian Institute for Substance Use Research, 2020

Hartmann A, Lisboa SF, Sonego AB, et al: Cannabidiol attenuates aggressive behavior induced by social isolation in mice: involvement of 5-HT1A and CB1 receptors. Prog Neuropsychopharmacol Biol Psychiatry 94:109637, 2019 31054943

Hasan A, von Keller R, Friemel CM, et al: Cannabis use and psychosis: a review of reviews. Eur Arch Psychiatry Clin Neurosci 270(4):403–412, 2020 31563981

Hasin DS, Shmulewitz D, Sarvet AL: Time trends in US cannabis use and cannabis use disorders overall and by sociodemographic subgroups: a narrative review and new findings. Am J Drug Alcohol Abuse 45(6):623–643, 2019 30870044

Hermush V, Ore L, Stern N, et al: Effects of rich cannabidiol oil on behavioral disturbances in patients with dementia: a placebo controlled randomized clinical trial. Front Med (Lausanne) 9:951889, 2022 36148467

Hillis S, Mercy J, Amobi A, et al: Global prevalence of past-year violence against children: a systematic review and minimum estimates. Pediatrics 137(3):e20154079, 2016 26810785

Huang WJ, Chen WW, Zhang X: Endocannabinoid system: role in depression, reward and pain control (review). Mol Med Rep 14(4):2899–2903, 2016 27484193

Ilgen MA, Burnette ML, Conner KR, et al: The association between violence and lifetime suicidal thoughts and behaviors in individuals treated for substance use disorders. Addict Behav 35(2):111–115, 2010 19800173

Jacobus J, Tapert SF: Effects of cannabis on the adolescent brain. Curr Pharm Des 20(13):2186–2193, 2014 23829363

Johnson RM, LaValley M, Schneider KE, et al: Marijuana use and physical dating violence among adolescents and emerging adults: a systematic review and meta-analysis. Drug Alcohol Depend 174:47–57, 2017 28314193

Joyal CC, Putkonen A, Paavola P, et al: Characteristics and circumstances of homicidal acts committed by offenders with schizophrenia. Psychol Med 34(3):433–442, 2004 15259828

Kaur N, Bastien G, Gagnon L, et al: Variations of cannabis-related adverse mental health and addiction outcomes across adolescence and adulthood: a scoping review. Front Psychiatry 13:973–988, 2022 36299544

Kedia SK, Dillon PJ, Jiang Y, et al: The association between substance use and violence: results from a nationally representative sample of high school students in the United States. Community Ment Health J 57(2):294–306, 2021 32500451

Kimbrel NA, Newins AR, Dedert EA, et al: Cannabis use disorder and suicide attempts in Iraq/Afghanistan-era veterans. J Psychiatr Res 89:1–5, 2017 28129565

Kimbrel NA, Meyer EC, DeBeer BB, et al: The impact of cannabis use disorder on suicidal and nonsuicidal self-injury in Iraq/Afghanistan-era veterans with and without mental health disorders. Suicide Life Threat Behavior 48(2):140–148, 2018

Kokkevi A, Richardson C, Olszewski D, et al: Multiple substance use and self-reported suicide attempts by adolescents in 16 European countries. Eur Child Adolesc Psychiatry 21(8):443–450, 2012 22535305

Koren G, Cohen R, Sachs O: Use of cannabis in fetal alcohol spectrum disorder. Cannabis Cannabinoid Res 6(1):74–76, 2021 33614955

Kouri EM, Pope HG Jr, Lukas SE: Changes in aggressive behavior during withdrawal from long-term marijuana use. Psychopharmacology (Berl) 143(3):302–308, 1999 10353434

Krug EG, Dahlberg LL, Mercy J, et al: World Report on Violence and Health. Geneva, World Health Organization, 2002

Kuhns JB, Wilson DB, Maguire ER, et al: A meta-analysis of marijuana, cocaine and opiate toxicology study findings among homicide victims. Addiction 104(7):1122–1131, 2009 19438418

Lake S, Kerr T, Werb D, et al: Guidelines for public health and safety metrics to evaluate the potential harms and benefits of cannabis regulation in Canada. Drug Alcohol Rev 38(6):606–621, 2019 31577059

Lamsma J, Cahn W, Fazel S: Use of illicit substances and violent behaviour in psychotic disorders: two nationwide case-control studies and meta-analyses. Psychol Med 50(12):2028–2033, 2020 31462346

Lee D, Schroeder JR, Karschner EL, et al: Cannabis withdrawal in chronic, frequent cannabis smokers during sustained abstinence within a closed residential environment. Am J Addict 23(3):234–242, 2014 24724880

Leite RT, Nogueira SdeO, do Nascimento JP, et al: The use of cannabis as a predictor of early onset of bipolar disorder and suicide attempts. Neural Plast 2015:434127, 2015 26097750

Levin KH, Copersino ML, Heishman SJ, et al: Cannabis withdrawal symptoms in non-treatment-seeking adult cannabis smokers. Drug Alcohol Depend 111(1–2):120–127, 2010 20510550

Little R, D'Mello D: A cannabinoid hypothesis of schizophrenia: pathways to psychosis. Innov Clin Neurosci 19(7–9):38–43, 2022 36204167

Lopez-Morinigo JD, Di Forti M, Ajnakina O, et al: Insight and risk of suicidal behaviour in two first-episode psychosis cohorts: effects of previous suicide attempts and depression. Schizophr Res 204:80–89, 2019 30253893

Lowe DJE, Sasiadek JD, Coles AS, et al: Cannabis and mental illness: a review. Eur Arch Psychiatry Clin Neurosci 269(1):107–120, 2019 30564886

Maldonado R, Cabañero D, Martín-García E: The endocannabinoid system in modulating fear, anxiety, and stress. Dialogues Clin Neurosci 22(3):229–239, 2020 33162766

Mannekote Thippaiah S, Iyengar SS, Vinod KY: Exo- and endo-cannabinoids in depressive and suicidal behaviors. Front Psychiatry 12:636228, 2021 33967855

Marconi A, Di Forti M, Lewis CM, et al: Meta-analysis of the association between the level of cannabis use and risk of psychosis. Schizophr Bull 42(5):1262–1269, 2016 26884547

McDonald J, Schleifer L, Richards JB, et al: Effects of THC on behavioral measures of impulsivity in humans. Neuropsychopharmacology 28(7):1356–1365, 2003 12784123

McGinty EE, Choksy S, Wintemute GJ: The relationship between controlled substances and violence. Epidemiol Rev 38(1):5–31, 2016 26905893

Mennis J, Stahler GJ, Mason MJ: Cannabis legalization and the decline of cannabis use disorder (CUD) treatment utilization in the US. Curr Addict Rep 10:38–51, 2023

Meruelo AD, Castro N, Cota CI, et al: Cannabis and alcohol use, and the developing brain. Behav Brain Res 325(Pt A):44–50, 2017

Miller NS, Gold MS, Mahler JC: Violent behaviors associated with cocaine use: possible pharmacological mechanisms. Int J Addict 26(10):1077–1088, 1991 1683859

Miller NS, Ipeku R, Oberbarnscheidt T: A review of cases of marijuana and violence. Int J Environ Res Public Health 17(5):1578, 2020 32121373

Mills R, Kisely S, Alati R, et al: Child maltreatment and cannabis use in young adulthood: a birth cohort study. Addiction 112(3):494–501, 2017 27741369

Moore TM, Stuart GL: A review of the literature on marijuana and interpersonal violence. Aggress Violent Behav 10(2):171–192, 2005

Morgan CJ, Noronha LA, Muetzelfeldt M, et al: Harms and benefits associated with psychoactive drugs: findings of an international survey of active drug users. J Psychopharmacol 27(6):497–506, 2013 23438502

Moulin V, Baumann P, Gholamrezaee M, et al: Cannabis, a significant risk factor for violent behavior in the early phase psychosis: two patterns of interaction of factors increase the risk of violent behavior: cannabis use disorder and impulsivity; cannabis use disorder, lack of insight and treatment adherence. Front Psychiatry 9:294, 2018 30022956

Moulin V, Alameda L, Framorando D, et al: Early onset of cannabis use and violent behavior in psychosis. Eur Psychiatry 63(1):e78, 2020 32669157

Mueller A, Fixen DR: Use of cannabis for agitation in patients with dementia. Sr Care Pharm 35(7):312–317, 2020 32600509

Murnan AW, Keim SA, Yeates KO, et al: Behavioral and cognitive differences in early childhood related to prenatal marijuana exposure. J Appl Dev Psychol 77:77, 2021 34840377

Murnan A, Keim S, Klebanoff M: Understanding relationships between fetal health locus of control (FHLC) and maternal marijuana use during pregnancy. Clin Nurs Res 31(5):968–974, 2022 35075917

Myerscough R, Taylor S: The effects of marijuana on human physical aggression. J Pers Soc Psychol 49(6):1541–1546, 1985 3003332

Myran DT, Staykov E, Cantor N, Taljaard M, et al: How has access to legal cannabis changed over time? An analysis of the cannabis retail market in Canada 2 years following the legalisation of recreational cannabis. Drug Alcohol Rev 41(2):377–385, 2022

National Center for Injury Prevention and Control: National Violent Death Reporting System (NVDRS). Washington, DC, Division of Violence Prevention, Centers for Disease Control and Prevention, 2021

National Institute on Drug Abuse: Synthetic Cannabinoids (k2/Spice) Drug Facts. Washington, DC, National Institute on Drug Abuse, 2018. Available at: https://nida.nih.gov/publications/drugfacts/synthetic-cannabinoids -k2spice. Accessed June 25, 2023.

Nguyen N, Holmes LM, Pravosud V, et al: Changes in perceived harms of tobacco and cannabis and their correlations with use: a panel study of young adults 2014–2020. Addict Behav 144:107758, 2023 37263178

Nordentoft M, Madsen T, Fedyszyn I: Suicidal behavior and mortality in first-episode psychosis. J Nerv Ment Dis 203(5):387–392, 2015 25919385

Norström T, Rossow I: Alcohol consumption as a risk factor for suicidal behavior: a systematic review of associations at the individual and at the population level. Arch Suicide Res 20(4):489–506, 2016 26953621

Ortiz-Peregrina S, Ortiz C, Anera RG: Aggressive driving behaviours in cannabis users: the influence of consumer characteristics. Int J Environ Res Public Health 18(8):3911, 2021 33917856

Østergaard MLD, Nordentoft M, Hjorthøj C: Associations between substance use disorders and suicide or suicide attempts in people with mental illness: a Danish nation-wide, prospective, register-based study of patients diagnosed with schizophrenia, bipolar disorder, unipolar depression or personality disorder. Addiction 112(7):1250–1259, 2017 28192643

Pajević I, Hasanović M, Žigić N, et al: Do cannabis and cannabinoids have a psychopharmacotherapeutic effect? Psychiatr Danub 33(Suppl 4):1196–1203, 2021 35354187

Palmieri B, Vadalà M: Oral THC: CBD cannabis extract in main symptoms of Alzheimer disease: agitation and weight loss. Clin Ter 174(1):53–60, 2023 36655645

Pistis M, Perra S, Pillolla G, et al: Adolescent exposure to cannabinoids induces long-lasting changes in the response to drugs of abuse of rat midbrain dopamine neurons. Biol Psychiatry 56(2):86–94, 2004 15231440

Rafiei D, Kolla NJ: Fact or faction regarding the relationship between cannabis use and violent behavior. J Am Acad Psychiatry Law 50(1):44–55, 2022 34893489

Ramesh D, Schlosburg JE, Wiebelhaus JM, et al: Marijuana dependence: not just smoke and mirrors. ILAR J 52(3):295–308, 2011 23382144

Reingle JM, Staras SA, Jennings WG, et al: The relationship between marijuana use and intimate partner violence in a nationally representative, longitudinal sample. J Interpers Violence 27(8):1562–1578, 2012 22080574

Rocca G, Verde A, Gatti U: Impact of alcohol and cannabis use on juvenile delinquency: results from an international multi-city study (ISRD3). Eur J Crim Policy Res 25(3):259–271, 2019

Rodríguez-Arias M, Roger-Sánchez C, Vilanova I, et al: Effects of cannabinoid exposure during adolescence on the conditioned rewarding effects of WIN 55212-2 and cocaine in mice: influence of the novelty-seeking trait. Neural Plast 2016:6481862, 2016 26881125

Roque-Bravo R, Silva RS, Malheiro RF, et al: Synthetic cannabinoids: a pharmacological and toxicological overview. Annu Rev Pharmacol Toxicol 63:187–209, 2023 35914767

Saez TM, Aronne MP, Caltana L, et al: Prenatal exposure to the CB1 and CB2 cannabinoid receptor agonist WIN 55,212–2 alters migration of early born glutamatergic neurons and GABAergic interneurons in the rat cerebral cortex. J Neurochem 129(4):637–648, 2014 24329778

Sánchez-Gutiérrez T, Barbeito S, Gómez-Juncal R, et al: Neuropsychological functioning and suicidal behaviours in patients with first-episode psychosis: a systematic review. Acta Psychiatr Scand 146(6):515–528, 2022 36153777

Sardinha L, Maheu-Giroux M, Stöckl H, et al: Global, regional, and national prevalence estimates of physical or sexual, or both, intimate partner violence against women in 2018. Lancet 399(10327):803–813, 2022 35182472

Schoeler T, Theobald D, Pingault JB, et al: Continuity of cannabis use and violent offending over the life course. Psychol Med 46(8):1663–1677, 2016 26961342

Sheikh NK, Dua A: Cannabinoids. Treasure Island, FL, StatPearls Publishing, 2023. Available at: https://www.ncbi.nlm.nih.gov/books/NBK556062. Accessed June 9, 2023.

Shorey RC, Stuart GL, Moore TM, et al: The temporal relationship between alcohol, marijuana, angry affect, and dating violence perpetration: a daily diary study with female college students. Psychol Addict Behav 28(2):516–523, 2014 24274434

Shorey RC, Haynes E, Brem M, et al: Marijuana use is associated with intimate partner violence perpetration among men arrested for domestic violence. Transl Issues Psychol Sci 4(1):108–118, 2018 30829345

Silva EAD, Medeiros WMB, Torro N, et al: Cannabis and cannabinoid use in autism spectrum disorder: a systematic review. Trends Psychiatry Psychother 44:e20200149, 2022 34043900

Smith PH, Homish GG, Leonard KE, et al: Marijuana withdrawal and aggression among a representative sample of U.S. marijuana users. Drug Alcohol Depend 132(1–2):63–68, 2013 23380439

Sontate KV, Rahim Kamaluddin M, Naina Mohamed I, et al: Alcohol, aggression, and violence: from public health to neuroscience. Front Psychol 12:699726, 2021 35002823

Sorkhou M, Johnstone S, Kivlichan AE, et al: Does cannabis use predict aggressive or violent behavior in psychiatric populations? A systematic review. Am J Drug Alcohol Abuse 48(6):631–643, 2022 36137273

Spidel A, Lecomte T, Greaves C, et al: Early psychosis and aggression: predictors and prevalence of violent behaviour amongst individuals with early onset psychosis. Int J Law Psychiatry 33(3):171–176, 2010 20546896

Tatar O, Abdel-Baki A, Wittevrongel A, et al: Reducing cannabis use in young adults with psychosis using iCanChange, a mobile health app: protocol for a pilot randomized controlled trial (ReCAP-iCC). JMIR Res Protoc 11(11):e40817, 2022 36427227

Taylor SP, Vardaris RM, Rawtich AB, et al: The effects of alcohol and delta-9-tetrahydrocannabinol on human physical aggression. Aggress Behav 2(2):153–161, 1976

Testa M, Derrick JL, Wang W, et al: Does marijuana contribute to intimate partner aggression? Temporal effects in a community sample of marijuana-using couples. J Stud Alcohol Drugs 79(3):432–440, 2018 29885151

Turna J, MacKillop J: Cannabis use among military veterans: a great deal to gain or lose? Clin Psychol Rev 84:101958, 2021 33486280

United Nations: Drug Market Trends of Cannabis and Opioids. Vienna, Office on Drugs and Crime, United Nations, 2022a

United Nations: Global Overview on Drug Demand and Drug Supply. Vienna, Office on Drugs and Crime, United Nations, 2022b

Volkow ND, Baler RD, Compton WM, et al: Adverse health effects of
    marijuana use. N Engl J Med 370(23):2219–2227, 2014 24897085
Volkow ND, Hampson AJ, Baler RD: Don't worry, be happy:
    endocannabinoids and cannabis at the intersection of stress and reward.
    Annu Rev Pharmacol Toxicol 57:285–308, 2017 27618739
Wadsworth E, Driezen P, Chan G, et al: Perceived access to cannabis and ease
    of purchasing cannabis in retail stores in Canada immediately before
    and one year after legalization. Am J Drug Alcohol Abuse 48(2):195–205,
    2022 35157544
Watkins KE, Ober AJ, Lamp K, et al: Collaborative care for opioid and alcohol
    use disorders in primary care: the summit randomized clinical trial.
    JAMA Intern Med 177(10):1480–1488, 2017 28846769
West ML, Sharif S: Cannabis and psychosis. Child Adolesc Psychiatr Clin N
    Am 32(1):69–83, 2023 36410907
White CM: A review of human studies assessing cannabidiol's (CBD) therapeutic
    actions and potential. J Clin Pharmacol 59(7):923–934, 2019 30730563
Williams AR: Cannabis as a gateway drug for opioid use disorder. J Law Med
    Ethics 48(2):268–274, 2020 32631185
Wilson J, Freeman TP, Mackie CJ: Effects of increasing cannabis potency on
    adolescent health. Lancet Child Adolesc Health 3(2):121–128, 2019 30573419
Witt K, van Dorn R, Fazel S: Risk factors for violence in psychosis: systematic
    review and meta-regression analysis of 110 studies. PLoS One 8(2):e55942,
    2013 23418482
Wordefo DK, Kassim FM, Birhanu E, et al: Suicidal behaviors and associated
    factors among patients attending an emergency department: a facility-
    based cross-sectional study. BMC Psychiatry 23(1):462, 2023 37357261
World Health Organization: Suicide Worldwide in 2019. Geneva, World
    Health Organization, 2021
World Health Organization: Violence Against Children Online. Geneva,
    World Health Organization, 2022
Wrege J, Schmidt A, Walter A, et al: Effects of cannabis on impulsivity:
    a systematic review of neuroimaging findings. Curr Pharm Des
    20(13):2126–2137, 2014 23829358
Wright MJ Jr, Vandewater SA, Taffe MA: Cannabidiol attenuates deficits of
    visuospatial associative memory induced by D(9) tetrahydrocannabinol.
    Br J Pharmacol 170(7):1365–1373, 2013 23550724
Young MM, Jesseman R: The Impact of Substance Use Disorders on Hospital
    Use: Technical Report. Ottawa, ON, Canadian Centre on Substance
    Abuse, 2014
Zhong S, Yu R, Fazel S: Drug use disorders and violence: associations with
    individual drug categories. Epidemiol Rev 42(1):103–116, 2020 33005950
Zuardi AW, Shirakawa I, Finkelfarb E, et al: Action of cannabidiol on the
    anxiety and other effects produced by delta 9-THC in normal subjects.
    Psychopharmacology (Berl) 76(3):245–250, 1982 6285406

10

Cannabis Use and Driving Risk

Jonathan Chevinsky, M.D.

David Gorelick, M.D., Ph.D.

Kevin P. Hill, M.D., M.H.S.

According to the National Survey on Drug Use and Health (NSDUH), cannabis is the most commonly used federally illegal substance in the United States, with more than 50 million users in 2021 (U.S. Department of Health and Human Services 2023). As the rates of cannabis use have climbed in the United States in recent years, bolstered by medicinal and recreational cannabis legalization at the state level, one effect of cannabis that warrants consideration is its effect on driving. An understanding of the current literature on the effects of cannabis on driving is crucial to inform policy decisions and clinician recommendations alike. This chapter reviews several aspects of the association between cannabis use and driving—or driving under the influence of cannabis (DUIC)—including the evidence for cannabis-associated driving impairment, risk factors associated with rates of DUIC, self-perception of DUIC, the influence of concurrent alcohol use on the risk from DUIC, the current state of roadside cannabis testing, and the effectiveness of prevention and educational strategies. The term *driving under the influence of cannabis* may be considered a misnomer of sorts, because in many studies it refers to driving with cannabinoids in the body, not driving while impaired by cannabis. For the purposes of this review, *cannabis* refers to products containing Δ^9-tetrahydrocannabinol (Δ^9-THC), the main constituent of cannabis responsible for its cognitive- and psychomotor-impairing effects. Cannabidiol (CBD), another important cannabis constituent, does not have such impairing effects and is not associated with driving impairment in laboratory studies (Arkell et al. 2020a, 2020b).

Current State of Evidence

Factors That Increase Probability of Driving Under the Influence of Cannabis

Several driver-related factors have been associated with the probability of DUIC, ranging from cannabis use patterns to sociodemographic factors and attitudes toward cannabis. Although the data are often conflicting, they offer guidance for efforts to prevent DUIC.

One strong association is with the frequency of cannabis use and the recency of last use. The presence of cannabis use disorder (CaUD) or cannabis dependence increases the probability of DUIC by up to 60%, which may be an artifact of higher frequency and intensity of cannabis use in those with CaUD (Cantor et al. 2021; Dahlgren et al. 2020; Salas-Wright et al. 2021). The frequency of cannabis use is positively associated with an increased probability of DUIC (Whitehill et al. 2014, 2019). Some studies using driving simulators have yielded conflicting results. One study found that chronic cannabis use increased the probability of driving-related errors (Dahlgren et al. 2020), while another study found that chronic cannabis use might moderate the risk of cannabis-associated motor vehicle accidents (MVAs) due to a propensity for chronic cannabis users to drive more slowly (Miller et al. 2022). Tolerance to the acute impairing effects of cannabis in chronic users may also reduce the probability of cannabis-associated MVAs (Hartley et al. 2019).

Both past-month and past-year cannabis use have been shown to correlate with substantial increases in the probability of DUIC in multiple large-scale cross-sectional studies (Mann et al. 2010; Whitehill et al. 2014), as might be expected from temporal association. Although past-year cannabis users may not be more likely to report a past-year MVA as a result of recall bias, one study found that MVA risk still increased during that period (DiGuiseppi et al. 2019).

Several sociodemographic factors are associated with an increased probability of DUIC, including age and sex, although these associations may be confounded by an independent association with increased frequency of cannabis use. Males are at an increased risk of DUIC, although it is unclear if this effect may be mediated by heavier cannabis use (Asbridge et al. 2005; Korn et al. 2017; Lloyd et al. 2020). Among females, being a parent by age 21 seems to be an independent risk factor (Begg et al. 2003). Early age at first use of cannabis and early age of cannabis dependence have been implicated as risks for DUIC as well, although one study in particular found this trend to hold only for females (Begg et al. 2003; Dahlgren et al. 2020; Jones et al. 2008). DUIC in elderly individuals may increase the risk of an MVA compared with middle-aged individuals (Johnson et al. 2021).

Conversely, driving with a child seems to be inversely correlated with DUIC, although among those who do not view DUIC as dangerous, driving with a child while under the influence of cannabis still often occurs (Romano et al. 2019). Marriage tends to lower the risk across age groups (Terry-McElrath and O'Malley 2021). Location also seems to play a role. Whereas DUIC seems to be increased among those living in rural locales (Asbridge et al. 2005), rates of fatally injured drivers who tested positive for cannabis are higher in urban settings (Azagba et al. 2020). That being said, these findings do not control for possible locality differences in overall rates and intensity of cannabis use.

Many studies have found that DUIC willingness (i.e., predisposition to drive while using cannabis) and intention (i.e., the deliberate decision to DUIC) increase the probability of DUIC (Scott et al. 2021; Ward et al. 2018). This is also true of perceived peer acceptance, whereas perceptions of disappointing important others seem to have the opposite effect (McCarthy et al. 2007; Ward et al. 2018). Another interesting societal factor is economic demand, as measured by how much an individual is willing to pay for cannabis. As has been established for driving under the influence of alcohol (DUIA) and increased economic demand for alcohol, one study noted that DUIC is correlated with increased economic demand for cannabis (Patel and Amlung 2019).

One major cluster of personality traits that has been studied is impulsivity and risk-taking behavior. One study found that trait impulsivity was correlated with increased sensitivity to the impairing effects of cannabis and a compensatory response of slowing down while DUIC (Wickens et al. 2022). Other studies have found that those who engaged in DUIC were more reckless drivers and more likely to engage in numerous risky driving behaviors, such as negative emotional driving (i.e., driving while experiencing self-described strong negative emotions) and being a passenger while the driver is DUIC (Bergeron and Paquette 2014; Dahlgren et al. 2020; Korn et al. 2017; Richer and Bergeron 2009). Still, it is important to note that the association between such traits and MVAs (independent of cannabis use) and cannabis use (independent of MVAs) strongly confounds any observed association with cannabis-related MVAs.

Similarly, correlations have been drawn between DUIC and having committed crimes or misused illicit substances. Studies have found that prior convictions, police contact as a juvenile, and the use of fake identification to purchase alcohol are all independent risk factors for DUIC (Asbridge et al. 2005; Begg et al. 2003). Those who engaged in DUIC were also more likely to drive under the influence of other substances and were generally more likely to misuse other illicit substances (Salas-Wright et al. 2021). Notably, the use of alcohol ignition interlock devices seemed to decrease alcohol use but simultaneously increase cannabis use (Scherer et al. 2022). These increases in cannabis use persisted even after the device was removed, suggesting that those individuals required to use such devices may be at higher risk for DUIC.

Finally, it is worth delving into the effects of cannabis legalization on DUIC. Some studies have shown that legalization or decriminalization does increase the risk of DUIC (Pollini et al. 2015; Windle et al. 2021). This is unsurprising because this likely increases cannabis availability overall. A pro-legalization attitude is an independent risk factor as well (Cantor et al. 2021). Moreover, even medicinal cannabis use has been shown to increase the risk of DUIC (Lloyd et al. 2020; Tucker et al. 2019). This likely also owes to a similar trend in increased availability.

Lack of Insight Into Cannabis-Related Driving Impairment

One factor to consider in terms of the risk of driving while under the influence of any substance is whether the person using such substances recognizes the effects of intoxication on their driving ability. There is a gap in knowledge about whether those who engage in DUIC are aware of the potential risks and whether such self-perception alters driving behavior.

One study by Wickens et al. (2019), composed of semistructured interviews with a small group of participants in a remedial program for impaired drivers, found a common perception that DUIC was less dangerous than DUIA or other potentially impairing substances. These apparent perceptions that DUIC is safer than DUIA have been replicated in multiple college student samples, with one sample of young adults demonstrating that although alcohol was deemed to be universally impairing, the effect of cannabis was deemed to be mediated by individual characteristics and the cannabis itself (Greene 2018; McCarthy et al. 2007).

The Wickens et al. (2019) study also found trends of comparative optimism (i.e., perceptions that individuals themselves are less likely to be involved in an MVA than other cannabis users) and normative influence (i.e., that friends were viewed to be more accepting of DUIC than family, and that the opinions of others who used cannabis were more credible than the opinions of those who did not). Another community sample of regular cannabis users who were not seeking treatment had a similar association, with more peer disapproval and higher perceived dangerousness of DUIC leading to a lower frequency of DUIC overall (Aston et al. 2016). In terms of societal pressures, it is worth noting that recreational cannabis legalization seems to not have a significant impact on perceptions of cannabis impairment risk and risk of arrest for DUIC (Eichelberger 2019).

Another large study of college students created a four-profile model of low-level engagers in substance misuse: 1) low-level users, 2) alcohol-centric engagers (high alcohol use but low cannabis use), 3) cannabis-centric/simultaneous engagers (highest rates of cannabis use and simultaneous alcohol and cannabis use), and 4) concurrent engagers (high rates of cannabis and alcohol use but lower rates of simultaneous use than the cannabis-centric/simultaneous group) (Arterberry et al. 2017). This study found that participants in the cannabis-centric/simultaneous engager group were more likely to have a lower perceived dangerousness of DUIC and higher rates of DUIC, suggesting that the frequency of cannabis use is correlated with the frequency of DUIC, possibly mediated by this lower perceived risk. These results have been corroborated in additional college sample studies that have shown that a lower perceived risk of negative consequences is associated with higher rates of DUIC (McCarthy et al. 2007).

Borodovsky et al. (2020) demonstrated a clear correlation between the frequency of DUIC and the median cannabis intoxication perceived as safe while driving and suggested this as a potential screening metric. This low perceived risk of DUIC seems to extend to medicinal cannabis users as well, with more than one-third of medicinal cannabis users feeling comfortable driving within 3 hours of cannabis use (Arkell et al. 2020b). There are even data to suggest that some individuals believe that MVA risk is increased only in novice cannabis users (Wickens et al. 2019) or that some regular cannabis users perceive their driving to improve when under the influence of cannabis (Terry and Wright 2005).

Influence of Alcohol Use on Driving Under the Influence of Cannabis

Both cannabis and alcohol impair driving performance in experimental studies using driving simulators or closed-road courses. One recent systematic review and meta-analysis comparing cannabis with alcohol in terms of driving impairment found that the combination of cannabis and alcohol produced greater impairment than either substance alone on only two of the performance measures evaluated: time out of lane and lateral position variability (Simmons et al. 2022). There was no additive effect observed on any other measure. A systematic review and meta-analysis of on-road studies found no significant additive effect of combined alcohol and cannabis use on risk of MVAs compared with driving after using only alcohol (OR 1.3, range 0.9–1.8) (White and Burns 2023). A recent study of fatal MVAs in Washington State also found that both the combination of alcohol and THC and alcohol alone similarly increased risk and that both of those risks were greater than when only THC was found in the blood (Woo et al. 2023).

Both alcohol and cannabis misuse may increase the risk of riding with an impaired driver. More than 40% of drivers who reported using both alcohol and cannabis in the past year reported driving under the influence of one or both substances (Gonçalves et al. 2022). In one study of 408 young adults, using cannabis and alcohol during the same day increased the risk of driving under the influence and riding with an impaired driver compared with using either substance alone (Patrick et al. 2021). Compared with alcohol use alone, the combination of cannabis and alcohol use by college students significantly increased their risk of both driving under the influence and riding with an impaired driver (Hultgren et al. 2021). Increased frequency of simultaneous use of alcohol and cannabis was associated with an increased likelihood of unsafe driving compared with using either substance alone (Terry-McElrath et al. 2014).

Several factors may account for the effect of combined cannabis and alcohol on experimental driving performance. In particular, drivers may experience increased sedation from the additive effects of two

CNS depressants (Ronen et al. 2010), and it has been found that alcohol increases serum concentrations of THC when consumed prior to cannabis (Downey et al. 2013). Conversely, in a study by Wright and Terry (2002), alcohol use impaired psychomotor skills relevant to driving in infrequent cannabis users substantially more than in chronic cannabis users, which may help account for the failure to find an additive risk for MVAs from combined alcohol and cannabis use.

Deleterious Effects

Association Between Motor Vehicle Accidents and Driving Under the Influence of Cannabis

Evaluating the contribution of DUIC to the probability of MVAs or MVA-related fatalities is not straightforward. Two major challenges are distinguishing the presence of cannabinoids (primarily THC) in the body from actual cannabinoid-induced impairment and evaluating the varied testing and reporting procedures across studies (Berning and Smither 2014).

The most direct evidence for the association between cannabis use and MVAs comes from epidemiological studies of real-world drivers. Dozens of such studies have been published in the past four decades. These studies generate odds ratios for cannabis use (i.e., the change in probability of an MVA) ranging from 0.46 (95% CI 0.2–1.3) to 10.88 (95% CI 6.4–18.4) (White and Burns 2021). These studies also vary greatly in methodological rigor—that is, the degree to which they account for major sources of bias. These include the identification of cannabis use (self-report or identification of cannabinoids in a bodily fluid, including blood, urine, or oral fluid), the interval between the last cannabis use and the MVA, the presence of other psychoactive substances that might have contributed to the MVA, and the presence or absence of controlling for differences between drivers with and without cannabis use (e.g., age, urban vs. rural location) that might confound the analysis (Preuss et al. 2021). Studies also vary in their outcome measure (e.g., all MVAs, culpable MVAs, or fatal MVAs). Publication bias may play a role as well because evidence has shown that studies showing a strong positive association between cannabis use and MVAs are more likely to be published (Preuss et al. 2021). Meta-analysis is a useful approach to obtaining a valid estimate in the face of substantial variability across individual studies.

Recent high-quality meta-analyses that adjusted for confounds as much as possible showed a statistically significant, albeit modest, increase in the probability of an MVA in drivers using cannabis, with odds ratios of 1.36 (95% CI 1.15–1.61; Rogeberg and Elvik 2016) and 1.42 (95% CI 1.18–1.71; Hostiuc et al. 2018) for all MVAs and odds ratios of 1.42 (95% CI 1.11–1.75; Rogeberg and Elvik 2016) and 1.37 (95% CI 1.10–1.69; White and Burns 2021) for culpable MVAs. The overall MVA risk is comparable with the risk associated with a breath/blood alcohol concentration (BAC) of 0.05% (OR 1.38–1.75) but substantially less than the culpable MVA risk at that BAC (OR 2.2) (Arkell et al. 2021). This comparison based on real-world driving is consistent with experimental studies of performance in driving simulators or closed-road courses, in which cannabis-induced impairment is comparable with that induced by a BAC of 0.04%–0.06% (Simmons et al. 2022).

Beneficial Effects

There are no apparent beneficial effects of cannabis use on driving safety.

Clinical Significance and Recommendations

Current State of Cannabis Roadside Testing

Roadside testing of body fluids for cannabinoids is of little value in detecting impaired driving because of the poor correlation between THC or THC metabolite concentrations and driving impairment (Ginsburg 2019; McCartney et al. 2022; Wennberg et al. 2023). Oral fluid is the most practical matrix for roadside testing, and currently available portable devices have adequate sensitivity and specificity for cannabinoid detection, per se (Wennberg et al. 2023). Although standardized field sobriety tests have long been used by law enforcement to detect DUIA, no validated field sobriety test is available to detect DUIC.

Several other issues may confound the association between cannabinoid concentration and level of impairment. One key issue is delayed testing, which may result in lower concentrations than would be anticipated based on the observed level of impairment (Jones et al. 2008; Wood et al. 2016). Another issue is the duration of impairment after cannabis consumption. Some studies find impairment resolving 3–6 hours after consumption (Tank et al. 2019), while others find some individuals remaining impaired up to 9–10 hours after low-dose cannabis administration (Trojan et al. 2022). THC concentrations in any biological matrix correlate poorly with the degree of intoxication identified by observational tests such as field sobriety tests (Chow et al. 2019; Declues et al. 2016; Raikos et al. 2014), in part because THC can be detectable in blood in some individuals more than a month after last use (Bergamaschi et al. 2013; Karschner et al. 2016).

The question of what to use as a THC concentration threshold has been hotly contested in various countries and even from state to state within the United States. Five states (Illinois, Montana, Nevada, Ohio, and Washington) currently have *per se* laws (i.e., a prohibition against driving with a serum level above a certain threshold) with established THC serum limits ranging from 2 ng/mL to 5 ng/mL of THC on serum tests; 14 states have zero-tolerance laws; and most other states have driving under the influence laws as would be found for other impairing substances (Governors Highway Safety Association 2023). The only exception is Colorado, which uses a permissible inference law wherein a test result higher than 5 ng/mL does not inherently imply impairment but allows a jury to use this data point to determine whether cannabis caused impairment.

Data on the effectiveness of such thresholds are mixed. Some arguments have been made for zero-tolerance laws because of the decrease in tested THC levels by the time of sample collection, the inconsistent correlation between THC levels and impairment, and concerns about alterations in brain circuitry and cognition that occur at any level of cannabis use (Battistella et al. 2013; Jones et al. 2008). Contrarily, others have suggested poor efficacy of zero-limit laws in other countries (Jones 2005). Whereas most studies agree that very high levels of THC are likely to cause impairment (Del Balzo et al. 2018; Ramaekers et al. 2006), establishing a lower limit is challenging. Most studies did focus on the range of 2–5 ng/mL. Some small cross-sectional studies found impairment with THC cutoffs as low as 2 ng/mL (Doroudgar et al. 2018); other similar small samples found that values as high as 40 ng/mL were unreliable (Fabritius et al. 2014). In the absence of conclusive evidence, it seems challenging to establish a single, firm THC cutoff threshold.

Given the unreliability of measuring THC concentration, considerable research has gone into various field sobriety tests. Field sobriety tests perform poorly in most studies, with unacceptably high rates of false-positive identifications (i.e., participants given a placebo classified as impaired by cannabis) and difficulty distinguishing cannabis impairment from impairment due to other substances or conditions (Ginsburg 2019; Liguori et al. 2002; Marcotte et al. 2023; Papafotiou et al. 2005). One recent study, however, did find that combining a field sobriety test with oral fluid THC testing (2 ng/mL cutoff) eliminated all false-positive identifications (Fitzgerald et al. 2023).

In view of such uncertainty and the limited tools available for identifying cannabis-impaired driving, further research is urgently needed to inform public policy. Meanwhile, clinicians should provide evidence-based advice to their patients who use or plan to use cannabis and caution them about driving soon after cannabis use, especially in states with zero-tolerance or *per se* laws.

Prevention and Education Regarding Driving Under the Influence of Cannabis

Several strategies have been tested to prevent the public health concern of cannabis-impaired driving, including both direct roadside interventions (e.g., traffic stops) and educational campaigns. Educational campaigns can address the risks of DUIC, including the legal ramifications associated with this offense. Educational materials can be disseminated through various media, including smartphones, in-person educational or rehabilitation programs, advertising, and labeling of cannabis products.

Many interventions have focused on the route of information dissemination. Recent interventions using mobile-based strategies increased perceptions of dangerousness regarding DUIC among users through the use of personal feedback via text messages (Colonna et al. 2022; Teeters et al. 2021). Other studies found that formal substance use disorder rehabilitation programs decreased the incidence of DUIC following completion, likely mediated by decreased frequency of use (Macdonald et al. 2004).

A recent systematic review found that effective strategies for the deterrence of DUIC include cannabis packaging with health warnings and descriptions of the effects of driving under the influence, as well as either motivational interviewing or driver education programs for previous offenders or youth (Razaghizad et al. 2021). Roadside drug testing has also proven an effective deterrent among individuals who use cannabis (Mills et al. 2022; Razaghizad et al. 2021). Contrarily, state sanctions and driving laws seem to have a limited effect (Razaghizad et al. 2021).

The certainty of punishment is a more effective deterrent than the severity of punishment, which may inform messaging (Jones et al. 2006). Others simply postulate the importance of remediating gaps in knowledge about the dangerousness of DUIC (Lensch et al. 2020). In fact, one study suggested that safety risk was a stronger deterrent than legal risk (Davis et al. 2016). Still other studies found that any negative cannabis expectancies were associated with decreased risk of DUIC, suggesting the utility of general education about the risks of misusing cannabis (Arterberry et al. 2013). This accords well with the finding that negative pleasant affect regarding messaging tends to be a more effective deterrent (Stevens et al. 2019). One final point worth considering is whether effective strategies for DUIA may also be effective in curbing DUIC. Although interventions that have proven effective for alcohol should be considered, such as minimum-age laws and graduated driver licensing programs, more research into cannabis-specific deterrents is required before such policies can be implemented. Ultimately, clinician counseling of patients should focus on the substantially increased risk of MVAs with DUIC because some regular cannabis users lack such insight.

Conclusion

Cannabis impairs driving performance in driving simulators and significantly, albeit modestly, increases the probability of both nonlethal and lethal MVAs. THC concentrations in body fluids correlate poorly with the level of driving impairment, making it difficult to assess acute risk. Observational tests of impairment such as field sobriety tests are also not very effective. Future research is needed to improve roadside detection of cannabis-impaired driving and to develop more effective methods of prevention.

Key Points

- Cannabis use around the time of driving increases the risk of motor vehicle accidents (MVAs) by 30%–40%.
- Cannabinoid concentrations in body fluids (blood, oral fluid), particularly levels of Δ^9-tetrahydrocannabinol (Δ^9-THC), correlate poorly with the actual level of impairment, suggesting the importance of further research into observational tests such as field sobriety testing.
- Current field sobriety tests, adapted from those used for alcohol, have poor specificity.
- Factors that increase the risk of an individual driving under the influence of cannabis (DUIC) include male sex, increased frequency of use, early age at first use, and impulsivity and risk-taking behavior, including other substance use.
- Concurrent alcohol use is common among those who engage in DUIC and significantly increases MVA risk compared with cannabis use alone.
- Individuals with a lower perceived risk of DUIC are significantly more likely to do so, suggesting education on the risks of DUIC as a potential target for prevention.
- Interventions such as increased roadside testing and education focused more on safety than on legal risks of DUIC have been shown to reduce rates of DUIC.

References

Arkell TR, Lintzeris N, Mills L, et al: Driving-related behaviours, attitudes and perceptions among Australian medical cannabis users: results from the CAMS 18–19 survey. Accid Anal Prev 148:105784, 2020a 33017729

Arkell TR, Vinckenbosch F, Kevin RC, et al: Effect of cannabidiol and $\Delta 9$-tetrahydrocannabinol on driving performance: a randomized clinical trial. JAMA 324(21):2177–2186, 2020b 33258890

Arkell TR, McCartney D, McGregor IS: Medical cannabis and driving. Aust J Gen Pract 50(6):357–362, 2021 34059836

Arterberry BJ, Treloar HR, Smith AE, et al: Marijuana use, driving, and related cognitions. Psychol Addict Behav 27(3):854–860, 2013 23276319

Arterberry BJ, Treloar H, McCarthy DM: Empirical profiles of alcohol and marijuana use, drugged driving, and risk perceptions. J Stud Alcohol Drugs 78(6):889–898, 2017 29087824

Asbridge M, Poulin C, Donato A: Motor vehicle collision risk and driving under the influence of cannabis: evidence from adolescents in Atlantic Canada. Accid Anal Prev 37(6):1025–1034, 2005 15992751

Aston ER, Merrill JE, McCarthy DM, et al: Risk factors for driving after and during marijuana use. J Stud Alcohol Drugs 77(2):309–316, 2016 26997189

Azagba S, Shan L, Latham K: Rural-urban differences in cannabis detected in fatally injured drivers in the United States. Prev Med 132:105975, 2020 31899254

Battistella G, Fornari E, Thomas A, et al: Weed or wheel! FMRI, behavioural, and toxicological investigations of how cannabis smoking affects skills necessary for driving. PLoS One 8(1):e52545, 2013 23300977

Begg DJ, Langley JD, Stephenson S: Identifying factors that predict persistent driving after drinking, unsafe driving after drinking, and driving after using cannabis among young adults. Accid Anal Prev 35(5):669–675, 2003 12850067

Bergamaschi MM, Karschner EL, Goodwin RS, et al: Impact of prolonged cannabinoid excretion in chronic daily cannabis smokers' blood on per se drugged driving laws. Clin Chem 59(3):519–526, 2013 23449702

Bergeron J, Paquette M: Relationships between frequency of driving under the influence of cannabis, self-reported reckless driving and risk-taking behavior observed in a driving simulator. J Safety Res 49:19–24, 2014 24913481

Berning A, Smither DD: Understanding the Limitations of Drug Test Information, Reporting, and Testing Practices in Fatal Crashes: Traffic Safety Facts Research Note. Washington, DC, U.S. Department of Transportation, 2014

Borodovsky JT, Marsch LA, Scherer EA, et al: Perceived safety of cannabis intoxication predicts frequency of driving while intoxicated. Prev Med 131:105956, 2020 31863787

Cantor N, Kingsbury M, Hamilton HA, et al: Correlates of driving after cannabis use in high school students. Prev Med 150:106667, 2021 34081937

Chow RM, Marascalchi B, Abrams WB, et al: Driving under the influence of cannabis: a framework for future policy. Anesth Analg 128(6):1300–1308, 2019 31094805

Colonna R, Tucker P, Holmes J, et al: Mobile-based brief interventions targeting cannabis-impaired driving among youth: a Delphi study. J Subst Abuse Treat 141:108802, 2022 35599094

Dahlgren MK, Sagar KA, Smith RT, et al: Recreational cannabis use impairs driving performance in the absence of acute intoxication. Drug Alcohol Depend 208:107771, 2020 31952821

Davis KC, Allen J, Duke J, et al: Correlates of marijuana drugged driving and openness to driving while high: evidence from Colorado and Washington. PLoS One 11(1):e0146853, 2016 26800209

Declues K, Perez S, Figueroa A: A 2-year study of Δ9-tetrahydrocannabinol concentrations in drivers: examining driving and field sobriety test performance. J Forensic Sci 61(6):1664–1670, 2016 27479468

Del Balzo G, Gottardo R, Mengozzi S, et al: "Positive" urine testing for cannabis is associated with increased risk of traffic crashes. J Pharm Biomed Anal 151:71–74, 2018 29310049

DiGuiseppi CG, Smith AA, Betz ME, et al: Cannabis use in older drivers in Colorado: the LongROAD study. Accid Anal Prev 132:105273, 2019 31521874

Doroudgar S, Mae Chuang H, Bohnert K, et al: Effects of chronic marijuana use on driving performance. Traffic Inj Prev 19(7):680–686, 2018 30411981

Downey LA, King R, Papafotiou K, et al: The effects of cannabis and alcohol on simulated driving: influences of dose and experience. Accid Anal Prev 50:879–886, 2013 22871272

Eichelberger AH: Marijuana use and driving in Washington State: risk perceptions and behaviors before and after implementation of retail sales. Traffic Inj Prev 20(1):23–29, 2019 30822133

Fabritius M, Augsburger M, Chtioui H, et al: Fitness to drive and cannabis: validation of two blood THCCOOH thresholds to distinguish occasional users from heavy smokers. Forensic Sci Int 242:1–8, 2014 24999608

Fitzgerald RL, Umlauf A, Hubbard JA, et al: Driving under the influence of cannabis: impact of combining toxicology testing with field sobriety tests. Clin Chem 69(7):724–733, 2023 37228223

Ginsburg BC: Strengths and limitations of two cannabis-impaired driving detection methods: a review of the literature. Am J Drug Alcohol Abuse 45(6):610–622, 2019 31498702

Gonçalves PD, Gutkind S, Segura LE, et al: Simultaneous alcohol/cannabis use and driving under the influence in the U.S. Am J Prev Med 62(5):661–669, 2022 35459450

Governors Highway Safety Association: Drug Impaired Driving. Washington, DC, Governors Highway Safety Association, 2023. Available at: https://www.ghsa.org/state-laws/issues/Drug%20Impaired%20Driving. Accessed July 26, 2024.

Greene KM: Perceptions of driving after marijuana use compared to alcohol use among rural American young adults. Drug Alcohol Rev 37(5):637–644, 2018 29464852

Hartley S, Simon N, Larabi A, et al: Effect of smoked cannabis on vigilance and accident risk using simulated driving in occasional and chronic users and the pharmacokinetic-pharmacodynamic relationship. Clin Chem 65(5):684–693, 2019 30872375

Hostiuc S, Moldoveanu A, Negoi I, et al: The association of unfavorable traffic events and cannabis usage: a meta-analysis. Front Pharmacol 9:99, 2018 29487531

Hultgren BA, Waldron KA, Mallett KA, et al: Alcohol, marijuana, and nicotine use as predictors of impaired driving and riding with an impaired driver among college students who engage in polysubstance use. Accid Anal Prev 160:106341, 2021 34392006

Johnson MB, Mechtler L, Ali B, et al: Cannabis and crash risk among older drivers. Accid Anal Prev 152:105987, 2021 33549974

Jones AW: Driving under the influence of drugs in Sweden with zero concentration limits in blood for controlled substances. Traffic Inj Prev 6(4):317–322, 2005 16266940

Jones AW, Holmgren A, Kugelberg FC: Driving under the influence of cannabis: a 10-year study of age and gender differences in the concentrations of tetrahydrocannabinol in blood. Addiction 103(3):452–461, 2008 18190663

Jones C, Donnelly N, Swift W, et al: Preventing cannabis users from driving under the influence of cannabis. Accid Anal Prev 38(5):854–861, 2006 16574046

Karschner EL, Swortwood MJ, Hirvonen J, et al: Extended plasma cannabinoid excretion in chronic frequent cannabis smokers during sustained abstinence and correlation with psychomotor performance. Drug Test Anal 8(7):682–689, 2016 26097154

Korn L, Weiss Y, Rosenbloom T: Driving violations and health promotion behaviors among undergraduate students: self-report of on-road behavior. Traffic Inj Prev 18(8):813–819, 2017 28409675

Lensch T, Sloan K, Ausmus J, et al: Cannabis use and driving under the influence: behaviors and attitudes by state-level legal sale of recreational cannabis. Prev Med 141:106320, 2020 33161068

Liguori A, Gatto CP, Jarrett DB: Separate and combined effects of marijuana and alcohol on mood, equilibrium and simulated driving. Psychopharmacology (Berl) 163(3–4):399–405, 2002 12373440

Lloyd SL, Lopez-Quintero C, Striley CW: Sex differences in driving under the influence of cannabis: the role of medical and recreational cannabis use. Addict Behav 110:106525, 2020 32711286

Macdonald S, DeSouza A, Mann R, et al: Driving behavior of alcohol, cannabis, and cocaine abuse treatment clients and population controls. Am J Drug Alcohol Abuse 30(2):429–444, 2004 15230084

Mann RE, Stoduto G, Ialomiteanu A, et al: Self-reported collision risk associated with cannabis use and driving after cannabis use among Ontario adults. Traffic Inj Prev 11(2):115–122, 2010 20373229

Marcotte TD, Umlauf A, Grelotti DJ, et al: Evaluation of field sobriety tests for identifying drivers under the influence of cannabis: a randomized clinical trial. JAMA Psychiatry 80(9):914–923, 2023 37531115

McCarthy DM, Lynch AM, Pederson SL: Driving after use of alcohol and marijuana in college students. Psychol Addict Behav 21(3):425–430, 2007 17874895

McCartney D, Arkell TR, Irwin C, et al: Are blood and oral fluid Δ9-tetrahydrocannabinol (THC) and metabolite concentrations related to impairment? A meta-regression analysis. Neurosci Biobehav Rev 134:104433, 2022 34767878

Miller R, Brown T, Wrobel J, et al: Influence of cannabis use history on the impact of acute cannabis smoking on simulated driving performance during a distraction task. Traffic Injury Prevention 23(Suppl 1):S1–S7, 2022 35686998

Mills L, Freeman J, Parkes A, et al: Do they need to be tested to be deterred? Exploring the impact of exposure to roadside drug testing on drug driving. J Safety Res 80:362–370, 2022 35249616

Papafotiou K, Carter JD, Stough C: The relationship between performance on the standardised field sobriety tests, driving performance and the level of delta9-tetrahydrocannabinol (THC) in blood. Forensic Sci Int 155(2–3):172–178, 2005 16226154

Patel H, Amlung M: Elevated cannabis demand is associated with driving after cannabis use in a crowd-sourced sample of adults. Exp Clin Psychopharmacol 27(2):109–114, 2019 30475012

Patrick ME, Graupensperger S, Dworkin ER, et al: Intoxicated driving and riding with impaired drivers: comparing days with alcohol, marijuana, and simultaneous use. Drug Alcohol Depend 225:108753, 2021 34058538

Pollini RA, Romano E, Johnson MB, et al: The impact of marijuana decriminalization on California drivers. Drug Alcohol Depend 150:135–140, 2015 25765482

Preuss UW, Huestis MA, Schneider M, et al: Cannabis use and car crashes: a review. Front Psychiatry 12:643315, 2021 34122176

Raikos N, Schmid H, Nussbaumer S, et al: Determination of Δ9-tetrahydrocannabinolic acid A (Δ9-THCA-A) in whole blood and plasma by LC-MS/MS and application in authentic samples from drivers suspected of driving under the influence of cannabis. Forensic Sci Int 243:130–136, 2014 25173986

Ramaekers JG, Moeller MR, van Ruitenbeek P, et al: Cognition and motor control as a function of delta9-THC concentration in serum and oral fluid: limits of impairment. Drug Alcohol Depend 85(2):114–122, 2006 16723194

Razaghizad A, Windle SB, Gore G, et al: Interventions to prevent drugged driving: a systematic review. Am J Prev Med 61(2):267–280, 2021 34099354

Richer I, Bergeron J: Driving under the influence of cannabis: links with dangerous driving, psychological predictors, and accident involvement. Accid Anal Prev 41(2):299–307, 2009 19245889

Rogeberg O, Elvik R: The effects of cannabis intoxication on motor vehicle collision revisited and revised. Addiction 111(8):1348–1359, 2016

Romano E, Kelley-Baker T, Hoff S, et al: Use of alcohol and cannabis among adults driving children in Washington State. J Stud Alcohol Drugs 80(2):196–200, 2019 31014464

Ronen A, Chassidim HS, Gershon P, et al: The effect of alcohol, THC and their combination on perceived effects, willingness to drive and performance of driving and non-driving tasks. Accid Anal Prev 42(6):1855–1865, 2010 20728636

Salas-Wright CP, Cano M, Hai AH, et al: Prevalence and correlates of driving under the influence of cannabis in the U.S. Am J Prev Med 60(6):e251–e260, 2021 33726992

Scherer M, Romano E, King S, et al: Cannabis adaptation during and after alcohol ignition interlock device installation: a longitudinal study. J Stud Alcohol Drugs 83(4):486–493, 2022 35838425

Scott B, Ward N, Otto J, et al: Modeling the system of beliefs that influence driving under the influence of cannabis (DUIC) in Washington State. Accid Anal Prev 151:105988, 2021 33484972

Simmons SM, Caird JK, Sterzer F, et al: The effects of cannabis and alcohol on driving performance and driver behaviour: a systematic review and meta-analysis. Addiction 117(7):1843–1856, 2022 35083810

Stevens EM, Cohn AM, Villanti AC, et al: Perceived effectiveness of anti-marijuana messages in adult users and nonusers: an examination of responses to messages about marijuana's effects on cognitive performance, driving, and health. J Stud Alcohol Drugs 80(4):415–422, 2019 31495378

Tank A, Tietz T, Daldrup T, et al: On the impact of cannabis consumption on traffic safety: a driving simulator study with habitual cannabis consumers. Int J Legal Med 133(5):1411–1420, 2019 30701315

Teeters JB, King SA, Hubbard SM: A mobile phone-based brief intervention with personalized feedback and interactive text messaging is associated with changes in driving after cannabis use cognitions in a proof-of-concept pilot trial. Exp Clin Psychopharmacol 29(2):203–209, 2021 34043401

Terry P, Wright KA: Self-reported driving behaviour and attitudes towards driving under the influence of cannabis among three different user groups in England. Addict Behav 30(3):619–626, 2005 15718082

Terry-McElrath YM, O'Malley PM: Social role, behavior, and belief changes associated with driving after using marijuana among U.S. young adults, and comparisons with driving after 5+ drinking. J Stud Alcohol Drugs 82(5):584–594, 2021 34546904

Terry-McElrath YM, O'Malley PM, Johnston LD: Alcohol and marijuana use patterns associated with unsafe driving among U.S. high school seniors: high use frequency, concurrent use, and simultaneous use. J Stud Alcohol Drugs 75(3):378–389, 2014 24766749

Trojan V, Landa L, Hrib R, et al: Assessment of delta-9-tetrahydrocannabinol (THC) in saliva and blood after oral administration of medical cannabis with respect to its effect on driving abilities. Physiol Res 71(5):703–712, 2022 36121021

Tucker JS, Rodriguez A, Pedersen ER, et al: Greater risk for frequent marijuana use and problems among young adult marijuana users with a medical marijuana card. Drug Alcohol Depend 194:178–183, 2019 30447509

U.S. Department of Health and Human Services: SAMHSA announces National Survey on Drug Use and Health (NSDUH) results detailing mental illness and substance use levels in 2021. Washington, DC, U.S. Department of Health and Human Services, 2023. Available at: https://www.hhs.gov/about/news/2023/01/04/samhsa-announces-national-survey-drug-use-health-results-detailing-mental-illness-substance-use-levels-2021.html. Accessed July 26, 2024.

Ward NJ, Schell W, Kelley-Baker T, et al: Developing a theoretical foundation to change road user behavior and improve traffic safety: driving under the influence of cannabis (DUIC). Traffic Inj Prev 19(4):358–363, 2018 29337600

Wennberg E, Windle SB, Filion KB, et al: Roadside screening tests for cannabis use: a systematic review. Heliyon 9(4):e14630, 2023 37064483

White MA, Burns NR: The risk of being culpable for or involved in a road crash after using cannabis: a systematic review and meta-analyses. Drug Sci Policy Law 7:1–20, 2021

White MA, Burns NR: Does the co-use of cannabis exacerbate the effect of alcohol on the risk of crashing? A systematic review and meta-analysis. Drug Sci Policy Law 9(536):1–10, 2023

Whitehill JM, Rivara FP, Moreno MA: Marijuana-using drivers, alcohol-using drivers, and their passengers: prevalence and risk factors among underage college students. JAMA Pediatr 168(7):618–624, 2014 24820649

Whitehill JM, Rodriguez-Monguio R, Doucette M, et al: Driving and riding under the influence of recent marijuana use: risk factors among a racially diverse sample of young adults. J Ethn Subst Abuse 18(4):594–612, 2019 29432083

Wickens CM, Watson TM, Mann RE, et al: Exploring perceptions among people who drive after cannabis use: collision risk, comparative optimism and normative influence. Drug Alcohol Rev 38(4):443–451, 2019 30896069

Wickens CM, Mann RE, Brands B, et al: Influence of personality on acute smoked cannabis effects on simulated driving. Exp Clin Psychopharmacol 30(5):547–559, 2022 34291988

Windle SB, Eisenberg MJ, Reynier P, et al: Association between legalization of recreational cannabis and fatal motor vehicle collisions in the United States: an ecologic study. CMAJ Open 9(1):E233–E241, 2021 33731424

Woo Y, Willits D, Stohr MK, et al: Relative risk of cannabis, alcohol, and their combination on driver behavior in fatal crashes in Washington State. Journal of Crime and Criminal Behavior 3(1):33–59, 2023

Wood E, Brooks-Russell A, Drum P: Delays in DUI blood testing: impact on cannabis DUI assessments. Traffic Inj Prev 17(2):105–108, 2016 26066003

Wright A, Terry P: Modulation of the effects of alcohol on driving-related psychomotor skills by chronic exposure to cannabis. Psychopharmacology (Berl) 160(2):213–219, 2002 11875640

11

Cannabis, Pregnancy, and Infertility

Sarena Hayer, M.D.

Rahul J. D'Mello, M.D., Ph.D.

Jasper C. Bash, M.D.

Jason C. Hedges, M.D., Ph.D.

Olivia J. Hagen, B.S.

Benjamin J. Burwitz, Ph.D.

Jennifer A. Manuzak, Ph.D.

B. Adam Crosland, M.D., M.P.H.

Ava D. Mandelbaum, B.S.

Ashley E. Benson, M.D., M.Sc.

Jamie O. Lo, M.D., M.C.R.

Cannabis use continues to rise, especially among individuals of reproductive age, due in part to changing legal restrictions and heightened anxiety and stress from the coronavirus disease 2019 (COVID-19) pandemic (Imtiaz et al. 2021; Young-Wolff et al. 2021). In 2021, cannabis was the most commonly used illicit substance in the United States, and the percentage of use was highest among 18- to 25-year-old adults (35.4% or 11.8 million people), followed by adults age 26 or older (17.2%

or 37.9 million individuals) (Center for Behavioral Health Statistics and Quality 2021). Currently, in the United States, 37 states and the District of Columbia have legalized some form of medical cannabis, and almost half have legalized cannabis for adult recreational use, resulting in increased perceptions of safety, accessibility, and acceptability (National Conference of State Legislatures 2022). A 2017 national survey demonstrated that 81% of adults in the United States believed that cannabis use had at least one benefit, 9% believed there was no risk to using cannabis, 22% believed that cannabis was not addictive, and 7.3% agreed that prenatal cannabis use was somewhat or completely safe (Keyhani et al. 2018). This is concerning because 10% of regular cannabis users and up to 50% of chronic daily users can develop cannabis use disorder (CaUD), defined by cannabis use and signs and symptoms of functional impairment per the DSM-5 criteria (American Psychiatric Association 2022).

Studies have demonstrated the presence of cannabinoid receptors in the male and female reproductive tracts and the placenta (Dunne 2019; Uhlén et al. 2015), which suggests that the endocannabinoid system is involved in the regulation of reproductive functions (Aquila et al. 2010; Jensen et al. 2015). Despite the growing prevalence of cannabis use, there is a paucity of safety information regarding its impact on fertility and offspring outcomes. The limited available evidence suggests that paternal and maternal cannabis use preconception and/or during pregnancy can adversely affect reproductive health, perinatal and fetal outcomes, and longer-term offspring health and developmental trajectories (Conner et al. 2016; Lo et al. 2022, 2023; Marchand et al. 2022). Cannabis use has been associated with altered male and female reproductive hormones, menstrual cycle changes, affected semen parameters, offspring who are small for gestational age, and preterm births (Hedges et al. 2022; Lo et al. 2022, 2023; Ryan et al. 2021b). Thus, multiple national societies, including the American Society for Reproductive Medicine and the American College of Obstetricians and Gynecologists, currently recommend against cannabis use when intending to conceive or while pregnant (American College of Obstetricians and Gynecologists Committee on Obstetric Practice 2015; Practice Committee of the American Society for Reproductive Medicine 2022).

Most existing literature surrounding cannabis use and reproductive health was published in the 1980s with a focus on smoked cannabis. Since then, the potency of cannabis has increased more than threefold (ElSohly et al. 2021). Human studies are often limited by confounders such as polysubstance use, selection bias, patient self-report, retrospective or observational study design, and different modes, potency, and frequency of cannabis use among participants. Additionally, preclinical research has largely focused on the effects of acute cannabis exposure and used modes of cannabis delivery such as intraperitoneal injection or oral gavage that do not recapitulate typical human use (Ryan et al. 2021a). As a result of the limited evidence regarding the safety of cannabis use, health care providers are not comfortable counseling patients. In a recent cross-sectional patient survey study among past-year users, 72% had or would have disclosed the use of cannabis to their provider, but only 9.4% reported that their provider advised against use (Jordan et al. 2020).

As the incidence of cannabis use continues to increase, it is important to better understand the role and contributions of cannabis use on reproductive health and offspring outcomes in order to counsel patients and inform public health policies focused on cannabis use.

Cannabis and Male Fertility

Current State of Evidence

The 2021 National Survey on Drug Use and Health (NSDUH) estimated the U.S. prevalence of cannabis use in the past year among males age 18 or older to be 22.1% (~27.2 million) (Center for Behavioral Health Statistics and Quality 2021). Prevalence of use was highest among males ages 18–25 (36.6%, ~6.1 million). There is a high degree of variability in the existing literature on cannabis use and male fertility, but the data support an association between cannabis use and decreased libido, erectile dysfunction, orgasmic dysfunction, altered reproductive hormones, changes in semen parameters, and premature or delayed ejaculation (Lo et al. 2022; Ryan et al. 2021a). Variability in results is partly because participants in human studies are often recruited from assisted reproductive centers, and data are frequently confounded by polysubstance use and sociodemographic factors.

Deleterious Effects

Male Reproductive Hormones

Many studies have evaluated the impact of cannabis use on the male hypothalamic-pituitary-gonadal axis and have demonstrated conflicting results, in part because of small sample sizes. Largely, studies have not demonstrated an effect on follicle-stimulating hormone (FSH) levels except with heavy chronic use (Payne et al. 2019). Kolodny et al. (1974) compared FSH levels of male control subjects with those of males who smoked 5–9 cannabis cigarettes per week ($n=11$) and males who smoked 10 or more cannabis cigarettes per week ($n=9$). Males who smoked 10 or more cannabis cigarettes per week were found to have significantly lower levels of FSH ($P<0.01$). In contrast, in a nonhuman primate study of males ($N=6$) chronically exposed to 2.5 mg/7 kg/day of edible Δ^9-tetrahydrocannabinol (Δ^9-THC, the main component of cannabis), which is equivalent to a heavy medical cannabis dose, researchers observed a significant increase in FSH ($P=0.01$) during dosing and a significant decrease in FSH ($P=0.025$) after cessation for 4 months (Hedges et al. 2022, 2023).

The existing preclinical and human studies are also mixed regarding the effect of cannabis exposure on luteinizing hormone (LH) levels. Serum LH levels have been reported to be significantly lower in males after acute THC exposure from smoking a cannabis cigarette (Cone et al. 1986). Effects of THC on serum LH levels do not appear to be dose-dependent, however, with Kolodny et al. (1974) finding no significant difference in plasma LH levels after chronic cannabis exposure when comparing males who smoked 5–9 cannabis cigarettes per week with those who smoked 10 or more cannabis cigarettes weekly. In contrast, the nonhuman primate study of edible THC consumption mentioned earlier reported elevated LH levels following chronic THC exposure (Hedges et al. 2022).

Similarly, the impact of cannabis exposure on serum testosterone levels is also variable, as demonstrated by a systematic review of 91 studies (Rajanahally et al. 2019). Preclinical and human studies reported a range of findings, including decreased, increased, or no effect on testosterone levels (Ryan et al. 2021a). A large population study of 1,215 healthy Danish males ages 18–26 showed a 7% higher serum testosterone level in those who regularly smoked cannabis compared with nonusers (Gundersen et al. 2015). In contrast, a study of 2,074 European males undergoing evaluation for infertility noted that those with infertility and a history of cannabis use had significantly decreased total testosterone levels compared with nonusers ($P=0.03$; Belladelli et al. 2022). Similarly, Kolodny et al. (1974) found that plasma testosterone was significantly reduced between chronic and never cannabis users ($P<0.001$), which is consistent with more recent observations in the Hedges et al. (2022) nonhuman primate model of chronic cannabis consumption. However, a study of males in the United

States using data collected from the National Health and Nutrition Examination Survey was overall notable for showing no difference in serum testosterone levels between males who reported ever using cannabis and never users (Thistle et al. 2017). Serum testosterone levels were higher among males with more recent cannabis use, suggesting that the effects may be transient. Interestingly, this study also observed that serum testosterone level was inversely associated with the time since last regular cannabis use and that this showed the strongest correlation with testosterone levels, rather than the duration or frequency of cannabis use.

Effects on Semen and Sperm Parameters

A strong association between cannabis use and decreased sperm count and concentration has been demonstrated in animal and human studies (Kolodny et al. 1974; Payne et al. 2019; Ryan et al. 2021a). Several human studies demonstrated an association between cannabis use and decreased sperm count (Gundersen et al. 2015; Hembree et al. 1978; Kolodny et al. 1974) and lower sperm counts among weekly THC users compared with never-users (Gundersen et al. 2015; Murphy et al. 2018). Although the underlying etiology is not well defined, the observed cannabis-induced sperm count and concentration reduction has been linked with arrested spermatogenesis (Payne et al. 2019).

Existing studies also indicate that cannabis exposure alters sperm morphology. This is demonstrated in several rodent studies (Huang et al. 1978; Zimmerman et al. 1978) and human studies (Pacey et al. 2014). A prospective study of 1,700 males in the United Kingdom seeking care at fertility clinics found that those younger than 30 who used cannabis in the 3 months prior to semen sample collection were more likely to have abnormal (<4% normal) sperm morphology (OR 1.94; 95% CI 1.05–3.60) (Pacey et al. 2014). In contrast, the Hedges et al. (2023) nonhuman primate study of daily, chronic THC consumption noted no significant change in sperm morphology but did report a dose-dependent increase in sperm DNA fragmentation that partially reversed with at least 4 months' cessation (Hedges et al. 2023). A prior study of 498 mice given a high dose of THC (50 mg/kg) five times per week for 6 weeks did not record an increase in lethal mutations or heritable translocations in offspring (Generoso et al. 1985).

Along with changes in sperm count and morphology, cannabis exposure is associated with altered sperm motility. A prior study of 16 healthy chronic cannabis users exposed to 4 weeks of high-dose cannabis noted decreased sperm motility on semen analysis (Hembree et al. 1978). Similar findings were also observed in vitro when sperm was incubated with THC at therapeutic doses typically used for pain relief or to reduce spasticity in individuals with multiple sclerosis (Whan et al. 2006). The underlying mechanism for these findings is attributed to decreased mitochondrial transmembrane potential, mediated by cannabinoid 1 (CB_1) receptor activation (Barbonetti et al. 2010).

Testicular Size

Animal studies using rodent, canine, and nonhuman primate models demonstrate an association between cannabis use and testicular atrophy (Dixit et al. 1977; Hedges et al. 2022), as well as reduced prostate and seminal vesicle weight (Banerjee et al. 2011; Dixit et al. 1974; Fujimoto et al. 1982; Ryan et al. 2021a). Hedges et al. (2022) showed that chronic THC exposure in rhesus macaques resulted in significant testicular atrophy. After 7 months of daily THC exposure, total testicular volume of subjects was reduced by 58%, in part due to decreases in both seminiferous tubule diameter and germ cell layers on testicular histology (Hedges et al. 2022, 2023). Similarly, rodent studies of intraperitoneally injected THC also resulted in reduced seminiferous tubule diameter on testicular histology, with only partial recovery after cannabis cessation (Mandal and Das 2010; Ryan et al. 2021a). The underlying etiology for the observed testicular damage is unclear but may be secondary to oxidative stress (Alagbonsi et al. 2016; Mandal and Das 2010).

Erectile Function

There is emerging evidence that the endocannabinoid system is associated with erectile signaling and capacity (Payne et al. 2019) and that cannabis use is linked with erectile dysfunction (Cohen 1982; Kolodny et al. 1974; Ryan et al. 2021a). Although the underlying mechanism is not well understood, studies demonstrate that chronic THC use may induce erectile dysfunction through early endothelial damage (Aversa et al. 2008). Males who use cannabis are more commonly noted to have impaired endothelium-dependent vasodilation (Aversa et al. 2008) and poor orgasmic function (Elbendary et al. 2009). Prior rat studies linked the endocannabinoid system with erectile function by demonstrating that rimonabant, a cannabinoid receptor antagonist, can induce an erection (Succu et al. 2006). This effect is likely secondary to neuronal nitric oxide synthase activation by rimonabant (Melis et al. 2006). A systematic review and meta-analysis of five case-controlled studies focused on cannabis and erectile dysfunction and found that the prevalence of erectile dysfunction doubled in cannabis users compared with control subjects (Pizzol et al. 2019). Smith et al. (2010) also performed a computer-assisted telephone survey of 8,656 Australian males and found that frequent cannabis use was associated with difficulties in achieving orgasm. In this study, daily use compared with nonuse was associated with orgasmic disorders, including reaching orgasm too quickly (OR 2.68; 95% CI 1.41–5.08; $P < 0.01$) or too slowly (OR 2.05; 95% CI 1.02–4.12; $P = 0.04$) or the inability to orgasm (OR 3.94; 95% CI 1.71–9.07; $P < 0.01$).

Time to Conception

Existing studies investigating male cannabis use and time to conception, as well as fecundity, have reported conflicting results. Using data from the National Survey of Family Growth, a nationally representative population-based study of 121 geographical areas in the United States, Kasman et al. (2018) examined whether regular cannabis use affected time to pregnancy in participants actively trying to conceive. In 758 male participants ages 15–44 with past-year cannabis use, they found no association between cannabis use and time to conception in never-users versus daily cannabis users. Similarly, Wise et al. (2018) evaluated the relationship between male cannabis use and fecundability in a prospective North American cohort and reported little overall association. Fecundability ratios for male cannabis use less than once and greater than or equal to once per week relative to no cannabis use were 0.87 (95% CI 0.66–1.15) and 1.24 (95% CI 0.90–1.70), respectively.

Beneficial Effects

Overall, there are limited studies reporting benefits from cannabis use on male fertility, but some studies suggest that cannabis use may benefit sexual function.

The endocannabinoid system is known to play a role in male sexual function, but the effect of cannabis use on sexual function remains poorly understood. Cannabis use has been associated with increased coital frequency (8.8 events/month vs. 7.8 events/month; $P < 0.05$) (Shiff et al. 2021; Sun and Eisenberg 2017; Wise et al. 2018) and sexual satisfaction; however, no correlation has been seen with the method of cannabis exposure (e.g., edibles, smoking) or the cannabinoid used (cannabidiol or THC) (Bhambhvani et al. 2020; Halikas et al. 1982). The effects of cannabis on sexual behavior appear dose-dependent, with lower doses being associated with increased sexual desire and pleasure and higher doses being linked with decreased sexual potency (Abel 1981; Koff 1974). Daily cannabis use is also linked with having two or more sexual partners in the previous year (adjusted OR [AOR] 2.08; 95% CI 1.11–3.89; $P=0.02$) (Smith et al. 2010). In contrast, prior rodent studies have demonstrated decreased libido and copulatory behavior following acute and chronic cannabis administration (Dhawan and Sharma 2003; Murphy et al. 1994).

Clinical Significance and Recommendations

Because cannabis use is most prevalent among males of reproductive age, and the available evidence suggests an adverse impact on male reproductive health, cannabis use should be avoided preconception. For individuals with chronic, heavy cannabis use, the literature indicates that abstaining from cannabis for at least 4 months prior to conception will partially reverse cannabis-induced effects on testicular volume, sperm DNA methylation, male reproductive hormones, and key seminal fluid proteins related to fertility (Hedges et al. 2023).

Cannabis and Female Fertility

Current State of Evidence

The 2021 NSDUH estimated the U.S. prevalence of cannabis use in the past year among females age 18 or older to be 17.2% (~22.4 million) (Center for Behavioral Health Statistics and Quality 2021). Cannabis use was highest among females ages 18–25 (34.2%, ~5.7 million). A cross-sectional study of 270 infertility patients found that those with recent cannabis use were less likely to think that cannabis could adversely affect fertility (Jordan et al. 2020), possibly contributing to the high prevalence of use. This contradicts preclinical and human studies suggesting that cannabis use adversely affects female fertility and that it is associated with altered reproductive hormones and menstrual cyclicity and poorer in vitro fertilization (IVF) success (Corsi et al. 2021; Lo et al. 2022; Ryan et al. 2021a, 2021b).

Deleterious Effects

Menstrual Cycles and Ovulation

Preclinical and human studies consistently support an impact of THC on menstrual cyclicity and ovulation. A former study in rats showed that acute exposure to intraperitoneal THC (2 mg/rat) delayed ovulation by 24 hours (Ayalon et al. 1977). Several studies used a rhesus macaque model to better understand the implications of chronic THC exposure on female reproductive health (Asch et al. 1981; Smith and Asch 1984). The rhesus macaque is a relevant and translational model with a plasma disposition of THC (Grant et al. 2018) and menstrual cycle length (~28 days) similar to those of humans (Brenner and Slayden 2012; Brenner et al. 1990). In female rhesus macaques with regular menstrual cycles, Asch et al. (1981) demonstrated that daily intramuscular injection of THC during the first 18 days of their cycle was associated with an increased risk of anovulation. Similarly, Ryan et al. (2021b) administered a daily THC edible to female rhesus macaques (N=8) and observed increased menstrual cycle length and altered reproductive hormones suggestive of ovulatory dysfunction. Prior to THC administration, the average menstrual cycle length was 28.3 days (SD 2.8) but increased by more than 9 days to 37.8 days (SD 14) after 4 months of THC consumption (r=0.432; P=0.017). A previous study in humans found that females who smoked cannabis within a year of trying to conceive were twice as likely to have infertility secondary to ovulatory dysfunction compared with those who did not use cannabis (RR 2.1; 95% CI 1.1–4.0; Mueller et al. 1990).

Assisted Reproductive Technology Outcomes

Prior studies (Klonoff-Cohen et al. 2006; Ryan et al. 2021a) have demonstrated that cannabis use adversely affects assisted reproductive technology outcomes. A prospective study of 221 couples undergoing IVF and gamete intrafallopian transfer (GIFT) reported that lifetime heavy cannabis use negatively affected IVF/GIFT outcomes (Klonoff-Cohen et al. 2006). Females who smoked cannabis within a year prior to undergoing IVF/GIFT had 25% fewer oocytes retrieved (P=0.03), and couples had 28% (P=0.04) fewer oocytes fertilized (Klonoff-Cohen et al. 2006).

Time to Conception

There is a paucity of literature evaluating the relationship between regular female cannabis use and time to conception. A cross-sectional survey of past-year use in 1,076 females ages 15–44 participating in the National Survey of Family Growth reported no increased time to pregnancy between cannabis users and nonusers (Kasman et al. 2018). Similarly, Pregnancy Study Online, a prospective cohort study that included 4,200 North American couples, found little association between female cannabis use and spontaneous conception rates (Wise et al. 2018). Wise et al. (2018) showed that the fecundability ratio for females who used cannabis less than one time per week versus nonuse was 0.99 (95% CI 0.85–1.16). The fecundability ratio in females who used cannabis once per week or more versus nonuse was 0.98 (95% CI 0.80–1.20). Additionally, a prior retrospective review of cross-sectional survey data from female respondents did not report an impact of cannabis use on time to conception (Kasman et al. 2018).

In contrast, Mueller et al. (1990) found that females who reported smoking cannabis had a higher risk of infertility secondary to ovulatory dysfunction (RR 1.7; 95% CI 1.0–3.0), and the greatest risk was among females who smoked cannabis within 1 year of trying to conceive (RR 2.1; 95% CI 1.1–4.0). Most recently, a secondary analysis of a large prospective cohort study evaluating females with prior first-trimester pregnancy loss found that preconception cannabis use was associated with reduced fecundability (ratio 0.59; 95% CI 0.38–0.92) despite a greater frequency of intercourse (Mumford et al. 2021).

Female Reproductive Hormones

Overall, the literature suggests that cannabis exposure disrupts the hypothalamic-pituitary-gonadal axis in females via altered gonadotropin-releasing hormone, FSH, and LH secretion (Lo et al. 2022; Ryan et al. 2021a, 2021b). Preclinical rat models demonstrate that acute THC administration results in suppressed LH, FSH, and prolactin levels (Ayalon et al. 1977; Chakravarty et al. 1975; Dalterio et al. 1983). Chakravarty et al. (1975) showed that intraperitoneal high-dose THC significantly reduced serum LH and prolactin in rats. Another study in female rats reported an association between THC exposure and significantly decreased plasma concentrations of LH and FSH, whereas rats that had undergone ovariectomy had varying responses (Dalterio et al. 1983). Similarly, nonhuman primate studies of chronic

THC exposure reported altered female reproductive hormone levels, including increased FSH levels (Asch and Smith 1986; Asch et al. 1981; Besch et al. 1977; Ryan et al. 2021b). Compared with preclinical studies, results in humans using cannabis are more variable. Mendelson et al. (1986) examined the impact of acute THC exposure in 16 healthy adult females and found that smoking a single cannabis cigarette containing 1.8% THC resulted in a 30% suppression of plasma LH levels ($P<0.02$). In contrast, Block et al. (1991) investigated the effects of chronic cannabis use in 56 females and found no significant effect on LH, FSH, prolactin, or cortisol levels.

Beneficial Effects

There are limited data on the potential benefits of cannabis use on female fertility. Several studies report that female cannabis use is associated with increased sexual desire, orgasm, satisfaction, and improved dyspareunia (Lynn et al. 2019; Palamar et al. 2018). However, the existing literature largely suggests that cannabis exposure adversely affects female reproductive health.

Clinical Significance and Recommendations

Cannabis use is associated with altered female reproductive health, including menstrual cyclicity, ovulation, reproductive hormones, oocyte quality, and time to conception (Corsi et al. 2021; Klonoff-Cohen et al. 2006; Lo et al. 2022; Mumford et al. 2021; Ryan et al. 2021a). Consequently, individuals considering conception should abstain from cannabis use preconception.

Cannabis Use During Pregnancy

Current State of Evidence

Effects of Paternal Cannabis Use on Offspring Outcomes

Emerging data suggest that paternal cannabis exposure during spermatogenesis may alter epigenetic regulation and may affect short- and long-term offspring health, including brain and neurobehavioral development (Lo et al. 2022; Ross et al. 2015). A study in male rats demonstrated that cannabis-induced changes in sperm methylation were detected in offspring DNA and that these changes were functionally related to alterations in gene expression and cardiomegaly (Schrott et al. 2022). Additionally, paternal cannabis use during pregnancy has been linked with an increased risk of sudden infant death syndrome and poorer offspring mental health, specifically hyperactivity and ADHD (Easey and Sharp 2021).

Gestational Effects of Maternal Cannabis Use

The prevalence of prenatal cannabis use in the United States has nearly doubled in the past decade, and cannabis is now the most commonly used federally illicit substance in pregnancy (American College of Obstetricians and Gynecologists 2017; Martin et al. 2015; Volkow et al. 2019; Young-Wolff et al. 2021). Currently, the prevalence of past-month cannabis use is greater than 4.9% among pregnant females ages 15–44 and up to 8.5% in those ages 18–25 (McCance-Katz 2019). There has also been a rise in CaUD from 1.8 to 9.4 per 1,000 deliveries between 1993 and 2014 (Shi and Zhong 2018). According to Ko et al. (2015), 18.1% of pregnant individuals who used cannabis in the past year met the criteria for CaUD. Infants born to parents with CaUD are at increased risk of being small for gestational age, being born preterm, having low birth weight, and dying within 1 year of birth compared with infants born to parents without CaUD (Gabrhelík et al. 2021; Shi et al. 2021). Factors associated with increased cannabis use in pregnancy are single or unmarried status, younger age, low socioeconomic status, less education, and living with a partner who uses cannabis (Fried et al. 1980). Cannabis is commonly used in pregnancy for self-treatment of nausea and vomiting, especially during the first trimester when the fetus is most vulnerable to adversity (Beatty et al. 2012; Passey et al. 2014), as well as for stress, sleep, and appetite changes (Chang et al. 2019; Vanstone et al. 2021). Approximately half of females who use cannabis preconception will continue to use in pregnancy (Beatty et al. 2012; Passey et al. 2014). Smoking and edibles are the two most frequent methods of cannabis use during pregnancy (Young-Wolff et al. 2020a).

The American College of Obstetricians and Gynecologists (2017) and the American Academy of Pediatrics recommend that pregnant individuals should be counseled regarding the potential risks of prenatal cannabis use and encouraged to abstain from use in pregnancy and during lactation (Adams 2019; Ryan et al. 2018). However, the increasing prevalence of prenatal cannabis use is attributed to limited safety information due to the heterogeneity in the literature (Bayrampour et al. 2019), limited patient education (Barbosa-Leiker et al. 2021; Holland et al. 2016; Woodruff et al. 2021), and cannabis retailers promoting cannabis use as a safe, natural, and effective treatment for pregnancy symptoms (Chang et al. 2019; Dickson et al. 2018). A qualitative study of pregnant individuals using cannabis in California found consistent perceptions that legalization resulted in easier cannabis access, less stigma, fewer concerns about involvement of child protective services, and trust in product safety described by cannabis retailers and employees (Young-Wolff et al. 2022). Studies indicate increasing public interest in the impact of cannabis use before, during, and after pregnancy (Young-Wolff et al. 2020). Although some health care providers indicate that cannabis use during pregnancy and lactation is not safe, many are not discouraging use or appropriately counseling patients about the potential for adverse perinatal outcomes (Holland et al. 2016; Young-Wolff et al. 2020). The available literature suggests that THC crosses the placenta and binds to CB_1 and cannabinoid 2 (CB_2) receptors in the placenta and fetal organs (Cristino and Di Marzo 2014; Kenney et al. 1999; Lorenzetti et al. 2014; Marchand et al. 2022). In doing so, THC exposure during pregnancy is associated with adverse placental (Roberts et al. 2022) and offspring outcomes, including increased risk of preterm birth and of infants who are admitted to the neonatal intensive care unit (NICU), are small for gestational age, and have low birth weight (Conner et al. 2016; El Marroun et al. 2009; Fergusson et al. 2002; Gunn et al. 2016; Hurd et al. 2005; Marchand et al. 2022).

Deleterious Effects

Stillbirth and Miscarriage

At present, the existing literature suggests that maternal cannabis use is not associated with miscarriage or stillbirth. However, the literature is frequently confounded by polysubstance use and tobacco co-use, which are shown to independently increase the risk of stillbirth and pregnancy loss (Lo et al. 2022). In a retrospective cohort study of 1,228 females with a history of pregnancy loss, preconception cannabis use determined by urinary metabolite measurements and self-report suggested associations with anovulation (RR 1.92; 95% CI 0.88–4.18) and decreased live birth rate (42%, 19/45) versus nonusers (55%, 578/1,043; RR 0.8; 95% CI 0.57–1.12) (Mumford et al. 2021). No association was observed between preconception cannabis use and pregnancy loss (RR 0.81; 95% CI 0.46–1.42).

Neonatal Intensive Care Unit Admissions

Some studies have reported an increased risk of NICU admission for infants whose parent used cannabis during pregnancy (Lo et al. 2023; Marchand et al. 2022). A recent systematic review and meta-analysis by Lo et al. (2023) reported that prenatal cannabis exposure was associated with an increased neonatal risk of NICU admission (RR 1.38; 95% CI 1.18–1.62; $P<0.001$) but no significant differences in mean gestational age, 5-minute Apgar scores less than 7, or mean infant length.

Preterm Birth

The literature consistently demonstrates an increased risk of preterm birth (delivery before 37 weeks' gestation) with prenatal cannabis use (Conner et al. 2016; Lo et al. 2023; Marchand et al. 2022). Multiple systematic reviews and meta-analyses, including those adjusted for concomitant tobacco use, associate maternal cannabis use with increased risk of preterm delivery (Lo et al. 2023; Marchand et al. 2022). A recent systematic review and meta-analysis also noted that prenatal cannabis exposure increased the risk of preterm birth (AOR 1.42; 95% CI 1.10–1.69; $P<0.001$; Lo et al. 2023).

Low Birth Weight and Small for Gestational Age

The existing research on prenatal cannabis exposure and birth weight largely supports an association with low birth weight and small for gestational age infants (Conner et al. 2016; Lo et al. 2023), even after adjusting for nicotine use (Lo et al. 2023; Marchand et al. 2022). A systematic review and meta-analysis reported that cannabis use in pregnancy was associated with an increased risk of small for gestational age infants (AOR 1.76; 95% CI 1.52–2.05; $P<0.001$; Lo et al. 2023). The difference in birth weight between pregnancies exposed and not exposed to cannabis ranges from 84 g to 256 g (Lo et al. 2022; Marchand et al. 2022; Ryan et al. 2021a).

Congenital Anomalies

Few studies have evaluated prenatal cannabis use and major congenital anomalies. There are reports of acrania, gastroschisis, esophageal atresia, and congenital diaphragmatic hernia in offspring with prenatal cannabis exposure; however, these findings are not consistently demonstrated (Lo et al. 2022; Reece and Hulse 2021; van Gelder et al. 2014). A large population-based Canadian study recently found that cannabis use in the childbearing parent increased the likelihood of major congenital anomalies in the infant (AOR 1.32; 95% CI 1.23–1.42) (Luke et al. 2022).

Infant and Childhood Outcomes

Prenatal cannabis exposure has been associated with increased newborn withdrawal-like symptoms, sleep disturbances, and issues with self-soothing (Lo et al. 2022). It is also linked with increased aggression and attention deficits in the child, detected as early as 18 months of age. Preschool-aged children exposed to cannabis in utero have demonstrated poorer memory, verbal and visual reasoning skills, and attentiveness, in addition to increased impulsivity, hyperactivity, attention deficits, and symptoms of depression and anxiety. These findings, in addition to an increased risk of autism spectrum disorder and earlier experimentation with illicit drugs, are also observed in adolescents with prenatal cannabis exposure. A study in rats reported that adult rat offspring with prenatal THC exposure had enhanced heroin-seeking profiles and altered expression of cannabinoid, dopamine, and glutamate receptors in the striatum of the brain (Szutorisz et al. 2014). A large retrospective Canadian study by Corsi et al. (2020) noted that the prevalence of autism spectrum disorder was nearly twice as high in cannabis-exposed children versus unexposed children (4 vs. 2.42 per 1,000 person-years). In addition, offspring prenatally exposed to cannabis also had an increased prevalence of intellectual disability and learning disorders, although this was not adjusted for residual confounding.

Beneficial Effects

The reasons for cannabis use by pregnant or lactating individuals are dynamic and change across gestation due to perceptions of benefits and risks. Although not approved by the FDA for the following therapeutic uses, cannabis is often used in pregnancy for analgesia, muscle relaxation, anti-inflammation, stress, sedation, mood improvement, appetite stimulation, and antinausea effects (Barbosa-Leiker et al. 2020; Chang et al. 2019; National Academies of Sciences, Engineering, and Medicine 2017). A qualitative Canadian study by Vanstone et al. (2021) using both telephone and virtual interviews identified three categories of reasons for cannabis use in pregnancy and lactation: 1) sensation-seeking for fun and enjoyment, 2) managing symptoms of chronic or prenatal-related conditions, and 3) coping with life difficulties. During the preconception period, individuals endorsed these three categories equally as reasons for use. However, during pregnancy, the reasons for use were primarily for symptom management. During lactation, the reasons for use returned to those referenced preconception.

Clinical Significance and Recommendations

Data supporting the negative impact of cannabis use during pregnancy on perinatal outcomes continue to increase, and no cannabis dose is currently established to be safe in pregnancy. As a result, individuals who are pregnant should avoid cannabis use.

Conclusion

The use of cannabis continues to rise in the United States with increasing legalization, especially among individuals of reproductive age. Although there is a paucity of safety data, emerging data suggest that parental cannabis use preconception and during pregnancy adversely affects prenatal, short-term, and long-term offspring outcomes. This is concerning particularly because the potency and availability of cannabis products are increasing. More research is needed to develop evidence-based recommendations to guide public health measures and to aid health care providers in adequately counseling patients on cannabis-related risk mitigation.

Key Points

- Cannabis use is associated with an adverse impact on male and female fertility and reproductive capacity.
- Chronic cannabis use in males can negatively affect sexual function, semen parameters, reproductive hormones, testicular size, and spermatogenesis.
- Exposure to cannabis can alter sperm DNA methylation and potentially affect offspring health, including brain and neurobehavioral development.
- Chronic cannabis use can affect menstrual cyclicity and ovulation.

- Prenatal cannabis use is associated with an increased risk of a small for gestational age infant, preterm birth, and neonatal intensive care unit admission.
- Cannabis exposure in utero is linked with adverse long-term offspring outcomes, including an increased prevalence of autism spectrum disorder and addiction vulnerability.

References

Abel EL: Marihuana and sex: a critical survey. Drug Alcohol Depend 8(1):1–22, 1981 6271518

Adams J: U.S. Surgeon General's Advisory: Marijuana Use and the Developing Brain. Washington, DC, U.S. Department of Health and Human Services, 2019

Alagbonsi IA, Olayaki LA, Salman TM: Melatonin and vitamin C exacerbate cannabis sativa-induced testicular damage when administered separately but ameliorate it when combined in rats. J Basic Clin Physiol Pharmacol 27(3):277–287, 2016 26479341

American College of Obstetricians and Gynecologists: Marijuana Use During Pregnancy and Lactation (ACOG Committee Opinion No 637). Washington, DC, American College of Obstetricians and Gynecologists, 2017. Available at: https://www.acog.org/Clinical-Guidance-and -Publications/Committee-Opinions/Committee-on-Obstetric-Practice/ Marijuana-Use-During-Pregnancy-and-Lactation. Accessed July 15, 2024.

American College of Obstetricians and Gynecologists Committee on Obstetric Practice: Committee opinion no. 637: marijuana use during pregnancy and lactation. Obstet Gynecol 126(1):234–238, 2015 26241291

American Psychiatric Association: Diagnostic and Statistical Manual of Mental Disorders, 5th Edition, Text Revision. Washington, DC, American Psychiatric Association, 2022

Aquila S, Guido C, Santoro A, et al: Human sperm anatomy: ultrastructural localization of the cannabinoid1 receptor and a potential role of anandamide in sperm survival and acrosome reaction. Anat Rec (Hoboken) 293(2):298–309, 2010 19938110

Asch RH, Smith CG: Effects of delta 9-THC, the principal psychoactive component of marijuana, during pregnancy in the rhesus monkey. J Reprod Med 31(12):1071–1081, 1986 3025441

Asch RH, Smith CG, Siler-Khodr TM, et al: Effects of delta 9-tetrahydrocannabinol during the follicular phase of the rhesus monkey (Macaca mulatta). J Clin Endocrinol Metab 52(1):50–55, 1981 6256405

Aversa A, Rossi F, Francomano D, et al: Early endothelial dysfunction as a marker of vasculogenic erectile dysfunction in young habitual cannabis users. Int J Impot Res 20(6):566–573, 2008 18997809

Ayalon D, Nir I, Cordova T, et al: Acute effect of delta1-tetrahydrocannabinol on the hypothalamo-pituitary-ovarian axis in the rat. Neuroendocrinology 23(1):31–42, 1977 331132

Banerjee A, Singh A, Srivastava P, et al: Effects of chronic bhang (cannabis) administration on the reproductive system of male mice. Birth Defects Res B Dev Reprod Toxicol 92(3):195–205, 2011 21678546

Barbonetti A, Vassallo MR, Fortunato D, et al: Energetic metabolism and human sperm motility: impact of CB1 receptor activation. Endocrinology 151(12):5882–5892, 2010 20962050

Barbosa-Leiker C, Burduli E, Smith CL, et al: Daily cannabis use during pregnancy and postpartum in a state with legalized recreational cannabis. J Addict Med 14(6):467–474, 2020 32011411

Barbosa-Leiker C, Brooks O, Smith CL, et al: Healthcare professionals' and budtenders' perceptions of perinatal cannabis use. Am J Drug Alcohol Abuse 48(2):186–194, 2021 34779673

Bayrampour H, Zahradnik M, Lisonkova S, et al: Women's perspectives about cannabis use during pregnancy and the postpartum period: an integrative review. Prev Med 119:17–23, 2019 30552948

Beatty JR, Svikis DS, Ondersma SJ: Prevalence and perceived financial costs of marijuana versus tobacco use among urban low-income pregnant women. J Addict Res Ther 3(4):1000135, 2012 23858392

Belladelli F, Fallara G, Pozzi E, et al: Effects of recreational cannabis on testicular function in primary infertile men. Andrology 10(6):1172–1180, 2022 35868833

Besch NF, Smith CG, Besch PK, et al: The effect of marihuana (delta-9-tetrahydrocannabinol) on the secretion of luteinizing hormone in the ovariectomized rhesus monkey. Am J Obstet Gynecol 128(6):635–642, 1977 406789

Bhambhvani HP, Kasman AM, Wilson-King G, et al: A survey exploring the relationship between cannabis use characteristics and sexual function in men. Sex Med 8(3):436–445, 2020 32561331

Block RI, Farinpour R, Schlechte JA: Effects of chronic marijuana use on testosterone, luteinizing hormone, follicle stimulating hormone, prolactin and cortisol in men and women. Drug Alcohol Depend 28(2):121–128, 1991 1935564

Brenner RM, Slayden OD: Molecular and functional aspects of menstruation in the macaque. Rev Endocr Metab Disord 13(4):309–318, 2012 23108498

Brenner RM, West NB, McClellan MC: Estrogen and progestin receptors in the reproductive tract of male and female primates. Biol Reprod 42(1):11–19, 1990 2178696

Center for Behavioral Health Statistics and Quality: NSDUH Detailed Tables. Rockville, MD, Center for Behavioral Health Statistics and Quality, Substance Abuse and Mental Health Services Administration, 2021. Available at: https://www.samhsa.gov/data/sites/default/files/reports

/rpt39441/NSDUHDetailedTabs2021/NSDUHDetailedTabs2021/NSD
UHDetTabsSect1pe2021.htm. Accessed April 18, 2023.

Chakravarty I, Sheth AR, Ghosh JJ: Effect of acute delta9-tetrahydrocannabinol treatment on serum luteinizing hormone and prolactin levels in adult female rats. Fertil Steril 26(9):947–948, 1975 1237419

Chang JC, Tarr JA, Holland CL, et al: Beliefs and attitudes regarding prenatal marijuana use: perspectives of pregnant women who report use. Drug Alcohol Depend 196:14–20, 2019 30658220

Cohen S: Cannabis and sex: multifaceted paradoxes. J Psychoactive Drugs 14(1–2):55–58, 1982 7119944

Cone EJ, Johnson RE, Moore JD, et al: Acute effects of smoking marijuana on hormones, subjective effects and performance in male human subjects. Pharmacol Biochem Behav 24(6):1749–1754, 1986 3016764

Conner SN, Bedell V, Lipsey K, et al: Maternal marijuana use and adverse neonatal outcomes: a systematic review and meta-analysis. Obstet Gynecol 128(4):713–723, 2016 27607879

Corsi DJ, Donelle J, Sucha E, et al: Maternal cannabis use in pregnancy and child neurodevelopmental outcomes. Nat Med 26(10):1536–1540, 2020 32778828

Corsi DJ, Murphy MSQ, Cook J: The effects of cannabis on female reproductive health across the life course. Cannabis Cannabinoid Res 6(4):275–287, 2021 33998877

Cristino L, Di Marzo V: Fetal cannabinoid receptors and the "dis-joint-ed" brain. EMBO J 33(7):665–667, 2014 24631837

Dalterio SL, Mayfield DL, Bartke A: Effects of delta 9-THC on plasma hormone levels in female mice. Subst Alcohol Actions Misuse 4(5):339–345, 1983 6322366

Dhawan K, Sharma A: Restoration of chronic-delta 9-THC-induced decline in sexuality in male rats by a novel benzoflavone moiety from Passiflora incarnata Linn. Br J Pharmacol 138(1):117–120, 2003 12522080

Dickson B, Mansfield C, Guiahi M, et al: Recommendations from cannabis dispensaries about first-trimester cannabis use. Obstet Gynecol 131(6):1031–1038, 2018 29742676

Dixit VP, Sharma VN, Lohiya NK: The effect of chronically administered cannabis extract on the testicular function of mice. Eur J Pharmacol 26(1):111–114, 1974 4831978

Dixit VP, Gupta CL, Agrawal M: Testicular degeneration and necrosis induced by chronic administration of cannabis extract in dogs. Endokrinologie 69(3):299–305, 1977 913356

Dunne C: The effects of cannabis on female and male reproduction. B C Med J 61:282–285, 2019

Easey KE, Sharp GC: The impact of paternal alcohol, tobacco, caffeine use and physical activity on offspring mental health: a systematic review and meta-analysis. Reprod Health 18(1):214, 2021 34702308

Elbendary MA, El-Gamal OM, Salem KA: Analysis of risk factors for organic erectile dysfunction in Egyptian patients under the age of 40 years. J Androl 30(5):520–524, 2009 19234310

El Marroun H, Tiemeier H, Steegers EA, et al: Intrauterine cannabis exposure affects fetal growth trajectories: the Generation R Study. J Am Acad Child Adolesc Psychiatry 48(12):1173–1181, 2009 19858757

ElSohly MA, Chandra S, Radwan M, et al: A comprehensive review of cannabis potency in the USA in the last decade. Biol Psychiatry Cogn Neurosci Neuroimaging 6(6):603–606, 2021 33508497

Fergusson DM, Horwood LJ, Northstone K, et al: Maternal use of cannabis and pregnancy outcome. BJOG 109(1):21–27, 2002 11843371

Fried PA, Watkinson B, Grant A, et al: Changing patterns of soft drug use prior to and during pregnancy: a prospective study. Drug Alcohol Depend 6(5):323–343, 1980 7460764

Fujimoto GI, Morrill GA, O'Connell ME, et al: Effects of cannabinoids given orally and reduced appetite on the male rat reproductive system. Pharmacology 24(5):303–313, 1982 6285392

Gabrhelík R, Mahic M, Lund IO, et al: Cannabis use during pregnancy and risk of adverse birth outcomes: a longitudinal cohort study. Eur Addict Res 27(2):131–141, 2021 33040062

Generoso WM, Cain KT, Cornett CV, et al: Tests for induction of dominant-lethal mutations and heritable translocations with tetrahydrocannabinol in male mice. Mutat Res 143(1–2):51–53, 1985 2987686

Grant KS, Petroff R, Isoherranen N, et al: Cannabis use during pregnancy: pharmacokinetics and effects on child development. Pharmacol Ther 182:133–151, 2018 28847562

Gundersen TD, Jørgensen N, Andersson AM, et al: Association between use of marijuana and male reproductive hormones and semen quality: a study among 1,215 healthy young men. Am J Epidemiol 182(6):473–481, 2015 26283092

Gunn JK, Rosales CB, Center KE, et al: Prenatal exposure to cannabis and maternal and child health outcomes: a systematic review and meta-analysis. BMJ Open 6(4):e009986, 2016 27048634

Halikas J, Weller R, Morse C: Effects of regular marijuana use on sexual performance. J Psychoactive Drugs 14(1–2):59–70, 1982 6981694

Hedges JC, Hanna CB, Bash JC, et al: Chronic delta-9-tetrahydrocannabinol exposure impacts testicular volume and male reproductive health in rhesus macaques. Fertil Steril 117(4):698–707, 2022 35090702

Hedges JC, Hanna CB, Shorey-Kendrick LE, et al: Cessation of chronic delta-9-tetrahydrocannabinol use partially reverses impacts on male fertility and the sperm epigenome in rhesus macaques. Fertil Steril 120(1):163–174, 2023 36990913

Hembree WC III, Nahas GG, Zeidenberg P, et al: Changes in human spermatozoa associated with high dose marihuana smoking. Adv Biosci 22–23:429–439, 1978 574469

Holland CL, Rubio D, Rodriguez KL, et al: Obstetric health care providers' counseling responses to pregnant patient disclosures of marijuana use. Obstet Gynecol 127(4):681–687, 2016 26959210

Huang HF, Nahas GG, Hembree WC III: Effects of marihuana inhalation on spermatogenesis of the rat. Adv Biosci 22–23:419–427, 1978 756840

Hurd YL, Wang X, Anderson V, et al: Marijuana impairs growth in mid-gestation fetuses. Neurotoxicol Teratol 27(2):221–229, 2005 15734273

Imtiaz S, Wells S, Rehm J, et al: Cannabis use during the COVID-19 pandemic in Canada: a repeated cross-sectional study. J Addict Med 15(6):484–490, 2021 33323693

Jensen B, Chen J, Furnish T, et al: Medical marijuana and chronic pain: a review of basic science and clinical evidence. Curr Pain Headache Rep 19(10):50, 2015 26325482

Jordan T, Ngo B, Jones CA: The use of cannabis and perceptions of its effect on fertility among infertility patients. Hum Reprod Open 2020(1):hoz041, 2020 32072021

Kasman AM, Thoma ME, McLain AC, et al: Association between use of marijuana and time to pregnancy in men and women: findings from the National Survey of Family Growth. Fertil Steril 109(5):866–871, 2018 29555335

Kenney SP, Kekuda R, Prasad PD, et al: Cannabinoid receptors and their role in the regulation of the serotonin transporter in human placenta. Am J Obstet Gynecol 181(2):491–497, 1999 10454705

Keyhani S, Steigerwald S, Ishida J, et al: Risks and benefits of marijuana use: a national survey of U.S. adults. Ann Intern Med 169(5):282–290, 2018 30039154

Klonoff-Cohen HS, Natarajan L, Chen RV: A prospective study of the effects of female and male marijuana use on in vitro fertilization (IVF) and gamete intrafallopian transfer (GIFT) outcomes. Am J Obstet Gynecol 194(2):369–376, 2006 16458631

Ko JY, Farr SL, Tong VT, et al: Prevalence and patterns of marijuana use among pregnant and nonpregnant women of reproductive age. Am J Obstet Gynecol 213(2):201.e1–201.e10, 2015 25772211

Koff WC: Marijuana and sexual activity. J Sex Res 10(3):194–204, 1974 4469012

Kolodny RC, Masters WH, Kolodner RM, et al: Depression of plasma testosterone levels after chronic intensive marihuana use. N Engl J Med 290(16):872–874, 1974 4816961

Lo JO, Hedges JC, Girardi G: Impact of cannabinoids on pregnancy, reproductive health, and offspring outcomes. Am J Obstet Gynecol 227(4):571–581, 2022 35662548

Lo JO, Shaw B, Robalino S, et al: Cannabis use in pregnancy and neonatal outcomes: a systematic review and meta-analysis. Cannabis Cannabinoid Res 9(2):470–485, 2023 36730710

Lorenzetti V, Solowij N, Fornito A, et al: The association between regular cannabis exposure and alterations of human brain morphology: an updated review of the literature. Curr Pharm Des 20(13):2138–2167, 2014 23829361

Luke S, Hobbs AJ, Smith M, et al: Cannabis use in pregnancy and maternal and infant outcomes: a Canadian cross-jurisdictional population-based cohort study. PLoS One 17(11):e0276824, 2022 36417349

Lynn BK, López JD, Miller C, et al: The relationship between marijuana use prior to sex and sexual function in women. Sex Med 7(2):192–197, 2019 30833225

Mandal TK, Das NS: Testicular toxicity in cannabis extract treated mice: association with oxidative stress and role of antioxidant enzyme systems. Toxicol Ind Health 26(1):11–23, 2010 19942653

Marchand G, Masoud AT, Govindan M, et al: Birth outcomes of neonates exposed to marijuana in utero: a systematic review and meta-analysis. JAMA Netw Open 5(1):e2145653–e2145653, 2022 35084479

Martin CE, Longinaker N, Mark K, et al: Recent trends in treatment admissions for marijuana use during pregnancy. J Addict Med 9(2):99–104, 2015 25525944

McCance-Katz EF: The National Survey on Drug Use and Health: 2017. Rockville, MD, Substance Abuse and Mental Health Services Administration, 2019

Melis MR, Succu S, Mascia MS, et al: The cannabinoid receptor antagonist SR-141716A induces penile erection in male rats: involvement of paraventricular glutamic acid and nitric oxide. Neuropharmacology 50(2):219–228, 2006

Mendelson JH, Mello NK, Ellingboe J, et al: Marihuana smoking suppresses luteinizing hormone in women. J Pharmacol Exp Ther 237(3):862–866, 1986 3012072

Mueller BA, Daling JR, Weiss NS, et al: Recreational drug use and the risk of primary infertility. Epidemiology 1(3):195–200, 1990 2081252

Mumford SL, Flannagan KS, Radoc JG, et al: Cannabis use while trying to conceive: a prospective cohort study evaluating associations with fecundability, live birth and pregnancy loss. Hum Reprod 36(5):1405–1415, 2021 33421071

Murphy LL, Gher J, Steger RW, et al: Effects of delta 9-tetrahydrocannabinol on copulatory behavior and neuroendocrine responses of male rats to female conspecifics. Pharmacol Biochem Behav 48(4):1011–1017, 1994 7972278

Murphy SK, Itchon-Ramos N, Visco Z, et al: Cannabinoid exposure and altered DNA methylation in rat and human sperm. Epigenetics 13(12):1208–1221, 2018 30521419

National Academies of Sciences, Engineering, and Medicine: The Health Effects of Cannabis and Cannabinoids: The Current State of Evidence and Recommendations for Research. Washington, DC, National Academies Press, 2017

National Conference of State Legislatures: State medical marijuana laws. Denver, CO, National Conference of State Legislatures, 2022. Available at: http://www.ncsl.org/research/health/state-medical-marijuana-laws .aspx. Accessed January 5, 2023.

Pacey AA, Povey AC, Clyma JA, et al: Modifiable and non-modifiable risk factors for poor sperm morphology. Hum Reprod 29(8):1629–1636, 2014 24899128

Palamar JJ, Griffin-Tomas M, Acosta P, et al: A comparison of self-reported sexual effects of alcohol, marijuana, and ecstasy in a sample of young adult nightlife attendees. Psychol Sex 9(1):54–68, 2018 29430277

Passey ME, Sanson-Fisher RW, D'Este CA, et al: Tobacco, alcohol and cannabis use during pregnancy: clustering of risks. Drug Alcohol Depend 134:44–50, 2014 24095245

Payne KS, Mazur DJ, Hotaling JM, et al: Cannabis and male fertility: a systematic review. J Urol 202(4):674–681, 2019 30916627

Pizzol D, Demurtas J, Stubbs B, et al: Relationship between cannabis use and erectile dysfunction: a systematic review and meta-analysis. Am J Mens Health 13(6):1557988319892464, 2019 31795801

Practice Committee of the American Society of Reproductive Medicine: Optimizing natural fertility: a committee opinion. Fertil Steril 117(1):53–63, 2022 34815068

Rajanahally S, Raheem O, Rogers M, et al: The relationship between cannabis and male infertility, sexual health, and neoplasm: a systematic review. Andrology 7(2):139–147, 2019 30767424

Reece AS, Hulse GK: Epidemiological overview of multidimensional chromosomal and genome toxicity of cannabis exposure in congenital anomalies and cancer development. Sci Rep 11(1):13892, 2021 34230557

Roberts VHJ, Schabel MC, Boniface ER, et al: Chronic prenatal delta-9-tetrahydrocannabinol exposure adversely impacts placental function and development in a rhesus macaque model. Sci Rep 12(1):20260, 2022 36424495

Ross EJ, Graham DL, Money KM, et al: Developmental consequences of fetal exposure to drugs: what we know and what we still must learn. Neuropsychopharmacology 40(1):61–87, 2015 24938210

Ryan KS, Bash JC, Hanna CB, et al: Effects of marijuana on reproductive health: preconception and gestational effects. Curr Opin Endocrinol Diabetes Obes 28(6):558–565, 2021a 34709212

Ryan KS, Mahalingaiah S, Campbell LR, et al: The effects of delta-9-tetrahydrocannabinol exposure on female menstrual cyclicity and reproductive health in rhesus macaques. F S Sci 2(3):287–294, 2021b 34901892

Ryan SA, Ammerman SD, O'Connor ME, et al: Marijuana use during pregnancy and breastfeeding: implications for neonatal and childhood outcomes. Pediatrics 142(3):e20181889, 2018 30150209

Schrott R, Modliszewski JL, Hawkey AB, et al: Sperm DNA methylation alterations from cannabis extract exposure are evident in offspring. Epigenetics Chromatin 15(1):33, 2022 36085240

Shi Y, Zhong S: Trends in cannabis use disorder among pregnant women in the US, 1993–2014. J Gen Intern Med 33(3):245–246, 2018 29030807

Shi Y, Zhu B, Liang D: The associations between prenatal cannabis use disorder and neonatal outcomes. Addiction 116(11):3069–3079, 2021 33887075

Shiff B, Blankstein U, Hussaen J, et al: The impact of cannabis use on male sexual function: a 10-year, single-center experience. Can Urol Assoc J 15(12):E652–E657, 2021 34171210

Smith AM, Ferris JA, Simpson JM, et al: Cannabis use and sexual health. J Sex Med 7(2 Pt 1):787–793, 2010 19694929

Smith CG, Asch RH: Acute, short-term, and chronic effects of marijuana on the female primate reproductive function. NIDA Res Monogr 44:82–96, 1984 6090911

Succu S, Mascia MS, Sanna F, et al: The cannabinoid CB1 receptor antagonist SR 141716A induces penile erection by increasing extra-cellular glutamic acid in the paraventricular nucleus of male rats. Behav Brain Res 169(2):274–281, 2006 16516985

Sun AJ, Eisenberg ML: Association between marijuana use and sexual frequency in the United States: a population-based study. J Sex Med 14(11):1342–1347, 2017 29110804

Szutorisz H, DiNieri JA, Sweet E, et al: Parental THC exposure leads to compulsive heroin-seeking and altered striatal synaptic plasticity in the subsequent generation. Neuropsychopharmacology 39(6):1315–1323, 2014 24385132

Thistle JE, Graubard BI, Braunlin M, et al: Marijuana use and serum testosterone concentrations among U.S. males. Andrology 5(4):732–738, 2017 28395129

Uhlén M, Fagerberg L, Hallström BM, et al: Proteomics: tissue-based map of the human proteome. Science 347(6220):1260419, 2015 25613900

van Gelder MM, Donders AR, Devine O, et al: Using bayesian models to assess the effects of under-reporting of cannabis use on the association with birth defects, national birth defects prevention study, 1997–2005. Paediatr Perinat Epidemiol 28(5):424–433, 2014 25155701

Vanstone M, Taneja S, Popoola A, et al: Reasons for cannabis use during pregnancy and lactation: a qualitative study. CMAJ 193(50):E1906–E1914, 2021 34930765

Volkow ND, Han B, Compton WM, et al: Self-reported medical and nonmedical cannabis use among pregnant women in the United States. JAMA 322(2):167–169, 2019 31211824

Whan LB, West MC, McClure N, et al: Effects of delta-9-tetrahydrocannabinol, the primary psychoactive cannabinoid in marijuana, on human sperm function in vitro. Fertil Steril 85(3):653–660, 2006 16500334

Wise LA, Wesselink AK, Hatch EE, et al: Marijuana use and fecundability in a North American preconception cohort study. J Epidemiol Community Health 72(3):208–215, 2018 29273628

Woodruff K, Scott KA, Roberts SCM: Pregnant people's experiences discussing their cannabis use with prenatal care providers in a state with legalized cannabis. Drug Alcohol Depend 227:108998, 2021 34482037

Young-Wolff KC, Adams SR, Wi S, et al: Routes of cannabis administration among females in the year before and during pregnancy: results from a pilot project. Addict Behav 100:106–125, 2020a 31600645

Young-Wolff KC, Gali K, Sarovar V, et al: Women's questions about perinatal cannabis use and health care providers' responses. J Womens Health (Larchmt) 29(7):919–926, 2020b 32011205

Young-Wolff KC, Ray GT, Alexeeff SE, et al: Rates of prenatal cannabis use among pregnant women before and during the COVID-19 pandemic. JAMA 326(17):1745–1747, 2021 34570168

Young-Wolff KC, Foti TR, Green A, et al: Perceptions about cannabis following legalization among pregnant individuals with prenatal cannabis use in California. JAMA Netw Open 5(12):e2246912, 2022 36515947

Zimmerman AM, Zimmerman S, Raj AY: Effects of cannabinoids on spermatogenesis in mice. Adv Biosci 22–23:407–418, 1978 756839

Cannabis Impacts on the Cardiac and Respiratory Systems

Robert L. Page II, Pharm.D.

Onyedika J. Ilonze, M.D.

O ver the past two decades, attitudes toward and use of cannabis or marijuana have changed dramatically and continue to evolve within the United States. With the expansion of legalization at the state level and the advent of cannabis dispensaries on many street corners, the availability of medical and recreational cannabis has exploded. However, pharmacovigilance, safety, and efficacy of cannabis use have been limited by decades of worldwide illegality and by the ongoing classification of cannabis as a Schedule I controlled substance. These shifts in popular opinion, changes in state regulations, and increases in access now require clinicians to understand conflicting laws and health implications, as well as potential therapeutic but also hazardous effects. Within this chapter, we highlight each of these issues and explore the important clinical implications and recommendations for clinicians regarding cannabis use as it pertains to cardiovascular and respiratory health.

Background and Current State of Use

According to 2021 data from the Substance Abuse and Mental Health Services Administration (2023), cannabis was the most commonly used illicit substance, with 18.7% of people age 12 or older (52.5 million people) using it in the past year. Use was highest among young adults ages 18–25 (35.4% or 11.8 million people), followed by adults age 26 or older (17.2% or 37.9 million people), and then by adolescents ages 12–17 (10.5% or 2.7 million people). Based on these statistics, young adults, the population with the highest cannabis use, are also the most vulnerable because they may feel invincible to developing health issues and may not use the health care system for regular primary care and health maintenance. Another population-based concern lies in the lack of cannabis health literacy among not only patients but also clinicians because many practicing clinicians have not been exposed to cannabis pharmacology in their professional training (National Institutes of Health 2023). With these two issues in mind, a solid understanding of the evolution of cannabis from plant to product, regulation of its use at the state and federal levels, and its pharmacology is critical in ascertaining and understanding the potential health hazards of cannabis.

Definitions and Cannabis Formulations

Marijuana and hemp plants are cultivars of the genus *Cannabis*. The physiological effects of cannabis are derived primarily from its multiple compounds or cannabinoids, some of which are still being identified. Cannabidiol (CBD) and Δ^9-tetrahydrocannabinol (Δ^9-THC) are the best studied thus far; however, more than 100 different phytocannabinoids have been identified, including minor cannabinoids such as cannabigerol, cannabichromene, cannabinol, and tetrahydrocannabivarin (Health Canada 2018). As seen in Figure 12–1, commonly recognized strains of cannabis used recreationally and medically are *C. sativa*, *C. indica*, and *C. ruderalis* (National Academies of Sciences, Engineering, and Medicine 2017; Romero et al. 2020). These strains vary in THC and CBD content, which potentially reflects direction of use based on effect. Cannabis vendors characterize the strains as *sativa*, a high-THC-containing plant; *indica*, or a mixed THC-CBD plant; and *ruderalis*, a high-CBD-containing plant, although this method of characterization is rudimentary and often inaccurate. *C. sativa* appears to provide more

Sativa Strains

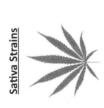

Plant Description
Plants grow tall and thin with fingerlike leaves; the plant can grow up to 12–20 feet.

Origins
Africa, Central America, Southeast Asia, portions of Western Asia.

CBD/THC Content
Often have lower doses of CBD and higher THC.

Associated Effects of Use
Produces a "cerebral high," or an energizing, anxiety-reducing effect.

Popular Strains
Acapulco Gold, Panama Red, and Durban Poison.

Indica Strains

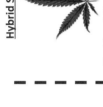

Plant Description
Plants are short and stocky with bushy greenery and chunky leaves that grow wide and broad.

Origins
Afghanistan, India, Pakistan, Turkey.

CBD/THC Content
Often have higher levels of CBD, but THC content isn't necessarily less.

Associated Effects of Use
Intensely relaxing effects; may help reduce nausea and pain and increase appetite.

Popular Strains
Hindu Kush, Afghan Kush, and Granddaddy Purple.

Hybrid Strains

Plant Description
Appearance depends on the combination of the parent plants.

Origins
Farms or in greenhouses from a combination of *C. sativa* and *C strains.*

CBD/THC Content
Grown to increase the THC percentage, but each type has a unique ratio of the two cannabinoids.

Associated Effects of Use
Can range from reducing anxiety and stress to decreasing insomnia and inflammation.

Popular Strains
Pineapple Express, Trainwreck, and Blue Dream.

Ruderalis Strains

Plant Description
Small, bushy plants that rarely grow taller than 12 inches and grow rapidly.

Origins
Eastern Europe, Himalaya, regions of India, Siberia, Russia.

CBD/THC Content
has little THC and higher amounts of CBD, but it may not be enough to produce any effects.

Associated Effects of Use
Low potency and not routinely used for medicinal or recreational purposes.

Popular Strains
Royal Haze, Haze Berry, and Hulkberry.

Figure 12–1. Description of various types of cannabis.
CBD = cannabidiol; THC = tetrahydrocannabinol.

Source. National Academies of Sciences, Engineering, and Medicine 2017.

stimulating, uplifting, and energizing effects, whereas *C. indica* provides a more relaxing, sedating, and pain-reducing effect (Page et al. 2020; Romero et al. 2020).

Cannabis plants are also classified on the basis of their ratio of THC to CBD, consisting of chemotype I or drug-type plants, which have a high THC:CBD ratio (>1.0); chemotype II or intermediate-type plants, which have a balanced THC:CBD ratio close to 1.0; and chemotype III or hemp-type plants, which have a low THC:CBD ratio (<1.0) and a THC percentage <0.30%, which is below the level of detectability (Hillig and Mahlberg 2004).

Loosely, cannabis can be considered as first or second generation. Compared with first-generation cannabis products (i.e., black-market products before 1996), second-generation, newer commercial products (i.e., state-permitted/unprosecuted products) that can be bought at any cannabis dispensary have a significantly higher average THC content. For example, between 1995 and 2021, the average THC concentration in a single leaf of cannabis increased almost fourfold from 3.96% to 15.34% (National Academies of Sciences, Engineering, and Medicine 2017; National Institute on Drug Abuse 2022). Second-generation products lack federal standardization in dose, concentration of cannabinoids, packaging, and labeling but are marketed in a large variety of formulations that can be combusted, vaped, or eaten (see Figure 12–2 and Table 12–1) (Page et al. 2020). For example, products purchased in a cannabis dispensary that claim a product contains pure CBD may still contain some amount of THC. Unfortunately, most of the published evidence is primarily based on first-generation cannabis that was combusted or smoked.

See Table 12–1 for explanation of synthetic cannabinoid types and cannabis-related terms.

Cannabis can also be classified as phyto-derived or synthetic. Unlike phytocannabinoids, synthetic cannabinoids are a class of molecules manufactured in a laboratory setting that can be arbitrarily divided into prescription and illicit cannabinoids. Initially developed to serve as pharmacological probes of the endogenous cannabinoid system, these synthetic illicit cannabinoids are now classified as new psychoactive drugs. In 2023, the Drug Enforcement Administration announced the proposal of new rules on the regulation of synthetic cannabinoids, including Δ^8- and Δ^9-THC ester, making these illegal as Schedule I controlled substances (Federal Register 2023). On the black

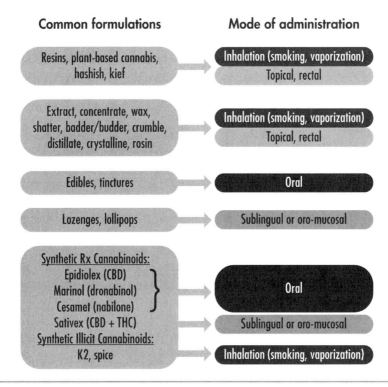

Figure 12–2. Summary of common formulations and modes of administration of cannabinoids.

Refer to Table 12–1 for common synthetic prescription cannabinoids and cannabis-releated terminology.

market, many of these compounds have been developed and marketed under various brand names, such as K2 and Spice, and may be adulterated (Drug Enforcement Administration 2022). Three synthetic prescription cannabinoids are currently marketed as Marinol (dronabinol) and Cesamet (nabilone) in the United States and Canada, and as Sativex (CBD + THC) in Canada. In the United States, Epidiolex (CBD) is the first and only purified phyto-derived CBD prescription drug approved by the FDA to treat seizures associated with Lennox-Gastaut syndrome, Dravet syndrome, or tuberous sclerosis complex in patients ages 1 year and older. Finally, depending on its use, cannabis is considered either medical or recreational, and the definition of each is based on specific individual state policies.

Table 12–1. Common types of cannabinoids and cannabis-related terminology

Synthetic prescription cannabinoids

Cesamet (nabilone)	Available in the United States and Canada and marketed by Bausch Health as a capsule. It is a Schedule II controlled substance in the United States. Mimics THC and is indicated for the management of severe nausea and vomiting associated with cancer chemotherapy in adults ≥18 years of age.
Epidiolex (CBD)	Available in the United States and marketed by Greenwich Biosciences as an oral solution. Epidiolex is the first and only purified plant-derived CBD prescription drug approved for the treatment of seizures associated with Lennox-Gastaut syndrome or Dravet syndrome in patients ≥1 year of age.
Marinol (dronabinol)	Available in the United States and Canada; marketed by AbbVie and as a generic capsule; labeled as a Schedule III controlled substance in the United States. Marinol (dronabinol) mimics THC and is indicated for anorexia associated with weight loss in adult patients with AIDS and nausea and vomiting associated with chemotherapy in adults who have failed conventional therapy.
Sativex (CBD + THC)	Available in Canada and marketed by GW Pharmaceuticals as an oromucosal spray. Sativex is a 1:1 ratio of CBD to THC and is a formulated extract from *Cannabis sativa*. It is approved for spasticity resulting from multiple sclerosis.

Cannabis-related terminology

Badder/budder	Cannabis concentrate whipped under heat to create a cake-like batter.
Concentrate	Product made from the cannabis plant that has been processed to keep only the most desirable plant compounds (primarily the cannabinoids and terpenes) while removing excess plant material and other impurities.

Table 12–1. Common types of cannabinoids and cannabis-related terminology (*continued*)

Cannabis-related terminology (*continued*)

Crumble	Dried cannabis oil with a honeycomb-like consistency. Concentrates made without the use of solvents are produced by mechanical or physical means to remove and gather trichomes.
Crystalline	Isolated cannabinoids in their pure crystal structure.
Distillate	Refined cannabinoid oil that is typically free of taste, smell, and flavor. It is the base of most edibles and vaporization cartridges.
Edible	Also known as a cannabis-containing food product, varying in concentrations of THC, CBD, or both. Examples include baked goods, powders, candies, popcorn, and drinks.
Extract	Cannabis concentrate created from solvents (e.g., alcohol, carbon dioxide) that essentially wash the trichomes off the cannabis plant.
Hash or hashish	Dried flower and buds from *Cannabis sativa* that are filtered and crushed into a powder and molded into a sticky ball or brick.
Kief	Most basic of THC concentrates; a powder-like substance found on cannabis flowers.
Resin	Trichome from cannabis flower or plant used to create hash.
Rosin	End product of cannabis flower that is squeezed under heat and pressure.
Shatter	Translucent, brittle, and often golden to amber concentrate used to make a solvent.
Tinctures (also known as green or golden dragon)	Alcohol-based cannabis extracts used to make edibles.

CBD = cannabidiol; THC = tetrahydrocannabinol.
Source.   Page et al. 2020.

State and Federal Policies Regulating Cannabis

In 1970, the Controlled Substances Act classified cannabis as a Schedule I substance, meaning it had no valid medical uses and a high potential for abuse, which significantly limited opportunities to study it clinically. However, in 2018, the Hemp Farming Act defined hemp as cannabis with less than 0.3% THC, thereby removing it from Schedule I status and allowing for the sale of CBD products outside of cannabis dispensaries. Per FDA regulations, manufacturers cannot make any claims for therapeutic or medical uses (Food and Drug Administration 2023). In 2014, Colorado was the first state to allow cannabis to be sold within a dispensary. Since that time, several states have either legalized or decriminalized cannabis, allowed it for medical use only, or made it fully legal (Mallinson and Hannah 2020). It is important to note that state policies on cannabis are specific to that state, and each state can individually establish definitions for medical use, labeling and packaging, possession and age limits, and medical versus recreational cannabis based on THC content (Page et al. 2020). Although these laws are rapidly changing and evolving, up-to-date resources are available and offer excellent information on current state laws and regulations and approved medical indications (DISA 2023; National Organization for the Reform of Marijuana Laws 2023). Regardless of state law, cannabis is still regulated by the Drug Enforcement Administration under Schedule I of the Controlled Substances Act, meaning interstate commerce of cannabis products is still considered a federal crime. However, in May 2024, the Department of Justice submitted a proposed rule to reschedule cannabis as a Schedule III drug, indicating a moderate to low risk of dependency, thus marking a significant move toward reducing federal limitations and recognizing the potential therapeutic benefits of cannabis.

Cannabis Pharmacology and Pharmacokinetics

The physiological effects of cannabis are derived from cannabinoids via their engagement with the endogenous endocannabinoid system, which is responsible for maintaining overall homeostasis (see Figure 12–2). Cannabinoids act through G protein–coupled receptors: cannabinoid 1 (CB_1) receptor and cannabinoid 2 (CB_2) receptor. CB_1 receptors are abundant in the mammalian brain and are primarily responsible for the psychotropic effects of cannabis. CB_1 receptors are also expressed in the myocardium, vascular endothelium, smooth muscle cells, and vagal afferents, while CB_2 receptors are predominantly found within macrophage-derived immune cells. THC is the primary psychoactive component of cannabis and a partial agonist of CB_1 and CB_2 receptors. However, CBD acts as a negative allosteric modulator of the CB_2 receptor, which in animal models has shown antioxidant and anti-inflammatory properties with limited psychoactive effect (Lu and Mackie 2021; Zou and Kumar 2018). Table 12–2 summarizes the pharmacology and pharmacokinetics of THC and CBD. The mode of administration is exceedingly important in terms of onset, bioavailability, and duration of effect, with inhalation having the shortest onset (within minutes) and duration (2–3 hours), and oral consumption having the longest onset (0.5–2 hours) and duration (5–8 hours) (Page et al. 2020).

Deleterious Effects on Cardiovascular and Respiratory Health

Many adverse effects have been reported with cannabis use, and observational and case report data have suggested that cannabis may trigger or potentiate major adverse cardiovascular events such as myocardial infarction, arrhythmias, and stroke, as well as serve as a cardiovascular risk factor for atherosclerotic cardiovascular disease (ASCVD). Although controversial, emerging data suggest that the negative effects of cannabis on the respiratory system and pulmonary function are mainly attributed to the smoke or aerosols produced when smoking or vaping cannabinoids, leading to potential pulmonary structural and cellular damage.

Cardiovascular Effects

When considering cardiovascular complications, much of the available published cannabis data are short term, observational, and retrospective in nature; lack exposure determination; exhibit recall bias; include minimal or variable cannabis exposure with no dose or product standardization; and typically evaluate low-risk cohorts. Additionally, the effect modification of mode of administration, dose, and chronicity of

Table 12–2. Pharmacology and pharmacokinetics of phytocannabinoids

Pharmacology and pharmacokinetics	Cannabinoids	
	CBD	**THC**
Mechanism of action	Activates CB_1 and CB_2	Activates CB_1
	Anandamide uptake inhibitor; $TRPV_1$, $TRPV_2$, $TRPA_1$, GPR_{55}, $5\text{-}HT_{1A}$, and $PPAR\gamma$ receptor activation	
	Inhibits adenosine uptake	
	Lowers FAAH levels and inhibits release of proinflammatory cytokines and expression of transcription factors ($IL\text{-}1\beta$, $IL\text{-}2$, $IL\text{-}6$, $IL\text{-}8$, $TNF\text{-}\alpha$, $IFN\text{-}\gamma$, CCL3, CCL4, $NF\text{-}\kappa B$)	
	Allosterically modulates other receptors: α_1-adrenoceptors, D_2, $GABA_A$, μ- and δ-opioid receptors (weak)	
	Inhibits calcium, potassium, and sodium channels by noncompetitive antagonism	
	Free radical scavenger	

Table 12–2. Pharmacology and pharmacokinetics of phytocannabinoids (*continued*)

Pharmacology and pharmacokinetics	Cannabinoids	
	CBD	**THC**
Absorption	Inhalation	Inhalation
	Onset: 3–5 mins	Onset: seconds–minutes
	Bioavailability: 11%–45%	Bioavailability: 2%–56%
	Duration: 2–3 hours	Duration: 2–3 hours
	Oral	Oral
	Onset: hours	Onset: 30 minutes–2 hours
	Bioavailability: 6%–33%	Bioavailability: 4%–20%
	Duration: 2–6 hours	Duration: 5–8 hours
		Transmucosal
		Onset: 15–40 minutes
		Bioavailability: Not known
		Duration: 45 minutes–2 hours
	Transdermal: Not known	Transdermal: Not known
	Transrectal: Not known	Transrectal: Not known

Table 12–2. Pharmacology and pharmacokinetics of phytocannabinoids (*continued*)

Pharmacology and pharmacokinetics	Cannabinoids	
	CBD	THC
Metabolism	Hepatic, via CYP1A1, 1A2, 2C8, 2C9, 2C19, 3A4, 2D6; UGT1A9, 2B7; undergoes hydroxylation	Hepatic, via CYP2C9, 2C19, 2D6, 3A4; UGT1A9, 2B7; undergoes glucuronidation
Distribution	Time dependent; fatty tissues and highly perfused organs such as brain, heart, lung, and liver	Time dependent; fatty tissues and highly perfused organs; protein binding: 97%
Elimination	Feces and urine: dependent on administration	Renal: 20%
		Feces: 65%
	Half-life: 18–32 hours	Half-life: 20–30 hours
	Preclinical and animal data suggest CBD may be a substrate and inhibitor of P-gp	THC may be a weak substrate and inhibitor of P-gp

CBD = cannabidiol; CB_1 = cannabinoid 1 receptor; CB_2 = cannabinoid 2 receptor; CCL = chemokine ligand; CYP = cytochrome P450; D_2 = dopamine receptor 2; FAAH = fatty acid amide hydrolase; GPR = G protein–coupled receptor; 5-HT = serotonin; IFN = interferon; IL = interleukin; mins = minutes; NF = nuclear factor; P-gp = P-glycoprotein; PPAR = peroxisome proliferator–activated receptors; secs = seconds; THC = tetrahydrocannabinol; TNF = tumor necrosis factor; TRPA = transient receptor potential ankyrin; TRPV = transient receptor potential vanilloid; UGT = uridine 5'-diphospho-glucuronosyltransferase.

Source. From Page RL, Allen LA, Kloner RA, et al: "Medical Marijuana, Recreational Cannabis, and Cardiovascular Health: A Scientific Statement From the American Heart Association. *Circulation* 142:e131–e152, 2020. Copyright ©2020 American Heart Association. Reprinted with permission.

use on these cardiovascular complications is scant (Pacher et al. 2018; Page et al. 2020). Nonetheless, based on the effects of exogenous cannabinoids at the receptor level and the differential expression of these receptors in certain tissues (e.g., myocyte, endothelium), potential cardiovascular complications can be postulated (Figure 12–3). The etiologies of such events may be due to activation of the sympathetic nervous system with parasympathetic nervous system inhibition, increased heart rate and supine blood pressure, increased platelet activation, and promotion of endothelial dysfunction and oxidative stress, which are all related to THC exposure (Figure 12–4). Alternatively, CBD may reduce heart rate and blood pressure, increase vasodilation, reduce inflammation, and lower vascular hyperpermeability, which could have beneficial cardiovascular effects (Pacher et al. 2018; Rezkalla and Kloner 2019). However, these benefits with CBD have not been documented in human trials.

A significant health concern is whether cannabis triggers or potentiates major adverse cardiovascular events and serves as a risk factor for ASCVD, similar to smoking tobacco. Although the data are conflicting, case series and observational and epidemiological studies suggest a temporal association between cannabis use and myocardial infarction, particularly in younger males without ischemic disease (DeFilippis et al. 2020; Pacher et al. 2018; Reis et al. 2017; Rezkalla and Kloner 2019).

Using U.S. adult survey data from the Behavioral Risk Factor Surveillance System, Ladha et al. (2021) evaluated the association between any recent cannabis use and myocardial infarction history using a weighted logistic regression model that adjusted for demographic factors, socioeconomic factors, health-related behaviors, concomitant substance use, and other comorbidities. Among 33,173 young adults (ages 18–44), 4,610 respondents reported recent cannabis use. Compared with nonusers, cannabis users had a higher risk for myocardial infarction (adjusted OR [AOR] 2.07; 95% CI 1.12–3.82). This association was similar in magnitude to associations found for current tobacco smoking (AOR 2.56; 95% CI 1.56–4.21) and smokeless tobacco use (AOR 1.88; 95% CI 1.00–3.50). Higher odds of myocardial infarction were associated with chronic cannabis use (more than four times per month; AOR 2.31; 95% CI 1.18–4.50) and smoking as a mode of administration (AOR 2.01; 95% CI 1.02–3.98) in those using cannabis compared with nonusers. Although a higher chance of myocardial infarction was associated with vaporization (AOR 2.26; 95% CI 0.58–8.82) and edible consumption (AOR 2.36; 95% CI 0.81–6.88) compared with nonusers, these findings were not statistically significant.

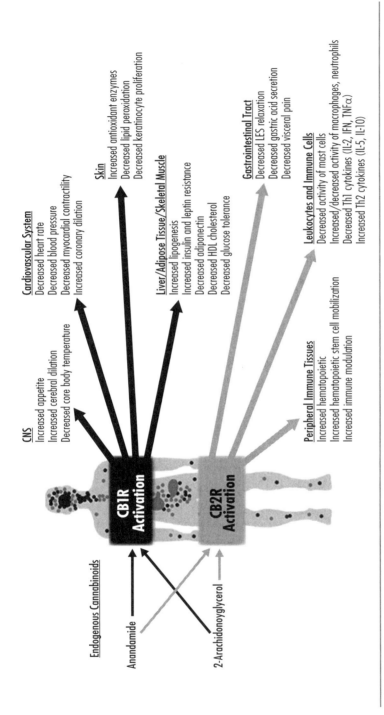

Figure 12–3. Physiological effects of endogenous cannabinoids.
CB1R = cannabinoid 1 receptor; CB2R = cannabinoid 2 receptor; HDL = high-density lipoprotein; IL = interleukin; IFN = interferon; LES = lower esophageal sphincter; Th = type; TNF = tumor necrosis factor.

Source.   Page et al. 2020.

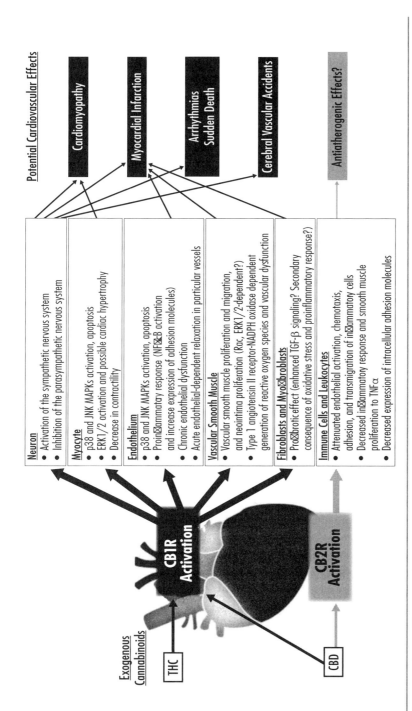

Figure 12–4. Effects of exogenous cannabinoids on the cardiovascular system.

? = questionable; CB1R = cannabinoid 1 receptor; CB2R = cannabinoid 2 receptor; CBD = cannabidiol; ERK = extracellular signal-regulated kinase; JNK = c-Jun N-terminal kinase; MAPK = mitogen-activated protein kinase; NADPH = nicotinamide adenine dinucleotide phosphate; NF = nuclear factor; TGF = transforming growth factor; THC = tetrahydrocannabinol; TNF = tumor necrosis factor.

Source. Page et al. 2020.

In a cross-sectional analysis using the 2014–2015 nationwide Veterans Affairs health care database and the Veterans wIth prema-Ture AtheroscLerosis (VITAL) registry, Mahtta et al. (2021) catego-rized patients as having premature (n=135,703), extremely premature (n=7,716), or nonpremature ASCVD (n=1,112,455); stratified each cohort based on the recreational substance used (e.g., tobacco, alcohol, cocaine, amphetamine, and cannabis); and evaluated the association with sub-stance use. Compared with patients with nonpremature ASCVD, patients with premature ASCVD had a higher use of cannabis (12.5% vs. 2.7%; $P<0.01$), and in adjusted models, cannabis use was indepen-dently associated with premature ASCVD (OR 2.65; 95% CI 2.59–2.7), and the association was stronger among females than males.

Similar associations have been documented between cannabis exposure and the risk of arrythmias and cerebrovascular accidents. Using the National Inpatient Sample database from 2010 to 2014, Desai et al. (2018) identified 2,459,856 hospitalized cannabis users, of whom 66,179 (2.7%) experienced arrhythmias, most commonly atrial fibrilla-tion. Using the 2016 Kids' Inpatient Database, Ramphul and Joynauth (2019) identified 68,793 cases of cannabis use, dependence, and abuse in teenagers ages 13–19. From this cohort, 26 patients had ventricular fibrillation (37.8 per 100,000 cases) and 96 patients reported palpita-tions (139.5 per 100,000 cases), whereas 57 had preexcitation syndrome (82.3 per 100,000 cases), 353 had long QT syndrome (513.1 per 100,000 cases), and 25 had atrial fibrillation (116.3 per 100,000 cases). The pos-sible mechanism lies in increased cannabis-related adrenergic stimula-tion and atrial ischemia that in turn lead to atrial arrhythmias, whereas catecholamine surges have been linked to ventricular fibrillation. Long QT syndrome may be due to the blocking of the human ether-à-go-go-related gene ($hERG$) channel (Rezkalla and Kloner 2019).

Finally, DeFilippis et al. (2020) estimated that 2 million (2.3%) of the 89.6 million U.S. adults who reported marijuana use had exist-ing cardiovascular disease, based on the 2005–2016 National Health and Nutrition Examination Survey. Taking this into account, cross-sectional data indicate that long-term (e.g., yearslong), continual can-nabis use is associated with an increased risk of metabolic syndrome compared with nonuse. However, conflicting studies have suggested that, compared with nonusers, those who use cannabis had a similar or reduced incidence of hyperglycemia, elevated fasting blood glu-cose, and diabetes mellitus, as well as lower BMI, total cholesterol, and low-density lipoprotein (DeFilippis et al. 2020; Rajavashisth et al. 2012; Vázquez-Bourgon et al. 2019).

Several case reports, case series, and observational studies (mostly in young adults) suggest a relationship between recent and heavy cannabis exposure and the risk of stroke. However, many of these studies are confounded by cigarette smoking, concomitant comorbidities leading to stroke, and other illicit substance use (Barber et al. 2013; Hemachandra et al. 2016; Simunek et al. 2018; Tirkey and Gupta 2016; Volpon et al. 2017). Nonetheless, in a retrospective evaluation of the Personality and Total Health Through Life study, which included participants ages 20–24 (*n*=2,383), 40–44 (*n*=2,532), and 60–64 (*n*=2,547) from 1999 to 2000, 2000 to 2001, and 2001 to 2002, respectively, Hemachandra et al. (2016) found a 3.3-fold risk of stroke/transient ischemic attack in cannabis users within the past year. However, this elevated risk was specific only to participants who used cannabis weekly or more often as opposed to those who used cannabis less often. Additionally, using weighted data from the National Inpatient Sample (2015–2017), Desai et al. (2018) identified hospitalizations among young patients (ages 18–44) with prior history of stroke/transient ischemic attack grouped into those with cannabis use disorder (CaUD; *n*=4,690) and those without CaUD (*n*=156,700) and evaluated the risk of recurrent stroke. Compared with those without CaUD, those with CaUD had higher odds of recurrent stroke (AOR 1.48; 95% CI 1.28–1.71).

Several postulated mechanisms for stroke include reversible cerebral vasoconstriction triggered by acute cannabis use; impairment in cerebrovascular function and cannabis-related angiopathy with chronic, heavy use; and an increase in procoagulant effects because THC increases the expression of glycoprotein IIb/IIIa and P-selectin on human platelets in a concentration-dependent manner based on in vitro data (Testai et al. 2022).

Athough the evidence is not concrete, both direct and secondhand exposure to cannabis smoke can affect endothelial function as well as arterial dilation, which can be assessed by flow-mediated dilation (FMD). FMD measures the extent to which arteries vasodilate in response to increased blood flow and is correlated with vascular health and endothelial function. In animal studies, 1 minute of exposure to secondhand cannabis smoke led to vasodilation that subsided within 25 minutes, whereas FMD remained impaired for at least 90 minutes (Wang et al. 2016). This effect may be in part due to reduced release of endothelial-derived nitric oxide, which is crucial to induce FMD, or through vascular structural changes such as greater arterial stiffness (Cheung et al. 2021; National Institutes of Health 2023). Whether this effect is also seen with edible forms of cannabis remains unknown.

However, emerging animal and in vitro models have suggested that reduced FMD may also be observed in high-THC, low-CBD edible products even though endothelial nitric oxide release was not attenuated (National Institutes of Health 2023).

Respiratory Effects

Smoke that is initially generated directly and inhaled from combusting or vaping cannabis and secondhand smoke that is produced on exhalation contain similar carcinogens as tobacco smoke (National Institutes of Health 2023). To this end, respiratory symptoms frequently associated with cannabis smoking include cough, increased sputum production, bronchitis, and wheezing (Gracie and Hancox 2021). On bronchoscopy and biopsy of the airway mucosa, people who habitually smoke cannabis frequently demonstrate histological changes, vascular hyperplasia, inflammation, and swelling of the airway epithelium, along with cellular disorganization and molecular dysregulation (Gracie and Hancox 2021; National Institutes of Health 2023). Additionally, instances of other pathologies linked with cannabis use include the development of chronic obstructive pulmonary disease (COPD), pulmonary bullae, spontaneous pneumothorax, pleuritic pain, pulmonary aspergillosis, hemoptysis, and pulmonary Langerhans cell histiocytosis (Vásconez-González et al. 2023).

In 2019, the Centers for Disease Control and Prevention found that vaping products containing THC were linked with cases of e-cigarette or vaping use–associated lung injuries (EVALI), which is possibly due to the vitamin E acetate that is often used as an oil-based solvent for THC (Krishnasamy et al. 2020). As a result of the vaping epidemic and surge in EVALI cases, cannabis research has now begun to evaluate the additives in cannabis products, which may also mediate adverse pulmonary effects (National Institutes of Health 2023).

However, smoking cannabis and its subsequent effects on lung function remain controversial because many cannabis users also smoke tobacco, which can confound overall conclusions (Gracie and Hancox 2021). A number of studies have suggested that smoking cannabis contributes to changes in lung function, but the pattern of these changes appears to be different from those of tobacco, and their clinical significance is uncertain (Gracie and Hancox 2021). Although cannabis use is associated with airway inflammation and symptoms of bronchitis, the evidence that persistent cannabis use causes airflow obstruction and COPD remains debatable. In some studies, cannabis has been associated with lower forced expiratory volume at 1 second (FEV1)/ forced vital capacity (FVC) ratios; however, this effect is mostly driven by an increase in FVC rather than a reduction in FEV1 (Gracie and Hancox 2021; Hancox et al. 2010; Kempker et al. 2015; Pletcher et al. 2012; Tashkin et al. 1987). Furthermore, people who smoke cannabis can have greater static lung volumes, suggesting hyperinflation and gas trapping, but there is no evidence of gas transfer impairment (Aldington et al. 2007; Tashkin et al. 1980, 1987). Another consistent finding is that cannabis users have higher large-airway resistance and lower conductance, which is compatible with the evidence that cannabis use causes bronchitis; however, considerable uncertainty exists about the effects of long-term cannabis use on lung function and whether these pulmonary changes are reversible upon cessation (Aldington et al. 2007; Gracie and Hancox 2021; Tashkin et al. 1980, 1987). One study suggested that the FEV1 of past cannabis users continued to decline after quitting; however, these data were generated from a very small number of heavy cannabis users, most of whom also smoked tobacco (Tan et al. 2019).

In a population-based cohort of 1,037 individuals born in 1972–1973 and followed to age 45, Hancox et al. (2022) evaluated cannabis and tobacco use at ages 18, 21, 26, 32, 38, and 45 and measured spirometry, plethysmography, and carbon monoxide transfer factor at age 45. On conclusion of the study, both cannabis use and tobacco use were associated with lower FEV1/FVC ratios; however, as found in previous studies, this effect was mostly owing to higher FVC values among cannabis users and with little difference in FEV1, whereas people who smoked tobacco had lower FEV1 values. In addition, both tobacco and cannabis use were associated with higher static lung volumes (e.g., total lung capacity, functional residual capacity, and residual volume) by plethysmography, indicating a tendency toward hyperinflation and gas trapping, but only cannabis was associated with increased ventilation air methane by gas dilution, suggesting a new finding of a lower gas transfer.

Because cannabis has been associated with an impairment in pulmonary immunity, the potential for infections has been reported, particularly in those with underlying pulmonary conditions such as chronic obstructive pulmonary disease or those who are immunosuppressed (Preteroti et al. 2023). *Aspergillus* is an invasive mold that can grow on cannabis plants, and although it is typically harmless in an immunocompetent patient, cannabis users who are immunocompromised, such as posttransplant patients or those who have a diagnosis of cancer or advanced HIV, have a higher risk for invasive aspergillosis, leading to pneumonia and possible death (Gwinn et al. 2023). In a survey of major transplant centers, Levi et al. (2019) found that of those centers reporting fungal infections associated with cannabis use, 67 (89%) reported infection associated with smoking, 11 (15%) with vape pens, and 3 (4%) with edibles. Although these infections have primarily been reported in patients obtaining cannabis on the black market, species of *Aspergillus* have been found in cannabis products sold in legitimate dispensaries (Arizona Department of Health Services 2023; California Department of Cannabis Control 2022; Colorado Department of Revenue 2022; Page et al. 2020).

Finally, because cannabis smoke and tobacco smoke contain similar carcinogens, the link between cannabis smoke exposure and the risk for lung cancer has been explored. Compared with people who smoke cigarettes, those who smoke cannabis tend to inhale more deeply and hold their breath longer, which leads to greater exposure per breath to tar and other carcinogens (Wu et al. 1988). Although studies have supported the biological plausibility of an association between cannabis smoking and lung cancer on the basis of molecular, cellular, and histopathological findings, observational studies suggest only a weak correlation between cannabis use and the development of lung or testicular cancer (Mehra et al. 2006; Solmi et al. 2023; Vásconez-González et al. 2023).

Drug-Medication Interactions

Because of the pharmacokinetic profile of cannabis, medication interactions with cannabis are highly variable in terms of clinical significance, given the variability in products, potencies, THC:CBD ratios, doses, routes of administration, and populations using cannabinoids (see Table 12–2). In vitro studies have suggested that THC may inhibit cytochrome P450 (CYP) 3A4/4, CYP2C9, CYP2C19, and CYP2D6, whereas CBD also may inhibit CYP3A4/5, CYP2C19, CYP2D6, and CYP1A2 (Bansal et al. 2020; Doohan et al. 2021; Nasrin et al. 2021). THC can induce CYP1A2, particularly with smoked cannabis. Preclinical and animal data suggest that cannabinoids can inhibit systemic transport proteins such as breast cancer–resistant protein (BCRP) and P-glycoprotein (P-gp) activity, decrease protein expression of P-gp, and increase protein expression of BCRP (Page et al. 2020). Therefore, cannabis can potentially interact with medications that are substrates of these enzymes and transport proteins, increasing their serum concentrations and leading to supratherapeutic effects, adverse effects, and the need for dosage adjustment. Such potential substrates include many commonly used cardiovascular medications, such as anticoagulants and antiplatelets (leading to increased bleeding), antiarrhythmics (prolonging the QTc interval), and statins (elevating the risk for myopathy and possible rhabdomyolysis). A free Web-based platform application, CANNabinoid Drug Interaction Review (CANN-DIR), can be used to detect potential drug-medication interactions (Kocis et al. 2023; Penn State College of Medicine 2020).

Beneficial Effects on Cardiovascular and Respiratory Health

Based on the evidence to date, cannabis in any of its formulations has not been shown to have any cardiovascular or respiratory benefits (Gracie and Hancox 2021; Page et al. 2020). As seen in Figure 12–4, by binding to the CB_2 receptor, CBD may potentially exert anti-inflammatory effects at the vascular endothelial level, which has been hypothesized to have a protective role in reducing ischemic damage and atherosclerotic disease (Dabiri and Kassab 2021). However, these hypotheses are generated solely through animal and in vitro models, not in humans or human trials.

Clinical Significance and Recommendations

With the advent of cannabis dispensaries and decreases in regulation at the state level in the United States, cannabis use, particularly among adolescents and young adults, continues to increase. Because of the status of cannabis as a Schedule 1 controlled substance, the science and outcomes associated with acute and chronic cannabis use have been slow to emerge but continue to be elucidated. Therefore, providers should always query patients at each encounter regarding potential cannabis use in a transparent, nonjudgmental fashion and incorporate shared decision-making between provider and patient, highlighting state and federal laws, possible risks and benefits of various forms of administration, and adverse effects. Patients should avoid all synthetic illicit cannabinoids because of the potential for contamination and adulteration, as well as avoid smoking or vaping cannabis because combusted cannabis has similar carcinogens to tobacco smoke.

From a cardiovascular standpoint, patients who are using cannabis, regardless of indication (medically or recreationally) or method of use (smoking, vaping, or consuming), should be informed about the potential risk of developing new cardiovascular events. This should be a focus of conversation, particularly with younger adult users who have significantly increased their cannabis use and people who have risk factors for ASCVD or already have established disease. The overall public perspective that cannabis is safer than smoking tobacco because it is natural should be dismissed (Gracie and Hancox 2021; Page et al. 2020). Although the published data only suggest an association, major negative signals suggest that cannabis exposure, regardless of the method or chronicity of use, could lead to the development of early ASCVD and may emerge in the future as a potentially modifiable risk factor for ASCVD, like tobacco smoking.

Unfortunately, regarding respiratory health, the data are not as clear-cut. However, patients with underlying pulmonary conditions such as asthma, COPD, and emphysema and those who are immunocompromised should avoid vaping or smoking cannabis due to the risk of worsening pulmonary function, disease exacerbation, and possible invasive fungal infections. Given the prevalence of cannabis smoking and the supporting biological plausibility of an association between cannabis smoking and lung cancer on a molecular, cellular, and histopathological basis, health care providers should advise patients about its potential cancer risks. Whether these respiratory issues are also seen with edible cannabis products remains unknown. Finally, as the hazardous effects of secondhand cannabis smoke are beginning to emerge, those with underlying pulmonary conditions should avoid cannabis smoke exposure as they would tobacco smoke.

Conclusion

With the rapidly changing landscape of cannabis laws and increased cannabis use, there is a pressing need to harmonize state and federal cannabis policies, provide high-quality education for clinicians and the public, warn of potential health hazards, and conduct prospective research on potential therapeutic benefits. From a pharmacovigilance perspective, safety signals have emerged regarding cannabis use and adverse cardiovascular events and pulmonary effects; however, there is a paucity of rigorously performed studies. Additional areas of research that are warranted include evaluation of the safety of first- versus second-generation cannabis products, chronicity and mode of use (particularly with edibles), and health impacts of secondhand cannabis smoke. Finally, based on the evidence to date, cannabis has not shown any beneficial effects on cardiovascular or pulmonary health in human subjects.

Key Points

- Attitudes toward recreational and medicinal use of cannabis have rapidly evolved. As of August 1, 2023, 49 U.S. states, the District of Columbia, and four of five U.S. territories allow some form of cannabis use. Cannabis use has risen considerably over the past decade in young adults ages 18–25.
- Safety signals have emerged regarding cannabis use and adverse cardiovascular outcomes; however, there is a paucity of rigorously performed studies. Observational and case report data suggest an association between cannabis use and the development of myocardial infarction, arrythmias, and stroke. Regardless of mode or chronicity of use, cannabis expsoure may be a potential risk factor for atherosclerotic cardiovascular disease.
- Δ^9-Tetrahydrocannabinol (Δ^9-THC) may stimulate the sympathetic nervous system while inhibiting the parasympathetic nervous system, increase heart rate and supine blood pressure, cause platelet activation, and promote endothelial dysfunction and oxidative stress. Cannabidiol may reduce heart rate and blood pressure, impove vasodilation, reduce inflammation, and lower vascular hyperpermability.
- Smoking cannabis has been reported to cause the following respiratory symptoms: cough, increased sputum production, bronchitis, and wheezing, which typically resolve upon cannabis discontinuation. Bronchoscopy and biopsy of airway mucosa suggest that people who habitually smoke cannabis demonstrate histological changes, vascular hyperplasia, inflammation, and swelling of airway epithelium, along with cellular disorganization and molecular dysregulation. Development of chronic obstructive pulmonary disease, pulmonary bullae, spontaneous pneumothorax, pleuritic pain, pulmonary aspergillosis, hemoptysis, and pulmonary Langerhans cell histiocytosis have been reported.

- Cannabis smoke contains many of the same carcinogens and mutagens as tobacco smoke and is associated with health risks. Until the pathophysiology of e-cigarette or vaping product use-associated lung injury (EVALI) is better understood, vaping cannabis should be avoided.
- Drug-medication interactions can exist and should be anticipated because THC and CBD have the potential to inhibit cytochrome P450 enzymes.
- No form of cannabis has yet been found to have any beneficial effects on cardiovascular or pulmonary health. Clinicians need more initial and continuing education about the various cannabis products and their health implications, particularly that the use of cannabis or its potent synthetic analogues might be the underlying cause of cardiovascular events and other respiratory issues.

References

Aldington S, Williams M, Nowitz M, et al: Effects of cannabis on pulmonary structure, function and symptoms. Thorax 62(12):1058–1063, 2007 17666437

Arizona Department of Health Services: Voluntary recall of certain marijuana products due to possible aspergillus contamination. Arizona Department of Health Services, June 14, 2023. Available at: https://www.azdhs.gov/director/public-information-office/index.php#news-release-061423. Accessed October 23, 2023.

Barber PA, Pridmore HM, Krishnamurthy V, et al: Cannabis, ischemic stroke, and transient ischemic attack: a case-control study. Stroke 44(8):2327–2329, 2013 23696547

Bansal S, Maharao N, Paine MF, et al. Predicting the potential for cannabinoids to precipitate pharmacokinetic drug interactions via reversible inhibition or inactivation of major cytochromes P450. Drug Metab Dispos 48(10):1008–1017, 2020 32587099

California Department of Cannabis Control: Mandatory recall: January 26, 2022. California Department of Cannabis Control, January 26, 2022. Available at: https://cannabis.ca.gov/resources/cannabis-recalls-and-safety-notices/mandatory-recall-2022–01–26/. Accessed October 23, 2023.

Cheung CP, Coates AM, Millar PJ, et al: Habitual cannabis use is associated with altered cardiac mechanics and arterial stiffness, but not endothelial function in young healthy smokers. J Appl Physiol 130(3):660–670, 2021 33444123

Colorado Department of Revenue: Health and safety advisory: SDJ LLC (DBA The Living Rose). Colorado Department of Revenue, October 26, 2022.

Available at: https://sbg.colorado.gov/sites/sbg/files/221026_SDJ_LLC _HSA.docx.pdf. Accessed October 23, 2023.

Dabiri AE, Kassab GS: Effects of cannabis on the cardiovascular system: the good, the bad, and the many unknowns. Med Cannabis Cannabinoids 4(2):75–85, 2021 35224427

DeFilippis EM, Bajaj NS, Singh A, et al: Marijuana use in patients with cardiovascular disease. J Am Coll Cardiol 75(3):320–332, 2020 31976871

Desai R, Patel U, Deshmukh A, et al: Burden of arrhythmia in recreational marijuana users. Int J Cardiol 264:91–92, 2018 29642998

DISA: Marijuana legality by state. DISA Global Solutions, August 1, 2023. Available at: https://disa.com/marijuana-legality-by-state. Accessed August 24, 2023.

Doohan P, Oldfield L, Arnold J, et al: Cannabinoid interactions with cytochrome p450 drug metabolism: a full-spectrum characterization. AAPS J 23:91, 2021 34181150

Drug Enforcement Administration: K2/Spice: Drug Fact Sheet. Springfield, VA, Drug Enforcement Administration, October 2022. Available at: https://www.dea.gov/sites/default/files/2023–04/K2-Spice%202022%2 0Drug%20Fact%20Sheet.pdf. Accessed August 28, 2023.

Federal Register: Schedules of controlled substances: temporary placement of MDMB-4en-PINACA, 4F-MDMB-BUTICA, ADB-4en-PINACA, CUMYL-PEGACLONE, 5F-EDMB-PICA, and MMB-FUBICA in Schedule I. Washington, DC, Federal Register, April 4, 2023. Available at: https:// www.federalregister.gov/documents/2023/04/04/2023–06893/schedules -of-controlled-substances-temporary-placement-of-mdmb-4en-pinaca- 4f-mdmb-butica. Accessed August 24, 2023.

Food and Drug Administration: FDA regulation of cannabis and cannabis- derived products, including cannabidiol (CBD). Food and Drug Administration, July 5, 2023. Available at: https://www.fda.gov/news -events/public-health-focus/fda-regulation-cannabis-and-cannabis -derived-products-including-cannabidiol-cbd. Accessed August 24, 2023.

Gracie K, Hancox RJ: Cannabis use disorder and the lungs. Addiction 116(1):182–190, 2021 32285993

Gwinn KD, Leung MC, Stephens AB, et al: Fungal and mycotoxin contaminants in cannabis and hemp flowers: implications for consumer health and directions for further research. Fron Microbiol 14:1278189, 2023 37928692

Hancox RJ, Poulton R, Ely M, et al: Effects of cannabis on lung function: a population-based cohort study. Eur Respir J 35(1):42–47, 2010 19679602

Hancox RJ, Gray AR, Zhang X, et al: Differential effects of cannabis and tobacco on lung function in mid-adult life. Am J Respir Crit Care Med 205(10):1179–1185, 2022 35073503

Health Canada: Information for health care professionals: cannabis (marihuana, marijuana) and the cannabinoids. Health Canada, October

12, 2018. Available at: https://www.canada.ca/en/health-canada/
    services/drugs-medication/cannabis/information-medical-practitioners
    /information-health-care-professionals-cannabis-cannabinoids.html.
    Accessed August 24, 2023.
Hemachandra D, McKetin R, Cherbuin N, et al: Heavy cannabis users at
    elevated risk of stroke: evidence from a general population survey. Aust
    N Z J Public Health 40(3):226–230, 2016 26558539
Hillig KW, Mahlberg PG: A chemotaxonomic analysis of cannabinoid
    variation in cannabis (Cannabaceae). Am J Bot 91(6):966–975, 2004
    21653452
Kempker JA, Honig EG, Martin GS: The effects of marijuana exposure
    on expiratory airflow: a study of adults who participated in the U.S.
    National Health and Nutrition Examination Study. Ann Am Thorac Soc
    12(2):135–141, 2015 25521349
Kocis PT, Wadrose S, Wakefield RL, et al: CANNabinoid Drug Interaction
    Review (CANN-DIR). Med Cannabis Cannabinoids 6(1):1–7, 2023
    36814686
Krishnasamy VP, Hallowell BD, Ko JY, et al: Characteristics of a nationwide
    outbreak of e-cigarette, or vaping, product use–associated lung injury—
    United States, August 2019–January 2020. MMWR Morb Mortal Wkly
    Rep 69(3):90–94, 2020 31971931
Ladha KS, Mistry N, Wijeysundera DN, et al: Recent cannabis use and
    myocardial infarction in young adults: a cross-sectional study. CMAJ
    193(35):E1377–E1384, 2021 34493564
Levi ME, Montague BT, Thurstone C, et al: Marijuana use in transplantation:
    a call for clarity. Clin Transplant 33(2):e13456, 2019 30506888
Lu HC, Mackie K: Review of the endocannabinoid system. Biol Psychiatry
    Cogn Neurosci Neuroimaging 6(6):607–615, 2021 32980261
Mahtta D, Ramsey D, Krittanawong C, et al: Recreational substance use
    among patients with premature atherosclerotic cardiovascular disease.
    Heart 107(8):650–656, 2021 33589427
Mallinson DJ, Hannah AL: Policy and political learning: the development of
    medical marijuana policies in the states. Publius 50:344–369, 2020
Mehra R, Moore BA, Crothers K, et al: The association between marijuana
    smoking and lung cancer: a systematic review. Arch Intern Med
    166(13):1359–1367, 2006 16832000
Nasrin S, Watson C, Perez-Paramo Y, et al: Cannabinoid metabolites as inhibitors
    of major hepatic CYP450 enzymes, with implications for cannabis-drug
    interactions. Drug Metab Dispos 49:1070–1080, 2021 34493602
National Academies of Sciences, Engineering, and Medicine: The Health
    Effects of Cannabis and Cannabinoids: The Current State of Evidence
    and Recommendations for Research. Washington, DC, National
    Academies Press, 2017

National Institute on Drug Abuse: Cannabis Potency Data. Rockville, MD, National Institutes of Health, November 23, 2022. Available at: https://nida.nih.gov/research/research-data-measures-resources/cannabis-potency-data. Accessed August 24, 2023.

National Institutes of Health: Cannabis and Cannabinoids in Heart, Lung, Blood, and Sleep. Rockville, MD, National Institutes of Health, June 2023. Available at: https://www.nhlbi.nih.gov/events/2023/cannabis-and-cannabinoids-heart-lung-blood-and-sleep. Accessed October 22, 2023.

National Organization for the Reform of Marijuana Laws: Medical Marijuana Laws. Washington, DC, National Organization for the Reform of Marijuana Laws, 2023. Available at: https://norml.org/laws/medical-laws. Accessed August 24, 2023.

Pacher P, Steffens S, Haskó G, et al: Cardiovascular effects of marijuana and synthetic cannabinoids: the good, the bad, and the ugly. Nat Rev Cardiol 15(3):151–166, 2018 28905873

Page RL, Allen LA, Kloner RA, et al: Medical marijuana, recreational cannabis, and cardiovascular health: a scientific statement from the American Heart Association. Circulation 142:e131–e152, 2020

Penn State College of Medicine: CANNabinoid Drug Interaction Review (CANN-DIR®), Version 3.0.1. Hershey, PA, Penn State College of Medicine, 2020. Available at: https://cann-dir.psu.edu. Accessed August 28, 2023.

Pletcher MJ, Vittinghoff E, Kalhan R, et al: Association between marijuana exposure and pulmonary function over 20 years. JAMA 307(2):173–181, 2012 22235088

Preteroti M, Wilson ET, Eidelman DH, et al: Modulation of pulmonary immune function by inhaled cannabis products and consequences for lung disease. Respir Res 24(1):95, 2023 36978106

Rajavashisth TB, Shaheen M, Norris KC, et al: Decreased prevalence of diabetes in marijuana users: cross-sectional data from the National Health and Nutrition Examination Survey (NHANES) III. BMJ Open 2(1):e000494, 2012 22368296

Ramphul K, Joynauth J: Cardiac arrhythmias among teenagers using cannabis in the United States. Am J Cardiol 124(12):1966, 2019 31653358

Reis JP, Auer R, Bancks MP, et al: Cumulative lifetime marijuana use and incident cardiovascular disease in middle age: the Coronary Artery Risk Development in Young Adults (CARDIA) study. Am J Public Health 107(4):601–606, 2017 28207342

Rezkalla S, Kloner RA: Cardiovascular effects of marijuana. Trends Cardiovasc Med 29(7):403–407, 2019 30447899

Romero P, Peris A, Vergara K, et al: Comprehending and improving cannabis specialized metabolism in the systems biology era. Plant Sci 298:110571, 2020 32771172

Simunek L, Krajina A, Herzig R, et al: Cerebral infarction in young marijuana smokers: case reports. Acta Medica (Hradec Kralove) 61(2):74–77, 2018 30216188

Solmi M, De Toffol M, Kim JY, et al: Balancing risks and benefits of cannabis use: umbrella review of meta-analyses of randomised controlled trials and observational studies. BMJ 382:e072348, 2023 37648266

Substance Abuse and Mental Health Services Administration: 2021 National Survey of Drug Use and Health releases. Rockville, MD, Substance Abuse and Mental Health Services Administration, January 4, 2023. Available at: https://www.samhsa.gov/data/release/2021-national-survey-drug-use-and-health-nsduh-releases. Accessed August 24, 2023.

Tan WC, Bourbeau J, Aaron SD, et al: The effects of marijuana smoking on lung function in older people. Eur Respir J 54(6):1900826, 2019 31537703

Tashkin DP, Calvarese BM, Simmons MS, et al: Respiratory status of seventy-four habitual marijuana smokers. Chest 78(5):699–706, 1980 7428453

Tashkin DP, Coulson AH, Clark VA, et al: Respiratory symptoms and lung function in habitual heavy smokers of marijuana alone, smokers of marijuana and tobacco, smokers of tobacco alone, and nonsmokers. Am Rev Respir Dis 135(1):209–216, 1987 3492159

Testai FD, Gorelick PB, Aparicio HJ, et al: Use of marijuana: effect on brain health: a scientific statement from the American Heart Association. Stroke 53(4):e176–e187, 2022 35142225

Tirkey NK, Gupta S: Acute antero-inferior wall ischaemia with acute ischaemic stroke caused by oral ingestion of cannabis in a young male. J Assoc Physicians India 64(9):93–94, 2016 27762529

Vásconez-González J, Delgado-Moreira K, López-Molina B, et al: Effects of smoking marijuana on the respiratory system: a systematic review. Subst Abus 44(3):249–260, 2023 37728136

Vázquez-Bourgon J, Setién-Suero E, Pilar-Cuéllar F, et al: Effect of cannabis on weight and metabolism in first-episode non-affective psychosis: results from a three-year longitudinal study. J Psychopharmacol 33(3):284–294, 2019 30702972

Volpon LC, Sousa CLMM, Moreira SKK, et al: Multiple cerebral infarcts in a young patient associated with marijuana use. J Addict Med 11(5):405–407, 2017 28614161

Wang X, Derakhshandeh R, Liu J, et al: One minute of marijuana secondhand smoke exposure substantially impairs vascular endothelial function. J Am Heart Assoc 5(8):e00385, 2016 27464788

Wu TC, Tashkin DP, Djahed B, et al: Pulmonary hazards of smoking marijuana as compared with tobacco. N Engl J Med 318(6):347–351, 1988 3340105

Zou S, Kumar U: Cannabinoid receptors and the endocannabinoid system: signaling and function in the central nervous system. Int J Mol Sci 19(3):833, 2018 29533978

13

Mechanisms, Efficacy, and Safety of Cannabinoids for Treating Chronic Pain

Mark K. Greenwald, Ph.D.

Chronic pain is a major personal, societal, and economic burden (U.S. Pain Foundation 2021); total annual costs in the United States due to health care and lost productivity approach $600 billion (Gaskin and Richard 2012). Approximately 20% of the U.S. population experiences chronic pain; however, disparities exist: chronic pain is more prevalent among females (Osborne and Davis 2022) and among adults who are unemployed, living at or below the poverty line, and living in rural areas (Kuehn 2018). Persons living with chronic pain are at elevated risk for anxiety, depression, and suicide (Petrosky et al. 2018) and live more years with disability (Rice et al. 2016). Pain conditions rank among the most common reasons for physician visits (St Sauver et al. 2013).

Besides nonsteroidal anti-inflammatory drugs (NSAIDs), paracetamol/acetaminophen, and aspirin for treating mild to moderate pain, prescription medications for treating moderate to severe pain include opioid agonists (e.g., morphine, hydrocodone, oxycodone, hydromor-phone, fentanyl); antiepileptics, including gabapentinoids (e.g., prega-balin, gabapentin); serotonin-norepinephrine reuptake inhibitors (SNRIs) and tricyclic antidepressants (e.g., duloxetine, amitriptyline); and local anesthetics such as lidocaine or capsaicin (Guerrero-Alba et al. 2019). Chronic use of these medications has limitations; for example, opi-oids can induce hyperalgesia, and gabapentinoids can lead to seda-tion and psychomotor impairment. These unwanted effects and the need for clinical monitoring stimulate demand for safer and effective alternatives.

Cannabis and plant-derived cannabinoids have been not only uncriti-cally accepted in American society for recreational use but also proposed for treating several medical conditions, including chronic pain. Although pain is the most common reason cited by patients for using cannabinoids (Turk and Rudy 1987), the seemingly attractive notion of using cannabis or cannabinoids as an analgesic must be approached with skepticism. First, cannabinoids are not FDA approved for treating any pain condition. Second, cannabis contains more than 500 chemical compounds, approxi-mately 125 of which are phytocannabinoids (Radwan et al. 2021; Rock and Parker 2021). Phytocannabinoids exert antinociceptive effects via sev-eral neuropharmacological mechanisms (Table 13–1). They can activate supraspinal and spinal G protein–coupled cannabinoid 1 (CB_1) or can-nabinoid 2 (CB_2) receptors that—given their location on presynaptic terminals of other neurons—modulate the release of neurotransmit-ters, including glutamate, GABA, serotonin, or noradrenaline (Bouchet and Ingram 2020; Dogrul et al. 2012; Milligan et al. 2020; Palazzo et al. 2010). Some phytocannabinoids can also indirectly modulate receptor function. For example, cannabidiol (CBD) is a negative allosteric mod-ulator at CB_1 receptors (Laprairie et al. 2015) and a positive allosteric modulator at CB_2 receptors and μ- and δ-opioid receptors (Kathmann et al. 2006). Phytocannabinoids can also indirectly enhance signal-ing at cannabinoid receptors and related sites (e.g., G protein–coupled receptor 55, transient receptor potential ion channels) by inhibiting the reuptake of endocannabinoids N-arachidonoylethanolamine (AEA, anandamide) or 2-arachidonoylglycerol (2-AG), or by inhibiting catabo-lism of anandamide by fatty acid amide hydrolase (FAAH) or inhib-iting catabolism of 2-AG by monoacylglycerol lipase (MAGL) (Pacher et al. 2006). Anandamide and 2-AG are degraded to arachidonic acid, which signals at cyclooxygenase and lipoxygenase receptors to influ-ence pain and inflammation (Donvito et al. 2018). Finally, cannabis contains terpenoids and flavonoids that can bind to cannabinoid and

Table 13–1. Summary of evidence for actions of phytocannabinoids at various signaling targets related to pain/analgesia

Phytocannabinoids	Molecular signaling targets							
	CB_1	CB_2	$5\text{-}HT_{1A}$	GPR_{18}	GPR_{55}	$TRPV_1$	$TRPA_1$	$TRPM_8$
Δ^9-THC	(+)	(+)		+	+		(+)	(+)
Δ^8-THC	(+)	(+)						
CBN	(+)	(+)/–					+	–
Δ^9-THCV	(+)/–	(+)	+		(+)	+	+	
CBD	NAM	(–)	+	–	–	+	+	–
CBDA	0		+			+	+	–
CBC	0	+					+	
CBG	(+)	(+)	–			+	+	–
CBDV	0				–	+	+	–

Table 13–1. Summary of evidence for actions of phytocannabinoids at various signaling targets related to pain/analgesia (*continued*)

Phytocannabinoids	Molecular signaling targets							
	FAAH	AEA reuptake	COX-2	PPAR (a/g)	TLR$_4$	Glycine	σ_1	μ opioid
Δ^9-THC				+		+		PAM
Δ^8-THC								
CBN								
Δ^9-THCV								
CBD	–	–		+		PAM	–	PAM
CBDA			–?	+				
CBC		–						
CBG		–						
CBDV					–			

For reviews, see Izzo et al. 2009; Morales et al. 2017; Pertwee 2008; Vučković et al. 2018; Woodhams et al. 2017; Zagzoog et al. 2020. AEA = anandamide (N-arachidonoylethanolamine); CB$_1$ = cannabinoid 1 receptor; CB$_2$ = cannabinoid 2 receptor; CBC = cannabichromene; CBD = cannabidiol; CBDA = cannabidiolic acid; CBDV = cannabidivarin; CBG = cannabigerol; CBN = cannabinol; COX-2 = cyclooxygenase-2; FAAH = fatty acid amide hydrolase; 5-HT$_{1A}$ = serotonin type 1A receptor; GPR = G protein–coupled receptor; NAM = negative allosteric modulator; PAM = positive allosteric modulator; PPAR = peroxisome proliferator-activated receptor; THC = tetrahydrocannabinol; THCV = tetrahydrocannabivarin; TLR$_4$ = Toll-like receptor 4; TRPA$_1$ = transient receptor potential ankyrin 1; TRPM$_8$ = transient receptor potential melastatin 8; TRPV$_1$ = transient receptor potential vanilloid 1.

other receptors, produce their own antinociceptive effects, and likely enhance the antinociceptive actions of cannabinoids, referred to as an entourage effect (Anand et al. 2021; LaVigne et al. 2021; Liktor-Busa et al. 2021; Rodriguez et al. 2022; Russo 2011).

Some evidence suggests that cannabinoids are potentially useful for the treatment of various chronic pain conditions. Herein, emphasis is placed on Δ^9-tetrahydrocannabinol (Δ^9-THC) and CBD due to a higher volume of research data for these compounds. However, data are also presented for other cannabinoids: Δ^8-THC, cannabinol, Δ^9-tetrahydrocannabivarin, cannabidiolic acid, cannabichromene, cannabigerol, and cannabidivarin. This chapter does not address specific synthetic cannabinoids that are used as experimental tools or are in pharmaceutical development (i.e., those that are not FDA approved), which produce pharmacological effects that mimic phytocannabinoids (i.e., "cannabimimetic"). To date, clinical research on cannabinoid analgesic efficacy has spanned various chronic pain conditions (e.g., low back pain, headache, fibromyalgia, orofacial pain, neuropathic pain, multiple sclerosis, sickle cell disease, spinal cord injury). The next section provides an overview of current evidence, with the goal of identifying promising therapeutic approaches and translating this knowledge into clinical practice.

Current State of Evidence

The antinociceptive effects of Δ^9-THC are primarily mediated by CB_1 receptors in the spinal cord dorsal horn, periaqueductal gray, dorsal raphe nucleus, and thalamus (Chiou et al. 2013). There is also limited evidence in rodent models for antinociceptive effects of cannabidiolic acid (Alegre-Zurano et al. 2020; Vigli et al. 2021; Zhu et al. 2020) and Δ^8-THC (Tagen and Klumpers 2022), and for anti-inflammatory effects of cannabigerol (Wen et al. 2023) and cannabichromene (DeLong et al. 2010; Wirth et al. 1980).

Substantial evidence supports a role of CB_2 receptors in mediating pain and inflammatory states. Activation of CB_2 receptors, which are located on several types of immune cells, suppresses proinflammatory cytokines and T cell proliferation (Cabral and Griffin-Thomas 2009). In animal models of inflammatory and neuropathic pain, systemic or peripheral administration of CB_2 agonists decreases hyperalgesia, which can be reversed selectively by CB_2 antagonists but not CB_1

antagonists (Guindon and Hohmann 2008). However, a clinical trial of a CB_2 agonist failed for osteoarthritis knee pain (Pereira et al. 2013).

FAAH inhibitors impede the breakdown of anandamide, which increases signaling at CB_1 and CB_2 receptors and transient receptor potential vanilloid 1 ($TRPV_1$) channels. FAAH inhibitors exhibit efficacy in animal models of nociceptive, neuropathic, and inflammatory pain (Pillarisetti et al. 2009). Although such data suggest these might be promising therapies in humans, to date, two clinical trials failed to demonstrate efficacy in chronic pain (Di Marzo 2012; Huggins et al. 2012). Other emerging approaches in animal models include MAGL inhibitors, which interfere with the breakdown of 2-AG and increase its signaling at CB_1 and CB_2 receptors, and $TRPV_1$ antagonists, which block signaling at pronociceptive (and prohypothermic) vanilloid channels on CB_1 receptors. However, $TRPV_1$ antagonists can induce hyperthermia, which led to a clinical trial failure (Gavva et al. 2008) and may limit the use of biosimilars as monotherapies.

Given the complexity of endocannabinoid signaling, how might we optimize analgesia and reduce side effects? Several research groups (e.g., Aiello et al. 2016; Grim et al. 2014; Maione et al. 2007; Malek and Starowicz 2016) have proposed leveraging this complexity using a multitargeting approach, with partially redundant components. Possible avenues include the combined inhibition of FAAH and cyclooxygenase-2 (COX-2) while activating $TRPV_1$ channels. Inhibition of FAAH leads to increased anandamide and decreased arachidonic acid signaling, inhibition of COX-2 increases anandamide and decreases prostaglandin signaling, and activation of vanilloid channels facilitates anandamide signaling. Additional strategies for improving the benefit/risk ratio are to administer cannabinoids via peripheral routes of administration (thus avoiding CB_1-associated side effects) and to use allosteric modulators that adjust activity-dependent endogenous signaling (Khurana et al. 2017; Slivicki et al. 2017).

In humans, open-label and retrospective studies are more likely to report evidence in favor of Δ^9-THC-related analgesia, whereas controlled studies are less likely to provide supportive evidence. Contemporary systematic reviews and meta-analyses of clinical trials (Giossi et al. 2022; Meng et al. 2017; Sainsbury et al. 2021; Wang et al. 2021) and other evidence reviews (e.g., Bialas et al. 2022; Canadian Agency for Drugs and Technologies in Health 2019; Pergolizzi et al. 2018; Shehata et al. 2022) have examined whether cannabinoids are effective for treating various types of chronic pain. Table 13–2 summarizes the conclusions from systematic reviews of the evidence regarding cannabinoid

Table 13–2. Summary of evidence for analgesic efficacy of phytocannabinoids in various chronic pain conditions, based on systematic reviews and unreviewed, prospective, controlled clinical studies

	Chronic pain conditions				
	Low back	Headache	Fibromyalgia	Orofacial	Neuropathic
Reviews	First et al. 2020; Kolber et al. 2021 Price et al. 2022	Baron 2015; Lochte et al. 2017; Okusanya et al. 2022; Poudel et al. 2021; Sherpa et al. 2022	Cameron and Hemingway 2020; Kurlyandchik et al. 2021; Walitt et al. 2016	Grossman et al. 2022; Votrubec et al. 2022	Cavaletti et al. 2021; Dykukha et al. 2021; McParland et al. 2023; Meng et al. 2017; Mücke et al. 2018; Sainsbury et al. 2021; Wong et al. 2020
Phytocannabinoids					
Δ^9-THC + CBD					++
Δ^9-THC		+			+
Δ^8-THC					
CBN					
Δ^9-THCV				+	
CBD	0				
CBDA					

Table 13–2. Summary of evidence for analgesic efficacy of phytocannabinoids in various chronic pain conditions, based on systematic reviews and unreviewed, prospective, controlled clinical studies (*continued*)

	Chronic pain conditions				
	Low back	Headache	Fibromyalgia	Orofacial	Neuropathic
Phytocannabinoids					
CBC					
CBG					
CBDV					0
Reviews	Multiple sclerosis Filippini et al. 2022; Haddad et al. 2022; Longoria et al. 2022	Sickle cell Argueta et al. 2020; Paulsingh et al. 2022	Spinal cord Ling et al. 2022; Nabata et al. 2021; Tsai et al. 2022	Cancer Häuser et al. 2019	
Phytocannabinoids					
Δ⁹-THC + CBD	+	0	0	0	
Δ⁹-THC	+		0	0	
Δ⁸-THC					
CBN					

Table 13–2. Summary of evidence for analgesic efficacy of phytocannabinoids in various chronic pain conditions, based on systematic reviews and unreviewed, prospective, controlled clinical studies (*continued*)

	Chronic pain conditions			
	Multiple sclerosis	Sickle cell	Spinal cord	Cancer
Phytocannabinoids				
Δ⁹-THCV				
CBD			0	
CBDA				
CBC				
CBG				
CBDV				

Note. PubMed article search strategy (limited to 2015–2023): "(Cannabis or cannabinoid) AND (pain condition)," filtered by "systematic review" or "meta-analysis" or "clinical trial" or "randomized clinical trial." 0 = tested in at least one trial but not effective; + = mild benefit > risk (e.g., analgesia with side effects such as somnolence, dizziness); ++ = moderate benefit > risk (e.g., analgesia relative to placebo [superiority] or comparator [non-inferiority] with minimal side effects). CBC = cannabichromene; CBD = cannabidiol; CBDA = cannabidiolic acid; CBDV = cannabidivarin; CBG = cannabigerol; CBN = cannabinol; THC = tetrahydrocannabinol; THCV = tetrahydrocannabivarin.

treatment of chronic pain conditions. Most studies compared cannabis or specific cannabinoids with placebo. However, there are difficulties in experimental blinding, and placebo effects have been noted (Gedin et al. 2022; Wilsey et al. 2016). Meta-analyses have concluded that most clinical studies have been generally of low (and moderate at best) quality, and many have been judged to have significant risk of bias.

Overall, results are complex but suggest a small benefit/risk ratio in pain relief for certain types of noncancer pain. Specifically, there is mild to moderate benefit for Δ^9-THC, alone or in combination with CBD, in the treatment of neuropathic pain and multiple sclerosis pain (see Table 13–2). Other reviews, which are based on very few well-controlled studies, have reported a modest benefit/risk ratio of oral Δ^9-THC for the treatment of headache (e.g., Pini et al. 2012) and transdermal CBD for treating orofacial pain (e.g., Nitecka-Buchta et al. 2019). In contrast, well-controlled studies have not demonstrated efficacy with Δ^9-THC, either alone or in combination with CBD, for treating sickle cell disease (e.g., Abrams et al. 2020), spinal cord injury, or cancer-related pain, and no efficacy of CBD was found for low back pain (e.g., Bebee et al. 2021). One well-controlled study failed to find a benefit of cannabidivarin for HIV-related neuropathic pain (Eibach et al. 2021).

Accordingly, the most important priority is conducting highly rigorous trials. Ideally, such controlled clinical trials will need to carefully define each treatment population, administer interventions over longer intervals (i.e., months rather than days or a few weeks), include positive and placebo control conditions, standardize doses or consider the virtues and challenges of flexible-dosing protocols (e.g., Zubcevic et al. 2023), measure cannabinoid concentrations to perform exposure-response analyses, examine biomarkers of improvement, control for use of concomitant medications, monitor analgesic and secondary outcomes over an adequate period following the intervention, and plan clinically meaningful efficacy and safety endpoints—all of which are highly relevant for FDA review. Also, during chronic treatment with Δ^9-THC, Tsagareli et al. (2021) found that mice developed tolerance to analgesic effects, but analgesic tolerance to repeated cannabinoid administration has not been determined in the clinical setting.

Very few analgesia trials with CBD have been published, and clinical trials for most other cannabinoids are severely lacking, including those for Δ^8-THC, cannabinol, Δ^9-tetrahydrocannabivarin, cannabidiolic acid, cannabichromene, cannabigerol, and cannabidivarin (see Table 13–2). Thus, it is not possible to make any recommendations in the absence of data.

Deleterious Effects

The adverse effects of cannabinoids are better understood for cannabis inhalation (i.e., smoking and vaping) as a route of administration and for the two most commonly studied phytocannabinoids, Δ^9-THC and CBD (in their plant-based or synthetic forms). There are too few studies of cannabinoids via non-inhaled routes of administration (e.g., topical/ transdermal, parenteral) and virtually none involving edible forms of cannabinoids.

The first concern is that CB_1 agonists such as Δ^9-THC are responsible for producing psychoactive effects (related to abuse potential) and for sedating and psychomotor-impairing effects. One systematic review of clinical trials for neuropathic pain found that 10% of participants receiving active cannabis, but only 5% receiving placebo cannabis, withdrew from the study due to adverse events such as sleepiness, dizziness, and confusion (Mücke et al. 2018).

Based on Table 13–1, one might expect some psychoactivity for Δ^8-THC (Tagen and Klumpers 2022) and possibly cannabigerol or cannabinol due to their CB_1 receptor partial agonist effects. In one survey study, most users of Δ^8-THC (who had also used Δ^9-THC and could compare their experiences) reported euphoria, relaxation, difficulty concentrating, and problems with short-term memory, in addition to pain relief (Kruger and Kruger 2022). In contrast, cannabidiolic acid (precursor to CBD), cannabidivarin, Δ^9-tetrahydrocannabivarin, and cannabichromene should be devoid of psychoactive effects.

A second possible concern is that some cannabinoids might worsen pain (i.e., cause hyperalgesia) or that placebo control might produce greater efficacy than active cannabinoids. Yet, based on meta-analyses that have presented effect sizes for individual studies (e.g., Meng et al. 2017; Sainsbury et al. 2021; Stockings et al. 2018; Wang et al. 2021; Wong et al. 2020), there is presently no evidence to support the idea that Δ^9-THC or CBD (alone or in combination) significantly worsens pain nor that placebo control produces superior analgesic efficacy than cannabinoids. These meta-analyses also indicate that these cannabinoids do not worsen secondary outcomes of physical function or sleep quality.

A third concern is that emerging data suggest cannabis strains with higher Δ^9-THC concentrations (at the same time often having lower CBD concentrations) can exacerbate psychotic and affective symptoms in vulnerable individuals (Petrilli et al. 2022; Sideli et al. 2020). These adverse effects are absent with CBD, which may attenuate some adverse effects of Δ^9-THC (García-Gutiérrez et al. 2020) and is the rationale for developing nabiximols (THC:CBD combinations). CB_2 agonists are not psychoactive and are not yet known to produce deleterious effects.

A fourth concern is that cannabis smoking (like tobacco smoking) is detrimental to respiratory function in several ways (Yayan and Rasche 2016). Vaping (cannabis or tobacco) has been found to produce pulmonary inflammation and alveolar damage, which has been attributed to the lipid-diluting agent vitamin E acetate in vaping fluid (Garg et al. 2022). Cannabis and Δ^9-THC consumption can also produce tachycardia, orthostatic hypotension, and—in the context of chronic use—potentially arrhythmias and stroke (Manolis et al. 2019).

Deleterious effects of smoking and vaping cannabinoids have led researchers to develop alternative cannabinoid formulations (e.g., oral, nasal, transmucosal, transdermal) for safer dosing. Also, because cannabinoids are fatty acids that are poorly absorbed via the oral route, various technologies are being pioneered to increase bioavailability for therapeutic applications (Palrasu et al. 2022; Reddy et al. 2023; Stella et al. 2021).

Thinking long term, it will be important to monitor the use of cannabinoids (by whichever route of administration) in combination with other psychoactive medications and substances because this could alter their safety profile.

Beneficial Effects

In this chapter, I focus on analgesia as a potential benefit of cannabinoid administration. As discussed in the section "Current State of Evidence," most published clinical study findings are typically based on low-quality and rarely moderate-quality evidence (e.g., case reports, retrospective studies), and most clinical trials clearly lack appropriate controls. Restricting conclusions to only those few studies with stronger methodology, the apparent analgesic benefits of THC, CBD, or THC+CBD combinations are circumscribed to neuropathic pain, multiple sclerosis pain, and potentially other conditions (e.g., headache, orofacial pain). Therapeutic (cannabinoid vs. placebo) effect sizes are small. Notably, psychiatric symptoms such as anxiety and depression may augment (or, at least, interact with) the experience of pain. However, current evidence that Δ^9-THC and CBD have anxiolytic or antidepressant effects is weak (Hasbi et al. 2023); if this were to hold true in future research, then any analgesic effect of these cannabinoids might be direct rather than indirectly mediated by the abatement of psychiatric symptoms.

As a result of the opioid crisis and the rising use of cannabinoids, there is keen interest in the ability of cannabinoid agonists to produce "opioid-sparing" effects (i.e., whether cannabinoids can reduce the analgesic dose of an opioid and thus improve safety). Data from observational and epidemiological studies are typically insufficient to draw conclusions due to inadequate controls. A systematic review and meta-analysis found that, despite evidence of opioid-sparing effects in 17 of 19 animal studies (yielding a 3.6-fold reduction in morphine equivalent dose), support for opioid-sparing effects was lacking across 9 clinical studies (Nielsen et al. 2017). A recent ecological momentary assessment that prospectively tracked pain and the use of cannabis and prescription opioids in patients with chronic pain also did not find evidence for opioid sparing (Mun et al. 2022). To date, there is no evidence that the combination of cannabinoids and opioids is associated with higher rates of adverse events. Thus, the combination of cannabinoids and opioids in clinical settings appears to be safe but has no opioid-sparing effect.

Clinical Significance and Recommendations

Clinicians must recognize that cannabinoids are not indicated for pain by the FDA. Only dronabinol/nabilone (synthetic Δ^9-THC to reduce nausea/vomiting and increase appetite) and CBD (for pediatric seizures) have received U.S. regulatory approvals. Nabiximols (Δ^9-THC + CBD combination) is still investigational; it has been studied for multiple sclerosis–related neuropathic pain but is not approved in the United States.

For patients who are already using cannabis or cannabinoids, clinicians can do the following:

1. Confirm with self-report (*why* the patient is taking cannabinoids, how *much*, how *often*) to monitor adverse events, which are more likely in combination with other medications or substance use, toward the goal of reducing risks.
2. Ask the patient whether they have accurate knowledge of THC and CBD content (but realize this is not reliable without a certificate of analysis).

3. Advise that cannabinoids, especially CB_1-acting compounds, have risks (e.g., sedation, cognitive impairment, worsening of psychiatric symptoms, pulmonary tissue inflammation caused by smoking and vaping), particularly in older patients.
4. Encourage and support safer alternative approaches that have demonstrated efficacy (e.g., exercise, meditation, and repetitive transcranial magnetic stimulation, which is cleared by the FDA for migraines with aura).

In addition to determining why and how a patient is using cannabinoids, it is important to understand the nature of the pain condition that is interacting with the patient's cannabinoid use. In this regard, it is worthwhile to conduct a functional analysis of pain/disability. The clinician should also evaluate sleep, fatigue, depression, and anxiety symptoms, which correlate with pain and may be altered by cannabinoids. If pain is intractable, the clinician should consider referral to a pain specialist, neurology, or physical medicine.

After careful assessment, if it is believed that the patient with pain is using cannabinoids responsibly, the clinician could consider whether analgesia might be augmented (or cannabinoid use reduced).

1. Adjust dosages of psychiatric medications such as serotonin type 1A agonists (e.g., buspirone) or SNRIs (e.g., duloxetine), because these may facilitate cannabinoid signaling in descending serotonin and norepinephrine circuitry, but consider whether sedation could be a side effect.
2. Recommend the use of lidocaine or capsaicin patches (peripheral targeting, better safety) in some cases of neuropathic pain, when appropriate.
3. Consider NSAIDs or COX-2 inhibitors because these can also produce synergism at non-cannabinoid receptors and are a safe option.

Based on these factors, some clinicians may advise patients not to use cannabinoids for pain (or other indications), whereas others may be comfortable allowing it but with caution. The key consideration, especially in the absence of definitive effectiveness data, is to promote safety for patients. Factors that clinicians might consider when offering advice are that the risk of complications increases when cannabinoids are used via the inhaled route of administration and when cannabinoids are used by patients who are using other substances or who have psychiatric or medical comorbidities.

Finally, it is important to read the scientific literature. The field is changing very rapidly, and clinicians can be responsible resources for educating, treating, and referring their patients to improve health care outcomes.

Conclusion

The National Academies of Sciences, Engineering, and Medicine (2017) reviewed and identified "conclusive or substantial evidence" for cannabinoids in treating chronic pain in adults; they recommended further research to determine how to improve efficacy and reduce side effects. A systematic review and meta-analysis of 374 studies involving 171 cannabinoid-based interventions in laboratory animal models found strong evidence for antinociceptive effects of CB_1, CB_2, nonselective CB_1/CB_2 (e.g., Δ^9-THC), and peroxisome proliferator–activated receptor (PPAR) α agonists in inflammatory and neuropathic pain models, and for CBD, FAAH inhibitors, and MAGL inhibitors in neuropathic pain models (Soliman et al. 2021). There is also evidence from animal models of opioid-sparing effects, such that CB_1 agonists seem to reduce the 50% effective dose of morphine for antinociception, whereas human study data are not supportive (Nielsen et al. 2017). Reviews and meta-analyses of clinical studies find weak evidence for analgesic effects of cannabis or cannabinoids in chronic pain. Evidence is most promising for neuropathic pain and perhaps fibromyalgia; however, there is a critical need for more rigorous trials. Cannabinoids are not supported for musculoskeletal or postoperative pain. Reviews have concluded that there is low-quality research evidence for cannabinoid analgesic effects because most studies involve case reports, retrospective studies, and clinical trials that lack appropriate controls.

Several critical challenges remain. First, researchers need to differentiate mechanisms of action—that is, disentangle direct and indirect therapeutic mechanisms/contributions from different cannabinoids and their metabolites ("endocannabinoidome") at a daunting array of molecular targets within and outside the endocannabinoid system. Second, if cannabinoids are found to be effective in certain types of chronic pain, then it follows that targets need to be reached to achieve adequate pharmaceutical exposure and that chronic dosing would be needed. Clinical trials will need to assess the development of tolerance to the antinociceptive effects of cannabinoids, as well as assess neural and behavioral adaptations that might pose safety risks. These include psychoactive effects and excessive use of cannabinoids that could lead to cannabis use disorder. Third, there are inevitable individual differences in cannabinoid response, including modulation by CNS and hepatic genes that lead to differences in analgesia, psychoactivity, and metabolism. Although some genetic differences have been identified in the context of acute cannabinoid administration, long-term studies are needed to understand response heterogeneity.

Key Points

- Given the complexity of the endocannabinoid system, cannabinoids that act on multiple endocannabinoid and other targets are likely to have superior efficacy and safety profiles for the treatment of chronic pain syndromes.
- Current evidence is most promising for cannabinoid efficacy in neuropathic pain, and preliminary signals from some studies (typically not well-controlled) suggest that patients with other types of pain could benefit as well.
- Rigorous clinical trials are needed to evaluate the analgesic efficacy of all cannabinoids, given the mixed literature on Δ^9-tetrahydrocannabinol and cannabidiol to date.
- Clinicians should carefully evaluate their patients with chronic pain (and typically other comorbid conditions) and can improve care by taking a cautious approach because cannabinoids are not FDA-approved for treating pain. They should ascertain which cannabinoids are being used, how much, and why; inform patients of cannabinoid risks; encourage alternative therapies; adjust dosages of psychiatric medications as needed; consider referrals for interdisciplinary care; and evaluate the evolving scientific literature to become trusted advisers to patients.

References

Abrams DI, Couey P, Dixit N, et al: Effect of inhaled cannabis for pain in adults with sickle cell disease: a randomized clinical trial. JAMA Netw Open 3(7):e2010874, 2020 32678452

Aiello F, Carullo G, Badolato M, et al: TRPV1-FAAH-COX: the couples game in pain treatment. ChemMedChem 11(16):1686–1694, 2016 27240888

Alegre-Zurano L, Martín-Sánchez A, Valverde O: Behavioural and molecular effects of cannabidiolic acid in mice. Life Sci 259:118271, 2020 32798553

Anand U, Pacchetti B, Anand P, et al: Cannabis-based medicines and pain: a review of potential synergistic and entourage effects. Pain Manag (Lond) 11(4):395–403, 2021 33703917

Argueta DA, Aich A, Muqolli F, et al: Considerations of cannabis use to treat pain in sickle cell disease. J Clin Med 9(12):3902, 2020 33271850

Baron EP: Comprehensive review of medicinal marijuana, cannabinoids, and therapeutic implications in medicine and headache: what a long strange trip it's been. Headache 55(6):885–916, 2015 26015168

Bebee B, Taylor DM, Bourke E, et al: The CANBACK trial: a randomised, controlled clinical trial of oral cannabidiol for people presenting to the emergency department with acute low back pain. Med J Aust 214(8):370–375, 2021 33846971

Bialas P, Fitzcharles M-A, Klose P, et al: Long-term observational studies with cannabis-based medicines for chronic non-cancer pain: a systematic review and meta-analysis of effectiveness and safety. Eur J Pain 26(6):1221–1233, 2022 35467781

Bouchet CA, Ingram SL: Cannabinoids in the descending pain modulatory circuit: role in inflammation. Pharmacol Ther 209:107495, 2020 32004514

Cabral GA, Griffin-Thomas L: Emerging role of the cannabinoid receptor CB2 in immune regulation: therapeutic prospects for neuroinflammation. Expert Rev Mol Med 11:e3, 2009 19152719

Cameron EC, Hemingway SL: Cannabinoids for fibromyalgia pain: a critical review of recent studies (2015–2019). J Cannabis Res 2(1):19, 2020 33526114

Canadian Agency for Drugs and Technologies in Health: Medical Cannabis for the Treatment of Chronic Pain: A Review of Clinical Effectiveness and Guidelines (CADTH Rapid Response Report: Summary With Critical Appraisal). Ottawa, ON, Canadian Agency for Drugs and Technologies in Health, 2019

Cavaletti G, Marmiroli P, Renn CL, et al: Cannabinoids: an effective treatment for chemotherapy-induced peripheral neurotoxicity? Neurotherapeutics 18(4):2324–2336, 2021 34668147

Chiou L-C, Hu SS-J, Ho Y-C: Targeting the cannabinoid system for pain relief? Acta Anaesthesiol Taiwan 51(4):161–170, 2013 24529672

DeLong GT, Wolf CE, Poklis A, et al: Pharmacological evaluation of the natural constituent of Cannabis sativa, cannabichromene and its modulation by Δ(9)-tetrahydrocannabinol. Drug Alcohol Depend 112(1–2):126–133, 2010 20619971

Di Marzo V: Inhibitors of endocannabinoid breakdown for pain: not so FA(AH)cile, after all. Pain 153(9):1785–1786, 2012 22785079

Dogrul A, Seyrek M, Yalcin B, et al: Involvement of descending serotonergic and noradrenergic pathways in CB1 receptor-mediated antinociception. Prog Neuropsychopharmacol Biol Psychiatry 38(1):97–105, 2012 22300745

Donvito G, Nass SR, Wilkerson JL, et al: The endogenous cannabinoid system: a budding source of targets for treating inflammatory and neuropathic pain. Neuropsychopharmacology 43(1):52–79, 2018 28857069

Dykukha I, Malessa R, Essner U, et al: Nabiximols in chronic neuropathic pain: a meta-analysis of randomized placebo-controlled trials. Pain Med 22(4):861–874, 2021 33561282

Eibach L, Scheffel S, Cardebring M, et al: Cannabidivarin for HIV-associated neuropathic pain: a randomized, blinded, controlled clinical trial. Clin Pharmacol Ther 109(4):1055–1062, 2021 32770831

Filippini G, Minozzi S, Borrelli F, et al: Cannabis and cannabinoids for symptomatic treatment for people with multiple sclerosis. Cochrane Database Syst Rev 5(5):CD013444, 2022 35510826

First L, Douglas W, Habibi B, et al: Cannabis use and low-back pain: a systematic review. Cannabis Cannabinoid Res 5(4):283–289, 2020 33381642

García-Gutiérrez MS, Navarrete F, Gasparyan A, et al: Cannabidiol: a potential new alternative for the treatment of anxiety, depression, and psychotic disorders. Biomolecules 10(11):1575, 2020 33228239

Garg I, Vidholia A, Garg A, et al: E-cigarette or vaping product use-associated lung injury: a review of clinico-radio-pathological characteristics. Respir Investig 60(6):738–749, 2022 35963780

Gaskin DJ, Richard P: The economic costs of pain in the United States. J Pain 13(8):715–724, 2012 22607834

Gavva NR, Treanor JJS, Garami A, et al: Pharmacological blockade of the vanilloid receptor TRPV1 elicits marked hyperthermia in humans. Pain 136(1–2):202–210, 2008 18337008

Gedin F, Blomé S, Pontén M, et al: Placebo response and media attention in randomized clinical trials, assessing cannabis-based therapies for pain: a systematic review and meta-analysis. JAMA Netw Open 5(11):e2243848, 2022 36441553

Giossi R, Carrara F, Padroni M, et al: Systematic review and meta-analysis seem to indicate that cannabinoids for chronic primary pain treatment have limited benefit. Pain Ther 11(4):1341–1358, 2022 36129666

Grim TW, Ghosh S, Hsu KL, et al: Combined inhibition of FAAH and COX produces enhanced anti-allodynic effects in mouse neuropathic and inflammatory pain models. Pharmacol Biochem Behav 124:405–411, 2014 25058512

Grossman S, Tan H, Gadiwalla Y: Cannabis and orofacial pain: a systematic review. Br J Oral Maxillofac Surg 60(5):e677–e690, 2022 35305839

Guerrero-Alba R, Barragán-Iglesias P, González-Hernández A, et al: Some prospective alternatives for treating pain: the endocannabinoid system and its putative receptors GPR18 and GPR55. Front Pharmacol 9:1496, 2019 30670965

Guindon J, Hohmann AG: Cannabinoid CB2 receptors: a therapeutic target for the treatment of inflammatory and neuropathic pain. Br J Pharmacol 153(2):319–334, 2008 17994113

Haddad F, Dokmak G, Karaman R: The efficacy of cannabis on multiple sclerosis-related symptoms. Life (Basel) 12(5):682, 2022 35629350

Hasbi A, Madras BK, George SR: Endocannabinoid system and exogenous cannabinoids in depression and anxiety: a review. Brain Sci 13(2):325, 2023 36831868

Häuser W, Welsch P, Klose P, et al: Efficacy, tolerability and safety of cannabis-based medicines for cancer pain: a systematic review with meta-analysis of randomised controlled trials. Schmerz 33(5):424–436, 2019 31073761

Huggins JP, Smart TS, Langman S, et al: An efficient randomised, placebo-controlled clinical trial with the irreversible fatty acid amide hydrolase-1 inhibitor PF-04457845, which modulates endocannabinoids but fails to induce effective analgesia in patients with pain due to osteoarthritis of the knee. Pain 153(9):1837–1846, 2012 22727500

Izzo AA, Borrelli F, Capasso R, et al: Non-psychotropic plant cannabinoids: new therapeutic opportunities from an ancient herb. Trends Pharmacol Sci 30(10):515–527, 2009 19729208

Kathmann M, Flau K, Redmer A, et al: Cannabidiol is an allosteric modulator at mu- and delta-opioid receptors. Naunyn Schmiedebergs Arch Pharmacol 372(5):354–361, 2006 16489449

Khurana L, Mackie K, Piomelli D, et al: Modulation of CB1 cannabinoid receptor by allosteric ligands: pharmacology and therapeutic opportunities. Neuropharmacology 124:3–12, 2017 28527758

Kolber MR, Ton J, Thomas B, et al: PEER systematic review of randomized controlled trials: management of chronic low back pain in primary care. Can Fam Physician 67(1):e20–e30, 2021 33483410

Kruger JS, Kruger DJ: Delta-8-THC: Delta-9-THC's nicer younger sibling? J Cannabis Res 4(1):4, 2022 34980292

Kuehn B: Chronic pain prevalence. JAMA 320(16):1632, 2018 30357307

Kurlyandchik I, Tiralongo E, Schloss J: Safety and efficacy of medicinal cannabis in the treatment of fibromyalgia: a systematic review. J Altern Complement Med 27(3):198–213, 2021 33337931

Laprairie RB, Bagher AM, Kelly MEM, et al: Cannabidiol is a negative allosteric modulator of the cannabinoid CB1 receptor. Br J Pharmacol 172(20):4790–4805, 2015 26218440

LaVigne JE, Hecksel R, Keresztes A, et al: Cannabis sativa terpenes are cannabimimetic and selectively enhance cannabinoid activity. Sci Rep 11(1):8232, 2021 33859287

Liktor-Busa E, Keresztes A, LaVigne J, et al: Analgesic potential of terpenes derived from Cannabis sativa. Pharmacol Rev 73(4):98–126, 2021 34663685

Ling H-Q, Chen Z-H, He L, et al: Comparative efficacy and safety of 11 drugs as therapies for adults with neuropathic pain after spinal cord injury: a Bayesian network analysis based on 20 randomized controlled trials. Front Neurol 13:818522, 2022 35386408

Lochte BC, Beletsky A, Samuel NK, et al: The use of cannabis for headache disorders. Cannabis Cannabinoid Res 2(1):61–71, 2017 28861505

Longoria V, Parcel H, Toma B, et al: Neurological benefits, clinical challenges, and neuropathologic promise of medical marijuana: a systematic review of cannabinoid effects in multiple sclerosis and experimental models of demyelination. Biomedicines 10(3):539, 2022 35327341

Maione S, De Petrocellis L, de Novellis V, et al: Analgesic actions of N-arachidonoyl-serotonin, a fatty acid amide hydrolase inhibitor with antagonistic activity at vanilloid TRPV1 receptors. Br J Pharmacol 150(6):766–781, 2007 17279090

Malek N, Starowicz K: Dual-acting compounds targeting endocannabinoid and endovanilloid systems: a novel treatment option for chronic pain management. Front Pharmacol 7:257, 2016 27582708

Manolis TA, Manolis AA, Manolis AS: Cannabis associated "high" cardiovascular morbidity and mortality: marijuana smoke like tobacco smoke? A déjà vu/déjà vécu story? Mini Rev Med Chem 19(11):870–879, 2019 30426899

McParland AL, Bhatia A, Matelski J, et al: Evaluating the impact of cannabinoids on sleep health and pain in patients with chronic neuropathic pain: a systematic review and meta-analysis of randomized controlled trials. Reg Anesth Pain Med 48(4):180–190, 2023 36598058

Meng H, Johnston B, Englesakis M, et al: Selective cannabinoids for chronic neuropathic pain: a systematic review and meta-analysis. Anesth Analg 125(5):1638–1652, 2017 28537982

Milligan AL, Szabo-Pardi TA, Burton MD: Cannabinoid receptor type 1 and its role as an analgesic: an opioid alternative? J Dual Diagn 16(1):106–119, 2020 31596190

Morales P, Hurst DP, Reggio PH: Molecular targets of the phytocannabinoids: a complex picture. Prog Chem Org Nat Prod 103:103–131, 2017 28120232

Mücke M, Phillips T, Radbruch L, et al: Cannabis-based medicines for chronic neuropathic pain in adults. Cochrane Database Syst Rev 3(3):CD012182, 2018 29513392

Mun CJ, Nordeck C, Goodell EMA, et al: Real-time monitoring of cannabis and prescription opioid co-use patterns, analgesic effectiveness, and the opioid-sparing effect of cannabis in individuals with chronic pain. J Pain 23(11):1799–1810, 2022 35817255

Nabata KJ, Tse EK, Nightingale TE, et al: The therapeutic potential and usage patterns of cannabinoids in people with spinal cord injuries: a systematic review. Curr Neuropharmacol 19(3):402–432, 2021 32310048

National Academies of Sciences, Engineering, and Medicine: The Health Effects of Cannabis and Cannabinoids: The Current State of Evidence and Recommendations for Research. Washington, DC, National Academies Press, 2017

Nielsen S, Sabioni P, Trigo JM, et al: Opioid-sparing effects of cannabinoids: a systematic review and meta-analysis. Neuropsychopharmacology 42(9):1752–1765, 2017 28327548

Nitecka-Buchta A, Nowak-Wachol A, Wachol K, et al: Myorelaxant effect of transdermal cannabidiol application in patients with TMD: a randomized, double-blind trial. J Clin Med 8(11):1886, 2019 31698733

Okusanya BO, Lott BE, Ehiri J, et al: Medical cannabis for the treatment of migraine in adults: a review of the evidence. Front Neurol 13:871187, 2022 35711271

Osborne NR, Davis KD: Sex and gender differences in pain. Int Rev Neurobiol 164:277–307, 2022 36038207

Pacher P, Bátkai S, Kunos G: The endocannabinoid system as an emerging target of pharmacotherapy. Pharmacol Rev 58(3):389–462, 2006 16968947

Palazzo E, Luongo L, Novellis V, et al: The role of cannabinoid receptors in the descending modulation of pain. Pharmaceuticals (Basel) 3(8):2661–2673, 2010 27713370

Palrasu M, Wright L, Patel M, et al: Perspectives on challenges in cannabis drug delivery systems: where are we? Med Cannabis Cannabinoids 5(1):102–119, 2022 36467783

Paulsingh CN, Mohamed MB, Elhaj MS, et al: The efficacy of marijuana use for pain relief in adults with sickle cell disease: a systematic review. Cureus 14(5):e24962, 2022 35706744

Pereira A, Chappell A, Dethy J, et al: A proof-of-concept (POC) study including experimental pain models (EPM) to assess the effects of a CB2 agonist (LY2828360) in the treatment of patients with osteoarthritic (OA) knee pain. Clin Pharmacol Ther 93:S56–S57, 2013

Pergolizzi JV Jr, Lequang JA, Taylor R Jr, et al: The role of cannabinoids in pain control: the good, the bad, and the ugly. Minerva Anestesiol 84(8):955–969, 2018 29338150

Pertwee RG: The diverse CB1 and CB2 receptor pharmacology of three plant cannabinoids: delta9-tetrahydrocannabinol, cannabidiol and delta9-tetrahydrocannabivarin. Br J Pharmacol 153(2):199–215, 2008 17828291

Petrilli K, Ofori S, Hines L, et al: Association of cannabis potency with mental ill health and addiction: a systematic review. Lancet Psychiatry 9(9):736–750, 2022 35901795

Petrosky E, Harpaz R, Fowler KA, et al: Chronic pain among suicide decedents, 2003 to 2014: findings from the National Violent Death Reporting System. Ann Intern Med 169(7):448–455, 2018 30208405

Pillarisetti S, Alexander CW, Khanna I: Pain and beyond: fatty acid amides and fatty acid amide hydrolase inhibitors in cardiovascular and metabolic diseases. Drug Discov Today 14(23–24):1098–1111, 2009 19716430

Pini LA, Guerzoni S, Cainazzo MM, et al: Nabilone for the treatment of medication overuse headache: results of a preliminary double-blind, active-controlled, randomized trial. J Headache Pain 13(8):677–684, 2012 23070400

Poudel S, Quinonez J, Choudhari J, et al: Medical cannabis, headaches, and migraines: a review of the current literature. Cureus 13(8):e17407, 2021 34589318

Price RL, Charlot KV, Frieler S, et al: The efficacy of cannabis in reducing back pain: a systematic review. Global Spine J 12(2):343–352, 2022 35128969

Radwan MM, Chandra S, Gul S, et al: Cannabinoids, phenolics, terpenes and alkaloids. Molecules 26(9):2774, 2021 34066753

Reddy TS, Zomer R, Mantri N: Nanoformulations as a strategy to overcome the delivery limitations of cannabinoids. Phytother Res 37(4):1526–1538, 2023 36748949

Rice ASC, Smith BH, Blyth FM: Pain and the global burden of disease. Pain 157(4):791–796, 2016 26670465

Rock EM, Parker LA: Constituents of Cannabis sativa. Adv Exp Med Biol 1264:1–13, 2021 33332000

Rodriguez CEB, Ouyang L, Kandasamy R: Antinociceptive effects of minor cannabinoids, terpenes and flavonoids in cannabis. Behav Pharmacol 33(2–3):130–157, 2022 33709984

Russo EB: Taming THC: potential cannabis synergy and phytocannabinoid-terpenoid entourage effects. Br J Pharmacol 163(7):1344–1364, 2011 21749363

Sainsbury B, Bloxham J, Pour MH, et al: Efficacy of cannabis-based medications compared to placebo for the treatment of chronic neuropathic pain: a systematic review with meta-analysis. J Dent Anesth Pain Med 21(6):479–506, 2021 34909469

Shehata I, Hashim A, Elsaeidy A, et al: Cannabinoids and their role in chronic pain treatment: concepts and a comprehensive review. Health Psychol Res 10(4):35848, 2022 36628124

Sherpa ML, Shrestha N, Ojinna BT, et al: Efficacy and safety of medical marijuana in migraine headache: a systematic review. Cureus 14(12):e32622, 2022 36660507

Sideli L, Quigley H, La Cascia C, et al: Cannabis use and the risk for psychosis and affective disorders. J Dual Diagn 16(1):22–42, 2020 31647377

Slivicki RA, Xu Z, Kulkarni PM, et al: Positive allosteric modulation of CB1 suppresses pathological pain without producing tolerance or dependence. Biol Psychiatry 84(10):722–733, 2017 28823711

Soliman N, Haroutounian S, Hohmann AG, et al: Systematic review and meta-analysis of cannabinoids, cannabis-based medicines, and endocannabinoid system modulators tested for antinociceptive effects in animal models of injury-related or pathological persistent pain. Pain 162(Suppl 1):S26–S44, 2021 33729209

Stella B, Baratta F, Della Pepa C, et al: Cannabinoid formulations and delivery systems: current and future options to treat pain. Drugs 81(13):1513–1557, 2021 34480749

Stockings E, Campbell G, Hall WD, et al: Cannabis and cannabinoids for the treatment of people with chronic noncancer pain conditions: a systematic review and meta-analysis of controlled and observational studies. Pain 159(10):1932–1954, 2018 29847469

St Sauver JL, Warner DO, Yawn BP, et al: Why patients visit their doctors: assessing the most prevalent conditions in a defined American population. Mayo Clin Proc 88(1):56–67, 2013 23274019

Tagen M, Klumpers LE: Review of delta-8-tetrahydrocannabinol (Δ8-THC): comparative pharmacology with Δ9-THC. Br J Pharmacol 179(15):3915–3933, 2022 35523678

Tsagareli M, Kvachadze I, Simone D: Antinociceptive tolerance to cannabinoids in adult male mice: a pilot study. Georgian Med News 320(320):148–153, 2021 34897062

Tsai SHL, Lin C-R, Shao S-C, et al: Cannabinoid use for pain reduction in spinal cord injuries: a meta-analysis of randomized controlled trials. Front Pharmacol 13:866235, 2022 35571093

Turk DC, Rudy TE: Towards a comprehensive assessment of chronic pain patients. Behav Res Ther 25(4):237–249, 1987 3662986

U.S. Pain Foundation: The financial and emotional cost of chronic pain. West Hartford, CT, U.S. Pain Foundation, 2021. Available at: https://uspainfoundation.org/news/the-financial-and-emotional-cost-of-chronic-pain. Accessed April 22, 2023.

Vigli D, Cosentino L, Pellas M, et al: Chronic treatment with cannabidiolic acid (CBDA) reduces thermal pain sensitivity in male mice and rescues the hyperalgesia in a mouse model of Rett syndrome. Neuroscience 453:113–123, 2021 33010341

Votrubec C, Tran P, Lei A, et al: Cannabinoid therapeutics in orofacial pain management: a systematic review. Aust Dent J 67(4):314–327, 2022 36082517

Vučković S, Srebro D, Vujović KS, et al: Cannabinoids and pain: new insights from old molecules. Front Pharmacol 9:1259, 2018 30542280

Walitt B, Klose P, Fitzcharles MA, et al: Cannabinoids for fibromyalgia. Cochrane Database Syst Rev 7(7):CD011694, 2016 27428009

Wang L, Hong PJ, May C, et al: Medical cannabis or cannabinoids for chronic non-cancer and cancer related pain: a systematic review and meta-analysis of randomised clinical trials. BMJ 374(1034):n1034, 2021 34497047

Wen Y, Wang Z, Zhang R, et al: The antinociceptive activity and mechanism of action of cannabigerol. Biomed Pharmacother 158:114163, 2023 36916438

Wilsey B, Deutsch R, Marcotte TD: Maintenance of blinding in clinical trials and the implications for studying analgesia using cannabinoids. Cannabis Cannabinoid Res 1(1):139-148, 2016 28861490

Wirth PW, Watson ES, ElSohly M, et al: Anti-inflammatory properties of cannabichromene. Life Sci 26(23):1991–1995, 1980 7401911

Wong SSC, Chan WS, Cheung CW: Analgesic effects of cannabinoids for chronic non-cancer pain: a systematic review and meta-analysis with meta-regression. J Neuroimmune Pharmacol 15(4):801–829, 2020 32172501

Woodhams SG, Chapman V, Finn DP, et al: The cannabinoid system and pain. Neuropharmacology 124:105–120, 2017 28625720

Yayan J, Rasche K: Damaging effects of cannabis use on the lungs. Adv Exp Med Biol 952:31–34, 2016 27573646

Zhu YF, Linher-Melville K, Niazmand MJ, et al: An evaluation of the anti-hyperalgesic effects of cannabidiolic acid-methyl ester in a preclinical model of peripheral neuropathic pain. Br J Pharmacol 177(12):2712–2725, 2020 31981216

Zagzoog A, Mohamed KA, Kim HJJ, et al: In vitro and in vivo pharmacological activity of minor cannabinoids isolated from Cannabis sativa. Sci Rep 10(1):20405, 2020 33230154

Zubcevic K, Petersen M, Bach FW, et al: Oral capsules of tetra-hydro-cannabinol (THC), cannabidiol (CBD) and their combination in peripheral neuropathic pain treatment. Eur J Pain 27(4):492–506, 2023 36571471

14

Special Issues in Adult Use

Tabitha E.H. Moses, M.S.

In this chapter, I focus on special issues in cannabis use that are not discussed elsewhere in this publication. Specifically, I focus on existing evidence for potential therapeutic uses of cannabis alongside potential misuse and harms of cannabis among adult populations, with an emphasis on cannabis-specific effects such as cannabis hyperemesis syndrome (CHS) and the effects of chronic cannabis use on responses to standard medical interventions, such as anesthesia and medication management. The potential psychoactive effects of cannabis and related compounds play a major role in their use, both recreationally and medically; however, the effects of cannabis are wide-ranging and not specific to one cognitive or physiological domain.

I begin by providing an overview of the current state of the evidence as it pertains to the therapeutic uses of cannabis, cannabis-specific disorders (e.g., CHS and cannabis withdrawal syndrome [CWS]), and the effects of cannabis use on medical management (e.g., anesthesia and medication pharmacokinetics). This is followed by a discussion of the relevant deleterious and therapeutic effects of cannabis and the mechanisms and frequency of these effects. Finally, I provide an overview of the clinical relevance of these special issues in cannabis use and any existing clinical recommendations.

Current State of Evidence

The potential therapeutic uses of cannabis underscore much of the drive and advocacy efforts toward legalizing it for medical use. Unfortunately, this advocacy has been associated with significant bias in both the conducting of scientific research and the reporting of those results; a 2015 review of randomized controlled trials (RCTs) of cannabis use in treating a range of medical conditions found that only 4 of the 79 evaluated trials were considered to have a low risk of bias (Whiting et al. 2015). This bias is further compounded by reporting in the local and national media, with more than 75% of news stories about medical cannabis providing misleading information about the results of reported studies, most of which appear to exaggerate its potential positive effects (Montané et al. 2005). The causes of this misinformation are multifaceted and often not the result of intentional malfeasance on the part of the researchers or physicians; nonetheless, significant harm can result from medical misinformation, particularly when it concerns the use of a substance with potentially harmful effects (Ishida et al. 2020; Wen et al. 2019). Despite the increasingly frequent references to cannabis as medicine, it is important to recognize that it is not the cannabis plant as a whole that specifically contributes to potential therapeutic effects but rather one or more of the more than 500 compounds within the *Cannabis* plant (Piomelli and Russo 2016). Cannabinoids are the most well-known active components, and more than 100 types of cannabinoids have been identified within cannabis (Pertwee 2014; Piomelli 2003; Shahbazi et al. 2020). The two most well-known cannabinoids are Δ^9-tetrahydrocannabinol (Δ^9-THC) and cannabidiol (CBD). The overall potency of any strain of cannabis is generally determined by the ratio of THC to CBD (Cash et al. 2020; Perisetti et al. 2020).

When researchers evaluate potential therapeutic uses and harms of cannabis and its related compounds, it is important that they are aware of the various absorption and distribution rates of these compounds, particularly because these rates may differ depending on the route of administration and the chronicity of use. Cannabis is most commonly consumed via either inhalation (e.g., smoking or vaping) or oral ingestion, and the bioavailability and absorption of cannabinoids vary considerably between these routes. Inhalation of cannabis typically results in the rapid onset of effects and peak plasma concentrations of THC within about 10 minutes of use. In contrast, oral ingestion typically results in delayed onset of effects, and peak THC plasma concentrations occur 1–5 hours after consumption (Huestis 2007). There is considerable interindividual variability in peak THC concentration, even in rigorously controlled experiments. In smoking studies, this variability appears to occur in part because of the length of inhalation and hold time; however, this variation still occurred in studies that controlled for these factors, so it is believed that the peak concentration differences may occur due to differences in the depth of inhalation (Chiang and Hawks 1990). This variation in peak concentration and onset time is an important factor to consider when evaluating seemingly contradictory evidence surrounding the potential effects of cannabis. Prior usage of cannabis may also affect physiological levels after use. Cannabinoids are highly lipophilic molecules that conjugate with fatty acids to be stored within fatty tissues, and they can remain stored in fatty tissues for many days or even weeks after cessation of use (Karschner et al. 2009; Kreuz and Axelrod 1973; Wong et al. 2013).

The cannabinoids found within cannabis primarily stimulate cannabinoid 1 (CB_1) and cannabinoid 2 (CB_2) receptors, which are part of the body's endocannabinoid system. These are G protein–coupled receptors, which normally respond to endogenous endocannabinoids and are involved in the regulation of a range of physiological processes, such as pain perception, appetite, memory, motor function, and bone health (Huestis 2007; Idris and Ralston 2012; Shahbazi et al. 2020). CB_1 receptors are predominantly found throughout the brain and CNS and play a key role in appetite, cognition, and motivation (Di Marzo et al. 2015). In contrast, although some CB_2 receptors are found in the brain, they are predominantly found in peripheral areas, where they play a key role in modulating responses related to pain and inflammation (Bie et al. 2018). Although CB_1 and CB_2 are the primary receptors that respond to them, cannabinoids can influence a range of receptors throughout the body (Perisetti et al. 2020), and the various compounds within cannabis plants also appear to have distinct and often divergent effects on these receptors. For example, THC is a CB_1 and CB_2 receptor agonist, whereas CBD may be a CB_1 and CB_2 receptor antagonist (Alexander and Joshi 2019). These divergent effects of cannabinoid compounds demonstrate another explanation for why researchers and clinicians might find seemingly contradictory results when examining the potential physiological effects of cannabis compounds.

Because the endogenous endocannabinoid system is integral in emesis, satiety, and inflammation, it makes sense that cannabis would also affect these systems, and certain potential therapeutic uses of cannabis have been theorized based on an understanding of the endogenous endocannabinoid system. Regarding therapeutic uses of cannabis, research most commonly focuses on a subset of compounds found in the cannabis plant. A wide range of RCTs, reviews, and meta-analyses have explored the varied potential therapeutic benefits of cannabis, and the results are generally not as promising as many believe. Some of the areas in which cannabinoids have been investigated for use include pain management, sleep disorders, spasticity, chemotherapy-induced nausea and vomiting (CINV), HIV-related weight loss, seizures, glaucoma, mood disorders, anxiety disorders, and psychosis (Allan et al. 2018; Colizzi and Bhattacharyya 2020; Gray et al. 2016; Sulak et al. 2017; Whiting et al. 2015). Results of these studies have varied, and although many individuals espouse the potential for cannabis to treat or even cure a range of disorders, the current evidence does not support the miracle-like properties of this substance. That is not to say that cannabis derivatives do not have potential therapeutic uses; there are indeed clear areas wherein the research does support a therapeutic role for cannabis. Additional therapeutic uses of cannabis are discussed later in this chapter.

Although the potential therapeutic uses of cannabis served to drive the legalization of cannabis for medical use, it was the supposed lack of potential harms that helped lay a foundation for the legalization of cannabis for recreational use. Other substances used recreationally (e.g., alcohol, cocaine) have more frequent and often more serious physiological and psychological harms than cannabis, but that does not mean cannabis does not have its own share of potentially harmful effects on those who use it. Previous chapters have focused on the psychological effects of cannabis and its effects in special populations (e.g., children, adolescents, and individuals who are pregnant), so here I focus primarily on the potential physiological benefits and harms of cannabis in healthy adult populations and on two cannabis-specific syndromes: CHS and CWS.

Deleterious Effects

Cannabis-Specific Syndromes

One often-overlooked consideration of the therapeutic uses of cannabis is that it is still a substance with whole-body impacts that can cause various side effects ranging from merely unpleasant to dangerous. Common side effects of cannabis use include dry mouth, nausea and vomiting, dizziness, loss of balance, fatigue and somnolence, and even hallucinations (Ashton 1999; Pratt et al. 2019; Wang et al. 2008). Although the use of any substance can lead to potential side effects, one reason the effects of cannabis may be more harmful than expected is due to the way cannabis is viewed by individuals who use it. To many users, cannabis is considered a "safe" and "natural" substance and a better alternative to the pharmaceuticals physicians usually prescribe (Piper et al. 2017; Townsend et al. 2022; Wen et al. 2019), a mindset that often lulls them into a false sense of security, leaving them unprepared for any adverse effects. The potential side effects of cannabis use are not pleasant, but they are usually transient and not more serious than those of many commonly used medications. If these were the only risks, perhaps there would not be much need for concern; however, increasing evidence shows harmful physiological effects associated with long-term or chronic cannabis use (Murray et al. 2017; Pratt et al. 2019; Wang et al. 2008).

Cannabis Hyperemesis Syndrome

CHS is a potential consequence of chronic cannabis use that was first identified in 2004 (Allen et al. 2004) and has been seen with increasing frequency in recent years. It is believed to be a variant of cyclic vomiting syndrome, and its symptoms overlap with various other conditions, including psychogenic vomiting, gastroenteritis, dyspepsia, and bulimia nervosa (Richards et al. 2018). The symptoms of CHS are often vague but usually consist of cyclical nausea, vomiting, and abdominal pain, and the syndrome is characterized by chronic cannabis use, severe cyclical nausea and vomiting, and reports of frequent hot bathing to relieve symptoms (Howard 2019). Symptoms typically develop over three stages. The prodromal phase occurs first and includes early symptoms such as morning nausea and abdominal discomfort. Next, the hyperemetic phase occurs, during which individuals experience severe nausea, vomiting, and abdominal pain. Finally, during the recovery phase, individuals typically experience relief from their symptoms; however, this relief is only temporary if they resume cannabis use.

Diagnosis of CHS usually occurs after the exclusion of other potential causes of vomiting, alongside self-report and toxicology results that indicate chronic cannabis use (Stanghellini et al. 2016). It should be noted that CHS does not only occur in people using cannabis recreationally. At least one case report described a patient who developed CHS after using cannabinoids as an antiemetic for chemotherapy-induced nausea and vomiting (Portman and Donovan 2018). Even though there are no specific laboratory, radiological, or endoscopic findings of CHS and no known physiological cause for the vomiting as of yet, physiological examination often identifies nonspecific electrolyte disturbances, highlighting a key concern in CHS (Dezieck et al. 2017; Perisetti et al. 2020). Vomiting with CHS can be so severe that it leads to dehydration, electrolyte imbalances, and kidney damage. Although unpleasant and potentially debilitating, CHS is not typically considered fatal; nonetheless, serious morbidity and even mortality reports have been directly attributed to it. Specifically, acute renal failure resulting from severe dehydration due to CHS is a real possibility (Habboushe and Sedor 2014), and as of 2023 at least three deaths in the United States had been attributed to CHS, with potential additional deaths overseas (Bouquet et al. 2023; Lathrop et al. 2023; Nourbakhsh et al. 2019; von Both and Santos 2021).

The precise cause of CHS is still unknown. Two popular theories focus on the main psychoactive component in cannabis: THC. The first hypothesis is that because THC sequesters in fat with slow rediffusion into serum plasma, individuals who use cannabis regularly may have a significant buildup of THC in their body that may lead to toxicity in predisposed individuals (Huestis 2007). The second hypothesis suggests that THC directly stimulates enteric nervous system cannabinoid receptors, which causes a reduction in gastric motility, leading to a proemetic state. Although at first glance this theory appears to contradict the use of cannabis as an antiemetic in chemotherapy, research in animals suggests a biphasic emetic/antiemetic response to THC, such that it has antiemetic properties at low doses and proemetic properties at high doses (Ruffle et al. 2015). This potential biphasic effect is further supported by the fact that slow rediffusion of lipophilic THC may result in higher plasma THC concentration in people who have been using cannabis regularly for a long period of time. The apparently contradictory emetic effects of cannabis can be explained by the varying locations of CB_1 and CB_2 receptors within the body. It is believed that the antiemetic properties of cannabis occur because of CB_1 receptors within the hypothalamus, whereas the proemetic properties seen in CHS are likely related to the CB_1 receptors found in the gastrointestinal system (Parvataneni et al. 2019). Understanding the various potential mechanisms for CHS may provide insight into why only some people develop symptoms and may provide a foundation for identifying which treatments might be most effective.

Cannabis Withdrawal Syndrome

CWS is also a relatively new diagnosis that has only recently been acknowledged as a problem associated with chronic cannabis use. DSM-5 (American Psychiatric Association 2022) describes symptoms associated with cannabis withdrawal, requiring three or more of the following to meet diagnostic criteria: irritability, anger or aggression, nervousness or anxiety, sleep difficulty, decreased appetite or weight loss, restlessness, and depressed mood. Additionally, at least one of the following physical symptoms must be present: abdominal pain, shakiness/tremors, sweating, fever, chills, or headache.

No predefined amount or frequency of cannabis use automatically results in CWS, which has made its recognition more difficult. Some individuals can use cannabis daily for years and not develop withdrawal symptoms, whereas others may use cannabis daily for only a couple of months before developing symptoms (Livne et al. 2019). This is further complicated by evidence suggesting that people using other substances regularly (e.g., opioids) appear to be spared symptoms of CWS, even after years of daily cannabis use. One potential reason for differing withdrawal outcomes may be associated with the frequency and type of cannabis compounds used. The exact clinical features of CWS appear to vary depending on the type of cannabinoid compounds and whether synthetic cannabinoids were used (Echeverria-Villalobos et al. 2019). Synthetic cannabinoids (e.g., Spice, K2) bind to the same receptors as natural cannabinoids, which can cause many of the same effects (Mills et al. 2015). Although CWS is not considered life-threatening, evidence suggests that those who primarily use synthetic cannabinoids may experience more severe symptoms, including seizures (Sampson et al. 2015).

Effects of Cannabis Use on Medical Management

In addition to clear side effects and syndromes directly associated with cannabis use, there are other necessary special considerations in medical settings, specifically regarding the use of anesthesia and other medications. Some evidence suggests that cannabis use, particularly chronic use, can impact an individual's response to anesthetics, and it seems that individuals with a history of regular cannabis use may present with altered physiology leading to increased risks of cardiovascular and respiratory complications during and after surgery (Copeland-Halperin et al. 2021; Heath et al. 2022; Lynn and Galinkin 2020). The highly lipophilic nature of cannabinoids results in their significant redistribution and accumulation, so they may remain in the body for days after the last consumption. Although the plasma half-life is usually 20–30 hours because of fat accumulation, the tissue half-life can be as long as 30 days in someone who uses cannabis regularly (Alexander and Joshi 2019). This prolonged presence and these potential physiological effects present a serious problem when managing anesthesia (Amornyotin 2022).

Evidence shows the effects of both acute and chronic cannabis use on response to anesthesia. Acute cannabis intoxication prior to surgery can contribute to more volatile and violent responses to anesthesia. Additionally, cannabis-induced psychosis can include fever, tachycardia, and hypertension, which can be mistaken for conditions such as malignant hyperthermia, serotonin syndrome, and neuroleptic malignant syndrome in the setting of general anesthesia (Alexander and Joshi 2019). Because of the potential effects of cannabis on the cardiovascular system, patients with additional risk factors may be at an increased risk of myocardial infarction during the first hour after last cannabis use (Abramovici et al. 2018; Aronow and Cassidy 1974). As a result of this increased risk, it may be prudent to delay anesthesia induction until this risk period has passed (Friedman et al. 1977; Mittleman et al. 2001). Although it is possible that these acute effects are blunted in people who use cannabis daily, chronic effects on the cardiovascular system are associated with increased heart rate and cardiac output, along with a possible increased risk of vasospasm and atherosclerosis, which can result in similar adverse responses (Brownlow and Sutherland 2002; Lee et al. 2024). Inhaled cannabis can also lead to bronchodilation and airway hyperreactivity like that seen in cigarette smoking. Some have theorized that cannabis may actually be more irritating to airways because it is often burned at higher temperatures than tobacco products, and there have been cases of uvular edema and diffuse alveolar hemorrhage following general anesthesia in patients with a recent cannabis smoking history (Alexander and Joshi 2019; Bucchino et al. 2019; Hernandez et al. 2005; Murray et al. 2014). Chapter 12, "Cannabis Impacts on the Cardiac and Respiratory Systems," presents a more detailed overview of the effects of cannabis on the cardiovascular and respiratory systems.

To date, most research examining the effects of acute or chronic cannabis administration on doses and effects of general anesthesia comes from animal models. These animal models have provided mixed evidence on the effects of cannabis on dose and length of anesthetic effects, but the general consensus is that cannabinoids may antagonize the effects of sedative hypnotics (Chesher et al. 1974; Paton and Temple 1972). This consensus aligns with data suggesting that chronic cannabis use and cannabis tolerance are associated with cross-tolerance to barbiturates, opioids, benzodiazepines, and phenothiazines (Ashton 1999; Garzón et al. 2009; Kumar et al. 2001). Studies in humans have been more limited, but existing evidence suggests that individuals who use cannabis regularly might have more variable needs for anesthesia, require higher doses, and be at increased risk of adverse responses (e.g., laryngospasm) (Alexander and Joshi 2019; Flisberg et al. 2009; Imasogie et al. 2021). However, some studies and reviews have also found limited or no effects of cannabis use on response to anesthesia (King et al. 2021). More research is needed into these potential effects.

The anesthetist's concerns do not end when the operation has concluded. Various potential postoperative complications should be considered in a patient with a recent history of cannabis use. One issue that has already been mentioned is the potential for cross-tolerance with postoperative pain medications (Ashton 1999; Garzón et al. 2009; Kumar et al. 2001). This cross-tolerance means that pain control in patients with a history of regular cannabis use should be closely monitored to ensure that medication dosages are adequate. Despite the potential for cannabis to be used to help manage pain, data suggest that, postoperatively, patients with a history of recent cannabis use report higher pain scores and greater analgesic use than those with no recent cannabis use (Alexander and Joshi 2019). CWS is also a concern for the hospitalized postoperative patient who had been using cannabis daily prior to admission. Withdrawal symptoms are most likely to appear in the postoperative period, and patients may require supportive care to help manage symptoms. Additionally, there are postoperative concerns related to healing across a variety of domains. For example, some evidence suggests that orthopedic medicine patients who endorse chronic cannabis use demonstrate delayed bone healing and are at increased risk of fractures, due in part to their having lower bone mineral density (Heath et al. 2022; Sophocleous et al. 2017). The data are mixed regarding the effects of cannabis on postsurgical wound healing itself (Copeland-Halperin et al. 2021). Cannabis use clearly modulates various aspects of the endocrine system and inflammatory response;

however, the research thus far does not provide clear answers for how cannabis use might impact postsurgical wound healing and whether the type of use (e.g., chronic, regular use vs. intermittent use) might modify these effects (Copeland-Halperin et al. 2021; Hillard 2015; Lee et al. 2024; Meah et al. 2022).

A related but distinct physiological effect of cannabis is its impact on the pharmacokinetics of various medications due to its ability to modulate enzymes involved in drug metabolism. The cannabinoids themselves are primarily metabolized by the cytochrome P450 (CYP) family of enzymes in the liver; the specific enzymes involved depend on the precise cannabinoid (Tapley and Kellett 2019). This means that any medications that affect CYP enzyme metabolism may modulate plasma concentrations of cannabinoids as well as the length of time they remain physiologically active. In addition, some cannabinoids themselves modulate the effects of certain CYP enzymes, which may, in turn, impact the concentrations of medications metabolized by those enzymes. One of the most notable examples is that CBD inhibits CYP3A4, which is an important enzyme in the metabolism of a wide range of medications (Lee et al. 2024). This inhibition can result in unexpectedly high or low levels of certain medications, which could be life-threatening. For example, warfarin, which is metabolized by CYP3A4, may be given to patients in the hospital setting, and evidence from case reports suggests that those using cannabis regularly may demonstrate higher than expected levels of warfarin and significant bleeding complications (Echeverria-Villalobos et al. 2019; Tapley and Kellett 2019). It is also important to be aware that heavy cannabis use can result in prolonged physiological levels of cannabis, which means that even after cessation of use, these effects may continue for longer than one might expect.

Beneficial Effects

Although the therapeutic effects of cannabis are considered controversial and are complicated by the fact that cannabis itself is composed of hundreds of different compounds with a wide range of physiological effects, there are some areas in which the evidence appears to support a therapeutic role for cannabinoids. These potential therapeutic effects have been reviewed by various national and governmental organizations to provide recommendations regarding the strongest evidence for the use of cannabis. In 2017, the Committee on the Health Effects of Marijuana of the National Academies of Sciences, Engineering, and Medicine published an important report providing an overview of the existing evidence surrounding cannabis use and potential therapeutic effects. The report summarized conclusive or substantial evidence to support therapeutic uses of cannabis for chronic pain, CINV, and muscle spasticity symptoms related to multiple sclerosis. Moderate evidence of the use of cannabis in the short-term treatment of certain sleep disturbances was also found. One of the most well-known uses of cannabis is to manage chronic pain, which is also the primary reason patients visit medical cannabis dispensaries in the United States; however, the evidence for this indication is still mixed (see Chapter 13, "Mechanisms, Efficacy, and Safety of Cannabinoids for Treating Chronic Pain"), and the efficacy of cannabis in pain management may depend on the context of the pain and the overall potency of the cannabis being consumed (Cash et al. 2020).

One of the first major therapeutic uses of cannabis was in the control of severe nausea, vomiting, and resultant appetite loss associated with chemotherapy (Smith et al. 2015). Multiple reviews and meta-analyses appear to support this use, suggesting that cannabinoids are more effective than placebo and may also be more effective than many existing antiemetics (Allan et al. 2018; Whiting et al. 2015). However, the existing reviews do not compare cannabinoids with steroids or serotonin antagonists, and there are still contradictory conclusions. Some reviews still state that the quality of evidence for this use is low (Smith et al. 2015; Whiting et al. 2015), whereas others state that there is substantial evidence for the utility of cannabinoids in this area (Abrams et al. 2011; Tapley and Kellett 2019).

The use of cannabinoids in the treatment of epilepsy is perhaps the most controversial because it is one of the only existing indications that appears to focus on pediatric patients (Sulak et al. 2017; Tapley and Kellett 2019). The FDA approved an oral CBD solution for the treatment of Lennox-Gastaut syndrome and Dravet syndrome in children older than 2 years. These rare forms of epilepsy previously had few effective treatments, and the ongoing seizures dramatically affect the children's quality of life. Thus far, the evidence is relatively strong, suggesting that CBD is effective for treating epilepsy in this specific pediatric population (Devinsky et al. 2016, 2018; Thiele et al. 2018), although the evidence for efficacy in other forms of epilepsy or in adult epilepsy is very limited (Abrams 2018; Koppel et al. 2014; Tapley and Kellett 2019).

Spasticity is not specific to multiple sclerosis and involves an abnormal increase in muscle tone, resulting in impaired movement and associated discomfort and pain (Otero-Romero et al. 2016). The general cause of spasticity is associated with damage to nerves within the CNS that control muscle movement. In multiple sclerosis, spasticity occurs due to disease-specific damage to the white matter tracts of those nerves. Typically, this damage cannot be reversed, but some medications may help alleviate the related symptoms. Spasticity in multiple sclerosis is progressive and often disabling, and it is not often alleviated by the medications used for other etiologies (Beard et al. 2003; Otero-Romero et al. 2016). However, several cannabinoid-based medications demonstrate efficacy in treating multiple sclerosis–associated spasticity and pain (Nielsen et al. 2018; Otero-Romero et al. 2016; Rice and Cameron 2018).

Finally, some evidence suggests that cannabinoids may be beneficial in the short-term treatment of certain sleep impairments. Nonetheless, it is important to be particularly cautious of this usage because cannabis use itself may impair sleep (Graupensperger et al. 2021; Winiger et al. 2021). The endogenous endocannabinoid system plays a role in sleep and circadian rhythms (Mondino et al. 2021; Sanford et al. 2008; Vaughn et al. 2010), and research suggests that cannabis and cannabinoid-based medications have varying effects depending on the type of sleep being measured and the potency of the products used (Babson et al. 2017; Mondino et al. 2021; Nicholson et al. 2004). Data thus far suggest that certain cannabinoids may play a role in improving sleep outcomes when used short-term for specific concerns such as insomnia, sleep impairment due to other symptoms (e.g., pain), and sleep apnea (Babson et al. 2017; Choi et al. 2020). Nonetheless, at this time, data are limited. Carefully controlled research is needed to examine which cannabinoids may be best for improving sleep outcomes and to ensure the substance is affecting sleep and not merely treating a separate symptom that causes sleep disturbances (e.g., pain).

Clinical Significance and Recommendations

Therapeutic Uses of Cannabis

Currently, the evidence for the therapeutic uses of cannabis is mixed and even conflicting in some areas. The most consistent results suggest that cannabinoids may be effective in treating specific types of pain, CINV, seizures associated with Lennox-Gastaut syndrome and Dravet syndrome in pediatric patients, spasticity associated with multiple sclerosis, and short-term relief of certain types of sleep disturbances (National Academies of Sciences, Engineering, and Medicine 2017; Tapley and Kellett 2019; Tramèr et al. 2001). In almost all cases, cannabis products should not be the first-line treatment for management of these disorders or symptoms, but they can be considered in appropriate circumstances. Given the increasing popularity of cannabis products and the increasing number of anecdotal reports regarding the therapeutic abilities of cannabis, it is probable that additional therapeutic benefits will be identified in the future, so clinicians should remain carefully informed of the literature in this area.

Although the potential therapeutic benefits of cannabis can be alluring, it is imperative to avoid overreliance on the results of case reports or anecdotal experiences. As with any substance used for treatment, carefully controlled studies are necessary prior to making assertions about any benefits of cannabis. To date, despite popular media attention and some positive individual reports, there is not yet sufficient evidence to support claims that cannabis may be an effective treatment for any form of cancer, gastrointestinal disorders (e.g., irritable bowel syndrome), glaucoma, or neurological disorders such as Huntington's disease, Parkinson's disease, dementia, or amyotrophic lateral sclerosis (National Academies of Sciences, Engineering, and Medicine 2017). As such, it is vital that the limited therapeutic uses of cannabis not stray into therapeutic misuse through the recommendation of cannabis for disorders for which evidence does not yet support its value (Felberbaum 2019; Macedo et al. 2022).

Despite some existing evidence for the potential therapeutic benefits of cannabis, one consistent concern is the lack of standardization of cannabis compounds and treatment regimens. The wide range of psychoactive compounds found in cannabis and the various potential effects that depend on varying concentrations of each compound create significant difficulties for researchers and health care professionals attempting to explore the benefits and harms of acute or chronic cannabis use (Cash et al. 2020). Furthermore, the most common method of cannabis consumption, inhalation via smoking or vaping, is associated with its own set of harms, and any physician focused on minimizing patient harm should avoid recommending treatments wherein the harms may outweigh the potential benefits. The harms specifically associated with inhaled cannabis administration can be mitigated via oral cannabis consumption or the use of specially formulated medical compounds that contain a known concentration of specific cannabinoids and can be carefully dosed and safely ingested.

Cannabis-Specific Syndromes

Cannabis Hyperemesis Syndrome

CHS is one of the most well-discussed physiological harms of cannabis use, and as such, distinct diagnostic criteria have been established and refined. The major and minor diagnostic criteria for CHS were proposed in 2012, and these were further refined in 2016 when it was categorized as a functional gastrointestinal disorder (Simonetto et al. 2012; Stanghellini et al. 2016). Despite a significant number of case reports and articles on the phenomenon of CHS, there is limited evidence for effective treatments beyond cessation of cannabis use. However, it should also be noted that some individuals will still argue that their cannabis use is not responsible for their symptoms, and they will not believe that cessation of cannabis use will relieve their symptoms (Collins et al. 2023). Immediate care of CHS is primarily supportive, focusing on providing intravenous fluids to treat volume depletion and monitoring electrolyte levels (Ruffle et al. 2015; Senderovich et al. 2022). Traditional antiemetic medications, those that focus on either gastrointestinal motility or the chemoreceptor trigger zone, appear to have no effect on CHS symptoms (Wallace et al. 2007). A few case studies have suggested that haloperidol may help manage nausea and vomiting symptoms, but more research is needed prior to confirming its efficacy (Inayat et al. 2017; Witsil and Mycyk 2017). Additionally, some studies have suggested that opioid medications may provide some benefit for associated abdominal pain, but their use is limited because opioids also contribute to symptoms of nausea and vomiting (Ruffle et al. 2015). Other potential treatments for CHS include the β-blocker propranolol, certain benzodiazepines, and the short-acting dopamine antagonist droperidol; however, limited reports are available regarding the efficacy of these medications, and more research is needed (Parvataneni et al. 2019; Perisetti et al. 2020; Senderovich et al. 2022).

One common finding in CHS is that patients obtain significant relief from symptoms by taking hot showers or baths (Perisetti et al. 2020). The mechanism behind the palliative effects of hot baths is not fully understood, but research supports their potential therapeutic value in providing temporary relief from symptoms. Cannabis can disrupt thermoregulation, and it is thought that the hot water causes a redirection of blood from the enteric system to the skin, resulting in a reduction in gastrointestinal symptoms. Additionally, the hot water may lead to the activation of transient receptor potential vanilloid 1 ($TRPV_1$) receptors, reducing levels of substance P, a neuropeptide commonly associated with inflammation and pain (Richards et al. 2018; Senderovich et al. 2022). Topical capsaicin applied to the abdomen also appears to show some efficacy in managing CHS symptoms, and it is believed to work through similar mechanisms as hot baths. Topical capsaicin causes both a redirection of blood flow to the skin and activation of $TRPV_1$ receptors (Dezieck et al. 2017; Richards et al. 2018; Senderovich et al. 2022). The neurokinin 1 (NK_1) receptor antagonist aprepitant shows some potential for treatment (Parvataneni et al. 2019; Senderovich et al. 2022). Aprepitant has been studied with some success in other cyclic vomiting syndromes, as well as CINV (Aapro et al. 2015; Cristofori et al. 2014). Substance P is the endogenous ligand of NK_1 receptors, and given the potential role of substance P in the therapeutic mechanisms of hot baths and topical capsaicin, it makes sense that an NK_1 antagonist may also be effective in treating CHS (Moon et al. 2018).

Cannabis Withdrawal Syndrome

In an acute care setting, it might not always be easy to initially distinguish CHS from CWS, particularly because abdominal pain and appetite changes are associated with both syndromes; nonetheless, a thorough history and physical examination should provide insight into the causative process (Razban et al. 2022). Almost half of individuals who use cannabis regularly or have cannabis use disorder will develop CWS when they initially stop all cannabis use (Bahji et al. 2020). The symptoms themselves can be wide-ranging and severe enough to impair functioning in regular daily activities, and they increase the risk of returning to cannabis use for people who are attempting to abstain (Allsop et al. 2012; Bahji et al. 2020; Livne et al. 2019). Given the increasing use and accessibility of cannabis and the considerable overlap between CWS and certain psychiatric symptoms (e.g., depression and anxiety), it is important that clinicians screen patients with these symptoms for current or previous cannabis use (Livne et al. 2019). Unlike many other substances whose withdrawal symptoms become apparent within a regular time frame shortly after cessation of use (e.g., opioid withdrawal within 2–3 days), the highly lipophilic nature of cannabinoids means that they may remain within the body for weeks after last consumption. This can result in a delayed onset of CWS, with some reports identifying symptom onset more than a month after the last consumption of any cannabis compounds (MacCamy and Hu 2021). Clinicians should be aware of this potential for delayed onset of symptoms in the development of differential diagnoses for a patient with unexplained physical and psychological symptoms alongside a history of heavy, regular cannabis use.

Unfortunately, the therapeutic options for CWS are even more limited than those for CHS. The use of cannabinoid agonists (e.g., THC or CBD) to manage symptoms appears to be well supported by both theory and evidence (Crippa et al. 2013; Razban et al. 2022); however, many who are experiencing CWS may not want to use cannabis-related products. There is also evidence that modulating the endocannabinoid system in other ways may mitigate CWS symptoms. One way in which this can be accomplished is through the inhibition of fatty acid amide hydrolase (FAAH), the enzyme involved in the degradation of the endocannabinoid anandamide; inhibition of this enzyme may reduce withdrawal symptoms in individuals with CWS (D'Souza et al. 2019). Outside of the endocannabinoid system, medications that dampen the responsiveness of the sympathetic nervous system may mitigate symptoms of withdrawal. Dexmedetomidine is a central α_2 agonist that has demonstrated some efficacy in managing symptoms associated with alcohol and opioid withdrawal. It has sedative and anxiolytic properties, which might help with some of the psychiatric symptoms of CWS. Dexmedetomidine has also been used to manage delirium symptoms in cases of severe cannabis intoxication and may show efficacy in managing CWS and withdrawal-associated hallucinations, which appear to occur in a few severe cases (MacCamy and Hu 2021).

All medical interventions for CWS are still under investigation, and evidence is still insufficient to recommend any first-line medication treatments. To date, most of the other therapeutic options for managing CWS have focused on behavioral therapies designed to help patients remain abstinent from cannabis despite their ongoing symptoms (Razban et al. 2022).

Effects of Cannabis Use on Medical Management

The main message surrounding the effects of cannabis use on medical management is the importance of asking patients about their cannabis (and any other substance) use prior to prescribing medications or initiating any other interventions. Whenever possible, if a surgery is elective and recent cannabis use is evident, the surgery should be rescheduled. Patients should be informed of the risks of cannabis use prior to surgery and reminded that information about any illicit substance use shared with health care providers is only collected in the interest of maintaining their health (Alexander and Joshi 2019). Patients should also be told about the potential risks of mixing cannabis with certain medications to elucidate why clinicians may be asking detailed questions about their use. In addition, given the ongoing research regarding the physiological effects of acute and chronic cannabis use, clinicians should ensure that they remain up to date on the literature in this area, particularly as it pertains to their specialty.

In the context of anesthesia, there are three main points of care at which cannabis use should be considered (Echeverria-Villalobos et al. 2019). Preoperative evaluations should always include an assessment of substance use and details about the duration, frequency, and route of administration, particularly because individuals who smoke cannabis may be at higher risk of adverse respiratory events due to airway hyperreactivity. The timing of the last use of cannabis is important due to the potential for an increased risk of myocardial infarction in the first hour following consumption. Understanding previous and current cannabis use will allow the health care team to anticipate any postoperative concerns related to cannabis use, such as withdrawal and increased agitation and anxiety. Intraoperatively, awareness should be maintained regarding the potential for cannabis cross-tolerance with other agents, including anesthetics, resulting in the potential need for higher doses (Echeverria-Villalobos et al. 2019). Careful monitoring for signs of potential subthreshold anesthesia should occur throughout all procedures. Finally, chronic cannabis use may contribute to postoperative cannabis withdrawal symptoms alongside potential cross-tolerance to analgesics and potentially heightened perception of pain and need for pain control (Lee et al. 2024). It is vital that clinicians remain aware of current clinical guidelines from relevant specialty organizations for specific care recommendations during anesthesia (Davidson et al. 2020). This is particularly important in the context of responding to adverse anesthesia events related to cannabis use because the correct responses and treatments are still not fully certain. For example, from the few cases of uvular edema in cannabis-related adverse anesthesia events, dexamethasone appears to be an effective treatment (Mallat et al. 1996); however, the evidence is sparse, so this recommendation may change in the future.

Conclusion

A wide range of topics in the field of therapeutic uses and medical effects of cannabis use has yet to be fully explored within the literature. Although some publications have demonstrated effects of cannabinoids in treating disorders not listed herein, larger meta-analyses and systematic reviews have not yet identified sufficient, high-quality evidence to support their use in those areas. In this chapter, I focused on a few of the most well-known and frequently occurring issues and provided a summary of the existing literature and clinical recommendations. It is likely that cannabinoids may demonstrate additional therapeutic effects in the future, but at this time, there is not sufficient evidence to make those claims in areas other than those discussed.

Both identified cannabis-specific syndromes, CHS and CWS, have clear diagnostic criteria and are seen in urgent care and primary care settings with increasing frequency. Evidence for effective first-line treatments for these syndromes is limited and mostly focuses on supportive care, but there is some clinical guidance for clinicians. In addition to the syndromes directly associated with cannabis use, people who use cannabis have the potential for an increased risk of adverse events in response to routine medical interventions, caused in part by cannabis-related pharmacokinetic alterations.

Despite these risks, cannabis use has some potential therapeutic benefits. At present, there are numerous potential therapeutic indications for cannabis, but only a few have sufficient evidence to support its use, including CINV, certain pain syndromes, spasticity associated with multiple sclerosis, specific pediatric seizure disorders, and short-term treatment of specific sleep issues. Overall, significant unknowns remain surrounding the potential uses and effects of cannabis, but the evidence to date demonstrates both potential benefits and harms and highlights the importance of ensuring both clinicians and patients are educated about the range of effects of cannabis use.

Key Points

- Cannabis hyperemesis syndrome is a potential serious consequence of regular, heavy cannabis use, although its exact precipitant is unclear.

- Cannabis withdrawal syndrome occurs in almost half of those who use cannabis regularly and can significantly impair daily functioning.
- Cannabis may interact negatively with certain prescription medications and anesthesia, altering the dosage required for effective treatment.
- Evidence regarding the therapeutic uses of cannabis is mixed and may be insufficient to make broad conclusions about its efficacy.
- Current evidence-based therapeutic uses of cannabis include the management of pain, spasticity in multiple sclerosis, chemo-therapy-associated nausea and vomiting, pediatric epilepsy, and short-term sleep disturbances.

References

Aapro M, Carides A, Rapoport BL, et al: Aprepitant and fosaprepitant: a 10-year review of efficacy and safety. Oncologist 20(4):450–458, 2015 25795636

Abramovici H, Lamour SA, Mammen G: For Health Care Professionals: Cannabis (Marihuana, Marijuana) and the Cannabinoids. Ottawa, ON, Health Canada, 2018. Available at: https://www.canada.ca/en /health-canada/services/drugs-medication/cannabis/information -medical-practitioners/information-health-care-professionals-cannabis -cannabinoids.html. Accessed March 25, 2023.

Abrams DI: The therapeutic effects of cannabis and cannabinoids: an update from the National Academies of Sciences, Engineering and Medicine report. Eur J Intern Med 49:7–11, 2018 29325791

Abrams DI, Couey P, Shade SB, et al: Cannabinoid-opioid interaction in chronic pain. Clin Pharmacol Ther 90(6):844–851, 2011 22048225

Alexander JC, Joshi GP: A review of the anesthetic implications of marijuana use. Proc Bayl Univ Med Cent 32(3):364–371, 2019 31384188

Allan GM, Finley CR, Ton J, et al: Systematic review of systematic reviews for medical cannabinoids: pain, nausea and vomiting, spasticity, and harms. Can Fam Physician 64(2):e78–e94, 2018 29449262

Allen JH, de Moore GM, Heddle R, et al: Cannabinoid hyperemesis: cyclical hyperemesis in association with chronic cannabis abuse. Gut 53(11):1566–1570, 2004 15479672

Allsop DJ, Copeland J, Norberg MM, et al: Quantifying the clinical significance of cannabis withdrawal. PLoS One 7(9):e44864, 2012 23049760

American Psychiatric Association: Diagnostic and Statistical Manual of Mental Disorders, 5th Edition, Text Revision. Washington, DC, American Psychiatric Association, 2022

Amornyotin S: Cannabis: what anesthesiologists need to know? Thai J Anesthesiol 48(3):3, 2022

Aronow WS, Cassidy J: Effect of marihuana and placebo-marihuana smoking on angina pectoris. N Engl J Med 291(2):65–67, 1974 4599385

Ashton CH: Adverse effects of cannabis and cannabinoids. Br J Anaesth 83(4):637–649, 1999 10673884

Babson KA, Sottile J, Morabito D: Cannabis, cannabinoids, and sleep: a review of the literature. Curr Psychiatry Rep 19(4):23, 2017 28349316

Bahji A, Stephenson C, Tyo R, et al: Prevalence of cannabis withdrawal symptoms among people with regular or dependent use of cannabinoids: a systematic review and meta-analysis. JAMA Netw Open 3(4):e202370, 2020 32271390

Beard S, Hunn A, Wight J: Treatments for spasticity and pain in multiple sclerosis: a systematic review. Health Technol Assess 7(40):1–111, 2003

Bie B, Wu J, Foss JF, et al: An overview of the cannabinoid type 2 receptor system and its therapeutic potential. Curr Opin Anaesthesiol 31(4):407–414, 2018 29794855

Bouquet E, Jouanjus E, Maryse Lapeyre-Mestre: Recreational cannabis use: French perspective of adverse effects, in Cannabis Use, Neurobiology, Psychology, and Treatment. Amsterdam, Elsevier Science, 2023, pp 127–138

Brownlow HA, Sutherland PD: Joint disagreement (letter). Anaesthesia 57(11):1142–1142, 2002 12392469

Bucchino L, Monzani A, Fracon S, et al: Cannabis-related diffuse alveolar hemorrhage in a 16-year-old patient: a case report. Front Pediatr 7:468, 2019 31799223

Cash MC, Cunnane K, Fan C, et al: Mapping cannabis potency in medical and recreational programs in the United States. PLoS One 15(3):e0230167, 2020 32214334

Chesher GB, Jackson DM, Starmer GA: Interaction of cannabis and general anaesthetic agents in mice. Br J Pharmacol 50(4):593–599, 1974 4280927

Chiang CN, Hawks RL: Research Findings on Smoking of Abused Substances. Washington, DC, U.S. Department of Health and Human Services, 1990

Choi S, Huang BC, Gamaldo CE: Therapeutic uses of cannabis on sleep disorders and related conditions. J Clin Neurophysiol 37(1):39–49, 2020 31895189

Colizzi M, Bhattacharyya S: Cannabis: neuropsychiatry and its effects on brain and behavior (editorial). Brain Sci 10(11):834, 2020 33182671

Collins AB, Beaudoin FL, Metrik J, et al: "I still partly think this is bullshit": a qualitative analysis of cannabinoid hyperemesis syndrome perceptions among people with chronic cannabis use and cyclic vomiting. Drug Alcohol Depend 246:109853, 2023 36996524

Copeland-Halperin LR, Herrera-Gomez LC, LaPier JR, et al: The effects of cannabis: implications for the surgical patient. Plast Reconstr Surg Glob Open 9(3):e3448, 2021 33747688

Crippa JAS, Hallak JEC, Machado-de-Sousa JP, et al: Cannabidiol for the treatment of cannabis withdrawal syndrome: a case report. J Clin Pharm Ther 38(2):162–164, 2013 23095052

Cristofori F, Thapar N, Saliakellis E, et al: Efficacy of the neurokinin-1 receptor antagonist aprepitant in children with cyclical vomiting syndrome. Aliment Pharmacol Ther 40(3):309–317, 2014 24898244

Davidson EM, Raz N, Eyal AM: Anesthetic considerations in medical cannabis patients. Curr Opin Anaesthesiol 33(6):832–840, 2020 33093301

Devinsky O, Marsh E, Friedman D, et al: Cannabidiol in patients with treatment-resistant epilepsy: an open-label interventional trial. Lancet Neurol 15(3):270–278, 2016 26724101

Devinsky O, Patel AD, Cross JH, et al: Effect of cannabidiol on drop seizures in the Lennox-Gastaut syndrome. N Engl J Med 378(20):1888–1897, 2018 29768152

Dezieck L, Hafez Z, Conicella A, et al: Resolution of cannabis hyperemesis syndrome with topical capsaicin in the emergency department: a case series. Clin Toxicol (Phila) 55(8):908–913, 2017 28494183

Di Marzo V, Stella N, Zimmer A: Endocannabinoid signalling and the deteriorating brain. Nat Rev Neurosci 16(1):30–42, 2015 25524120

D'Souza DC, Cortes-Briones J, Creatura G, et al: Efficacy and safety of a fatty acid amide hydrolase inhibitor (PF-04457845) in the treatment of cannabis withdrawal and dependence in men: a double-blind, placebo-controlled, parallel group, phase 2a single-site randomised controlled trial. Lancet Psychiatry 6(1):35–45, 2019 30528676

Echeverria-Villalobos M, Todeschini AB, Stoicea N, et al: Perioperative care of cannabis users: a comprehensive review of pharmacological and anesthetic considerations. J Clin Anesth 57:41–49, 2019 30852326

Felberbaum M: FDA warns company marketing unapproved cannabidiol products with unsubstantiated claims to treat cancer, Alzheimer's disease, opioid withdrawal, pain and pet anxiety. U.S. Food and Drug Administration, July 23, 2019. Available at: https://www.fda.gov/news-events/press-announcements/fda-warns-company-marketing-unapproved-cannabidiol-products-unsubstantiated-claims-treat-cancer. Accessed March 23, 2023.

Flisberg P, Paech MJ, Shah T, et al: Induction dose of propofol in patients using cannabis. Eur J Anaesthesiol 26(3):192–195, 2009

Friedman E, Gershon S, Hine B, et al: Cardiovascular effects of delta9-tetrahydrocannabinol in conscious and anaesthetized dogs. Br J Pharmacol 59(4):561–563, 1977 858008

Garzón J, de la Torre-Madrid E, Rodríguez-Muñoz M, et al: Gz mediates the long-lasting desensitization of brain CB1 receptors and is essential for cross-tolerance with morphine. Mol Pain 10(5):11, 2009

Graupensperger S, Fairlie AM, Vitiello MV, et al: Daily level effects of alcohol, marijuana, and simultaneous use on young adults' perceived sleep health. Sleep 44(12):zsab187, 2021 34291803

Gray DJ, Baker H, Clancy K, et al: Current and future needs and applications for cannabis. Crit Rev Plant Sci 35(5/6):425–426, 2016

Habboushe J, Sedor J: Cannabinoid hyperemesis acute renal failure: a common sequela of cannabinoid hyperemesis syndrome. Am J Emerg Med 32(6):690.e1–690.e2, 2014 24418446

Heath DM, Koslosky EJ, Bartush KC, et al: Marijuana in orthopaedics: effects on bone health, wound-healing, surgical complications, and pain management. JBJS Rev 10(2):e21.00184, 2022 35180183

Hernandez M, Birnbach DJ, Van Zundert AA: Anesthetic management of the illicit-substance-using patient. Curr Opin Anaesthesiol 18(3):315–324, 2005 16534357

Hillard CJ: Endocannabinoids and the endocrine system in health and disease. Handb Exp Pharmacol 231:317–339, 2015 26408166

Howard I: Cannabis hyperemesis syndrome in palliative care: a case study and narrative review. J Palliat Med 22(10):1227–1231, 2019 31084461

Huestis MA: Human cannabinoid pharmacokinetics. Chem Biodivers 4(8):1770–1804, 2007 17712819

Idris AI, Ralston SH: Role of cannabinoids in the regulation of bone remodeling. Front Endocrinol (Lausanne) 3:136, 2012 23181053

Imasogie N, Rose RV, Wilson A: High quantities: evaluating the association between cannabis use and propofol anesthesia during endoscopy. PLoS One 16(3):e0248062, 2021 33661987

Inayat F, Virk HUH, Ullah W, et al: Is haloperidol the wonder drug for cannabinoid hyperemesis syndrome? BMJ Case Rep 2017:bcr2016218239, 2017 28052951

Ishida JH, Zhang AJ, Steigerwald S, et al: Sources of information and beliefs about the health effects of marijuana. J Gen Intern Med 35(1):153–159, 2020 31637640

Karschner EL, Schwilke EW, Lowe RH, et al: Implications of plasma Δ9-tetrahydrocannabinol, 11-hydroxy-THC, and 11-nor-9-carboxy-THC concentrations in chronic cannabis smokers. J Anal Toxicol 33(8):469–477, 2009 19874654

King DD, Stewart SA, Collins-Yoder A, et al: Anesthesia for patients who self-report cannabis (marijuana) use before esophagogastroduodenoscopy: a retrospective review. AANA J 89(3):205–212, 2021 34042571

Koppel BS, Brust JCM, Fife T, et al: Systematic review: efficacy and safety of medical marijuana in selected neurologic disorders: report of the

Guideline Development Subcommittee of the American Academy of Neurology. Neurology 82(17):1556–1563, 2014 24778283

Kreuz DS, Axelrod J: Delta-9-tetrahydrocannabinol: localization in body fat. Science 179(4071):391–393, 1973 4682965

Kumar RN, Chambers WA, Pertwee RG: Pharmacological actions and therapeutic uses of cannabis and cannabinoids. Anaesthesia 56(11):1059–1068, 2001 11703238

Lathrop JR, Rosen SN, Heitkemper MM, et al: Cyclic vomiting syndrome and cannabis hyperemesis syndrome: the state of the science. Gastroenterol Nurs 46(3):208–224 2023

Lee BH, Sideris A, Ladha KS, et al: Cannabis and cannabinoids in the perioperative period. Anesth Analg 138(1):16–30, 2024 35551150

Livne O, Shmulewitz D, Lev-Ran S, et al: DSM-5 cannabis withdrawal syndrome: demographic and clinical correlates in U.S. adults. Drug Alcohol Depend 195:170–177, 2019 30361043

Lynn RSR, Galinkin JL: Cannabis, e-cigarettes and anesthesia. Curr Opin Anaesthesiol 33(3):318–326, 2020 32371642

MacCamy K, Hu D: Dexmedetomidine for treatment of delayed peak symptoms of cannabis withdrawal syndrome: a case report. Hosp Pharm 56(5):462–465, 2021 34720146

Macedo AC, de Faria AOV, Bizzi I, et al: Online information on medical cannabis is not always aligned with scientific evidence and may raise unrealistic expectations. J Cannabis Res 4(1):37, 2022 35820952

Mallat A, Roberson J, Brock-Utne JG: Preoperative marijuana inhalation: an airway concern. Can J Anaesth 43(7):691–693, 1996 8807175

Meah F, Lundholm M, Emanuele N, et al: The effects of cannabis and cannabinoids on the endocrine system. Rev Endocr Metab Disord 23(3):401–420, 2022 34460075

Mills B, Yepes A, Nugent K: Synthetic cannabinoids. Am J Med Sci 350(1):59–62, 2015 26132518

Mittleman MA, Lewis RA, Maclure M, et al: Triggering myocardial infarction by marijuana. Circulation 103(23):2805–2809, 2001 11401936

Mondino A, Cavelli M, González J, et al: Effects of cannabis consumption on sleep, in Cannabinoids and Sleep: Molecular, Functional and Clinical Aspects. Edited by Monti JM, Pandi-Perumal SR, Murillo-Rodríguez E. New York, Springer, 2021, pp 147–162

Montané E, Duran M, Capellà D, et al: Scientific drug information in newspapers: sensationalism and low quality: the example of therapeutic use of cannabinoids. Eur J Clin Pharmacol 61(5–6):475–477, 2005 15983825

Moon AM, Buckley SA, Mark NM: Successful treatment of cannabinoid hyperemesis syndrome with topical capsaicin. ACG Case Rep J 5:e3, 2018 29379817

Murray AW, Smith JD, Ibinson JW: Diffuse alveolar hemorrhage, anesthesia, and cannabis. Ann Am Thorac Soc 11(8):1338–1339, 2014 25343207

Murray RM, Englund A, Abi-Dargham A, et al: Cannabis-associated psychosis: neural substrate and clinical impact. Neuropharmacology 124:89–104, 2017 28634109

National Academies of Sciences, Engineering, and Medicine: The Health Effects of Cannabis and Cannabinoids: The Current State of Evidence and Recommendations for Research. Washington, DC, National Academies Press, 2017

Nicholson AN, Turner C, Stone BM, et al: Effect of Δ9-tetrahydrocannabinol and cannabidiol on nocturnal sleep and early morning behavior in young adults. J Clin Psychopharmacol 24(3):305–313, 2004 15118485

Nielsen S, Germanos R, Weier M, et al: The use of cannabis and cannabinoids in treating symptoms of multiple sclerosis: a systematic review of reviews. Curr Neurol Neurosci Rep 18(2):8, 2018 29442178

Nourbakhsh M, Miller A, Gofton J, et al: Cannabinoid hyperemesis syndrome: reports of fatal cases. J Forensic Sci 64(1):270–274, 2019 29768651

Otero-Romero S, Sastre-Garriga J, Comi G, et al: Pharmacological management of spasticity in multiple sclerosis: systematic review and consensus paper. Mult Scler 22(11):1386–1396, 2016 27207462

Parvataneni S, Varela L, Vemuri-Reddy SM, et al: Emerging role of aprepitant in cannabis hyperemesis syndrome. Cureus 11(6):e4825, 2019 31403013

Paton WD, Temple DM: Proceedings: effects of chronic and acute cannabis treatment upon thiopentone anaesthesia in rabbits. Br J Pharmacol 44(2):346P–347P, 1972 4668614

Perisetti A, Gajendran M, Dasari CS, et al: Cannabis hyperemesis syndrome: an update on the pathophysiology and management. Ann Gastroenterol 33(6):571–578, 2020 33162734

Pertwee R (ed): Handbook of Cannabis. Oxford, UK, Oxford University Press, 2014

Piomelli D: The molecular logic of endocannabinoid signalling. Nat Rev Neurosci 4(11):873–884, 2003 14595399

Piomelli D, Russo EB: The Cannabis sativa versus Cannabis indica debate: an interview with Ethan Russo, MD. Cannabis Cannabinoid Res 1(1):44–46, 2016 28861479

Piper BJ, Beals ML, Abess AT, et al: Chronic pain patients' perspectives of medical cannabis. Pain 158(7):1373–1379, 2017 28328576

Portman D, Donovan KA: Cannabinoid hyperemesis syndrome: a case report of a confounding entity in oncology care. J Oncol Pract 14(5):333–334, 2018 29543555

Pratt M, Stevens A, Thuku M, et al: Benefits and harms of medical cannabis: a scoping review of systematic reviews. Syst Rev 8(1):320, 2019 31823819

Razban M, Exadaktylos AK, Santa VD, et al: Cannabinoid hyperemesis syndrome and cannabis withdrawal syndrome: a review of the management of cannabis-related syndrome in the emergency department. Int J Emerg Med 15(1):45, 2022 36076180

Rice J, Cameron M: Cannabinoids for treatment of MS symptoms: state of the evidence. Curr Neurol Neurosci Rep 18(8):50, 2018 29923025

Richards JR, Lapoint JM, Burillo-Putze G: Cannabinoid hyperemesis syndrome: potential mechanisms for the benefit of capsaicin and hot water hydrotherapy in treatment. Clin Toxicol (Phila) 56(1):15–24, 2018 28730896

Ruffle JK, Bajgoric S, Samra K, et al: Cannabinoid hyperemesis syndrome: an important differential diagnosis of persistent unexplained vomiting. Eur J Gastroenterol Hepatol 27(12):1403–1408, 2015 26445382

Sampson CS, Bedy S-M, Carlisle T: Withdrawal seizures seen in the setting of synthetic cannabinoid abuse. Am J Emerg Med 33(11):1712.e3, 2015 25825034

Sanford AE, Castillo E, Gannon RL: Cannabinoids and hamster circadian activity rhythms. Brain Res 1222:141–148, 2008 18582849

Senderovich H, Patel P, Lopez BJ, et al: A systematic review on cannabis hyperemesis syndrome and management. Med Princ Pract 31(1):29–38, 2022 34724666

Shahbazi F, Grandi V, Banerjee A, et al: Cannabinoids and cannabinoid receptors: the story so far. iScience 23(7):101301, 2020 32629422

Simonetto DA, Oxentenko AS, Herman ML, et al: Cannabinoid hyperemesis: a case series of 98 patients. Mayo Clin Proc 87(2):114–119, 2012 22305024

Smith LA, Azariah F, Lavender VTC, et al: Cannabinoids for nausea and vomiting in adults with cancer receiving chemotherapy. Cochrane Database Syst Rev 2015(11):CD009464, 2015 26561338

Sophocleous A, Robertson R, Ferreira NB, et al: Heavy cannabis use is associated with low bone mineral density and an increased risk of fractures. Am J Med 130(2):214–221, 2017 27593602

Stanghellini V, Chan FKL, Hasler WL, et al: Gastroduodenal disorders. Gastroenterology 150(6):1380–1392, 2016 27147122

Sulak D, Saneto R, Goldstein B: The current status of artisanal cannabis for the treatment of epilepsy in the United States. Epilepsy Behav 70(Pt B):328–333, 2017 28254350

Tapley P, Kellett S: Cannabis-based medicines and the perioperative physician. Perioper Med (Lond) 8(1):19, 2019 31827774

Thiele EA, Marsh ED, French JA, et al: Cannabidiol in patients with seizures associated with Lennox-Gastaut syndrome (GWPCARE4): a randomised, double-blind, placebo-controlled phase 3 trial. Lancet 391(10125):1085–1096, 2018 29395273

Townsend CB, Liss F, Langman C, et al: Perspectives of orthopedic patients on medical cannabis: a survey of more than 2500 patients. Orthopedics 45(6):e309–e314, 2022 36098574

Tramèr MR, Carroll D, Campbell FA, et al: Cannabinoids for control of chemotherapy induced nausea and vomiting: quantitative systematic review. BMJ 323(7303):16–21, 2001 11440936

Vaughn LK, Denning G, Stuhr KL, et al: Endocannabinoid signalling: has it got rhythm? Br J Pharmacol 160(3):530–543, 2010 20590563

von Both I, Santos B: Death of a young woman with cyclic vomiting: a case report. Forensic Sci Med Pathol 17(4):715–722, 2021 34735682

Wallace D, Martin A-L, Park B: Cannabinoid hyperemesis: marijuana puts patients in hot water. Australas Psychiatry 15(2):156–158, 2007 17464661

Wang T, Collet J-P, Shapiro S, et al: Adverse effects of medical cannabinoids: a systematic review. CMAJ 178(13):1669–1678, 2008 18559804

Wen H, Hockenberry JM, Druss BG: The effect of medical marijuana laws on marijuana-related attitude and perception among US adolescents and young adults. Prev Sci 20(2):215–223, 2019 29767282

Whiting PF, Wolff RF, Deshpande S, et al: Cannabinoids for medical use: a systematic review and meta-analysis. JAMA 313(24):2456–2473, 2015 26103030

Winiger EA, Hitchcock LN, Bryan AD, et al: Cannabis use and sleep: expectations, outcomes, and the role of age. Addict Behav 112:106642, 2021 32949837

Witsil JC, Mycyk MB: Haloperidol, a novel treatment for cannabinoid hyperemesis syndrome. Am J Ther 24(1):e64–e67, 2017 25393073

Wong A, Montebello ME, Norberg MM, et al: Exercise increases plasma THC concentrations in regular cannabis users. Drug Alcohol Depend 133(2):763–767, 2013 24018317

Index

Page numbers in **boldface** font refer to figures and tables.

Gamete intrafallopian transfer
(GIFT), 259
García-Gutiérrez, MS, 180
Gastroschisis, 264
Gateway hypothesis, 15, 17, 20–24, 213
Gender, 9, 200, 233
Generalized anxiety disorder, 184
Generalized Anxiety Disorder–7, 176,
180
Genetic epidemiological studies, 96
Genetics and Psychosis case-control
study, 102, 106
Gibbs, M, **92**
Glaucoma, 332
Global Burden of Disease study,
198–199
Global Drug Survey, 164
Glutamate neurotransmission, 97
Gobbi, G, 148, 209
Gonadotropin-releasing hormone,
260
Gonçalves, PD, 67
Gorfinkel, LR, 149
G protein–coupled receptors, 331
G proteins, 96
Green, KM, 70, 73
Gruber, AJ, 160
Gukasyan, N, 144
Guttmannova, K, **156**

Halladay, JE, 148, **156**
Haloperidol, 94, 342
Hammersley, R, 47
Hancox, RJ, 295
Harm reduction approaches, 216
Hashish, **283**
Hasin, DS, 3–4
Headaches, 314
Hedges, JC, 254–256
Heitzeg, MM, 65, 67
Hemachandra, D, 293
Hemoptysis, 294
Hemp Farming Act, 284
Hemp plants, 278
Hengartner, MP, **157**
Heroin, 21
and THC, 19
High-potency cannabis, 102
High-risk behaviors, 11–12
Hippocampal abnormalities, 131
Histological changes, 294
HIV-related weight loss, 332
Hodgson, K, 151

Homicides, 197
Horwood, LJ, 11, 70, 72
Hospital admissions, 101
Hospital Anxiety and Depression
Scale, 185
Hot showers and baths, 342
Human ether-à-go-go-related gene
(hERG) channel, 292
Human laboratory studies, 94–95
Human studies, 252, 255
Hyggen, C, 72
Hyperalgesia, 315
Hyperglycemia, 292

Immunocompromised people, 295, 298
Impaired social functioning, 69
Impulsivity, 214, 233
Infertility, 259–260
Insomnia, 174, 180
IQ declines, 125, 127, 129
Irritability, 212, 214

Jackson, NJ, 127
Javanbakht, M, 39
Joynauth, J, 292

K2, 281
Kandel, DB, 7–8, 10
Kandel, ER, 10
Kasman, AM, 257
Kiburi, SK, **92**, 103
Kidney damage, 334
Kids' Inpatient Database, 292
Kief, **283**
Kolodny, RC, 254
Kraan, T, **89**
Kuhathasan, N, 180
Kuhns, L, 163

Lac, A, 76
Ladha, KS, 289
Lamarque, S, 19
Large, M, **90**
Lawn, W, 125
Lee, JO, 74
Lennox-Gastaut syndrome, 281, **282**,
339–340
Leon, V, 47
Lessem, JM, 15
Lev-Ran, S, 145
Libzon, S, 44
Lidocaine, 306
Lo, JO, 264